# Resolving Infertility

**RESOLVE co-editors**

**Diane N. Clapp, BSN, RN**
Medical Information Director
National RESOLVE

**Margaret R. Hollister, JD**
Director of HelpLine and Educational Services
National RESOLVE

# Resolving Infertility

THE STAFF OF RESOLVE,
WITH DIANE ARONSON, FORMER EXECUTIVE DIRECTOR

*Produced by Amaranth*

HarperResource
*An Imprint of HarperCollinsPublishers*

HarperCollins books may be purchased for educational, business, or sales promotional use. For information, please write: Special Markets Department, HarperCollins Publishers Inc., 10 East 53rd Street, New York, NY 10022.

*This book is intended as a general guide only. Consult your appropriate professional advisors before beginning a treatment program or other options described in this book.*

*All terms mentioned in this book that are known to be or are suspected to be trademarks or service marks have been appropriately capitalized. RESOLVE and HarperCollins cannot attest to the validity of this information. Use of a term in this book should not be regarded as affecting the validity of any trademark or service mark.*

*Page 370 constitutes an extension of the copyright page.*

First HarperResource Edition published 2001.

Produced by Amaranth
102 Factory Street, PO Box 156
Oxford, MD 21654

Design and Typesetting by RBDesign

Library of Congress Cataloging-in-Publication Data
Available upon request
Paperback ISBN 0-06-095799-9

04  05  ❖/RRD  10  9  8  7  6  5  4

# ACKNOWLEDGMENTS

This book is the gift of time, experience, and expertise from many. First, I want to thank the members of RESOLVE, chapter leaders, and volunteers, who have contributed through the telling and sharing of their infertility experiences. The personal accounts in *Resolving Infertility* set this book apart and help to focus on the challenges and the emotional aspects of medical treatment and all other resolutions for family building.*

Countless members of RESOLVE and others will be indebted forever to RESOLVE's founder, Barbara Eck Menning, for her vision in founding this unique and special organization. Through Barbara's fortitude and commitment, the psychological aspects of the infertility experience were given greater attention. Through her writing, education, and advocacy, its emotional impact became better understood.

*Resolving Infertility* has been greatly enriched through the contributions of dedicated professionals who work on a daily basis to assist individuals who are striving to accomplish their dream of a family. The following have offered their assistance to review chapters and/or provided their counsel and wisdom: G. David Adamson, MD[†]; Linda D. Applegarth, EdD[†]; Robert Barbieri, MD; Peg Beck, LICSW[†]; Kenneth Burry, MD; Maria Bustillo, MD; Sandra Carson, MD; Sharon Covington, MSW; Joann P. Galst, PhD; Marc Goldstein, MD; Arthur Haney, MD; Joseph A. Hill, MD; Robert B. Hunt, MD; Mary Ann Jablonski; Larry I. Lipshultz, MD[†]; Joe B. Massey, MD[†]; Selwyn P. Oskowitz, MD; Veronica Ravnikar, MD; Zev Rosenwaks, MD; Kaylen M. Silverberg, MD; Michael Soules, MD; Brian C. Su, MD[†]; Eric Surrey, MD; Dan Tulchinsky, MD; J. David Wininger, PhD[†]; Bill Yee, MD[†]; and Shirley M. Zager.

I would like to thank the current and past board members and chapter leaders of RESOLVE. Chapter leaders offer quality service through peer support, educational meetings and personal commitment, often in the midst of their own infertility experiences. The expertise and wisdom of members of the board of directors over the years have contributed to the success of RESOLVE today. This book was conceived during the tenure of the immediate past Chair of RESOLVE's board, Mary Beth Grady. Her many contributions to RESOLVE live on. RESOLVE's 25 years of service have been made possible through the exceptional assistance of the

*The names of interviewees for this book, and in many cases identifying details of their stories, have been changed to protect individual privacy.

[†]Our special gratitude to these individuals who gave extensively of their expertise, time, and resources in the production of *Resolving Infertility*.

many members of its national board. Linda Applegarth, EdD, the current national Chair, is a dedicated professional who has contributed generously of her time and support to RESOLVE. She also served as an astute reviewer for many book chapters. The Executive Committee (G. David Adamson, MD, Linda Applegarth, EdD, Carol Jones, and Cecile Lampton) and the entire board are helping RESOLVE address the critical issues for the millennium.

To Patty Leasure, Linda Cunningham, Tricia Medved, Lois Brown, Carl Mark Raymond, and Greg Chaput of HarperCollins, thank you for inspiring *Resolving Infertility* and for your work in bringing it to the thousands who will benefit from its thorough presentation.

Lee Ann Chearney, creative director of Amaranth, and her entire staff embody professionalism. Thanks to copyeditors Candace B. Levy, PhD, ELS; and Mary L. Tod; PhD, ELS; proofreaders Elizabeth LaManna and Bill Trudell; researcher Debby Young; indexer Dave Prout; typesetter/designer Rhea Braunstein; illustrator Wendy Frost; graphic artist Kathleen Edwards; and editorial assistant Alice Lane. They worked tirelessly to ensure that deadlines were met and that quality was assured. Their dedication to the project and attention to detail were extraordinary.

A special thank you to Deborah S. Romaine and Suzanne LeVert for their assistance with research and writing. The research confirmed the complexity of the subject and helped to provide the voices in this comprehensive guide to the options and the emotional and financial concerns of family building.

Colleen Mohyde of the Doe Cover Agency was a patient agent throughout, responding to our requests for periodic negotiations and interceding when needed. Attorney Suzanne Glassburn provided cautious, considerate, and excellent legal counsel as we ventured into the new world of book publishing.

Thanks to all the staff of National RESOLVE for providing proofreading, word processing, and moral support to this project. To Deborah Wachenheim, RESOLVE's Government Affairs Director, thank you for your incredible dedication to advocacy on behalf of those experiencing infertility. RESOLVE is only hampered by its financial resources in its efforts to accomplish equitable insurance coverage, more research, and better adoption benefits. Deborah's oversight and management of legislative and research concerns have made a difference to the lives of many.

Without the contributions of Diane Clapp, the Medical Information Director at RESOLVE, this book would not have been possible. Diane has been a valued and treasured member of the staff since the early days of RESOLVE's founding. Diane's expertise as a nurse and counselor, and her years of staffing the Medical Call-In Hours at the national office, have enriched this process with reliable, sound information. Diane devoted priority time, creative energy, and writing and editing skills to ensure an end product of quality. For the many who have spoken with Diane through the years, they will be reminded of her caring manner and her careful assistance to so many who have called in crisis.

This entire book project was managed within the RESOLVE office by Margaret Hollister, the Director of the HelpLine and Educational Services. Margaret committed hundreds of hours to overseeing the project to completion. When we faced what appeared to be insurmountable deadlines, Margaret encouraged the whole team, and we were able to move forward with renewed determination and continuing efficiency. Margaret's legal and management expertise has contributed enormous value to RESOLVE and to this project. Margaret has an incredible grasp of the volume of information available to support the dedicated HelpLine staff and those who call, e-mail, or write for RESOLVE's help and resources. All her tasks are accomplished with great aplomb and respect for and from others, and in her cheerful and witty manner.

To Diane and Margaret—what a team! My days at RESOLVE are enriched by your presence. The administration of RESOLVE is enhanced by your expertise. I am indebted to you both for your commitment to RESOLVE and to all who contact us in need. RESOLVE is made unique through your ongoing contributions. You, and the entire staff, continue the pursuit of excellence in all of the services RESOLVE provides.

To Jan Surrey, thank you for your valued friendship, the times we were able to share and compare our infertility journeys, and the foresight in suggesting my post-infertility reconnection with RESOLVE.

Finally, I would like to thank my personal infertility team—my husband and daughter—for their patience and understanding when my duties have included extensive travel and schedules and job-related work that stretched long past the normal 9 to 5 day and into the weekends. Carl and Rachal know firsthand what can happen through contact with RESOLVE and the gathering of quality information and support. To you both, and to my entire family, thank you.

DIANE D. ARONSON
Executive Director
RESOLVE, The National Infertility Association
October 1999

# CONTENTS

# Introduction: When You're Wishing for a Baby

*RESOLVE's mission is to provide timely, compassionate support and information to people who are experiencing infertility and to increase awareness of infertility issues through public education and advocacy.*

Twenty-five years ago, RESOLVE was founded by Barbara Eck Menning, a nurse who was experiencing infertility. She recognized the deep, often hidden, need for support to those wishing to build families but facing the life crisis of infertility. Her efforts began at her kitchen table in Belmont, Massachusetts, where she and a small group of volunteers created and answered a local HelpLine and mailed out fact sheets about treatment options, adoption, and coping with the emotional roller coaster of the infertility experience.

Today, RESOLVE reaches hundreds of thousands a year through its chapter network, national and chapter HelpLines, e-mail service, Web site, and business office. Our services now include chapter peer connection, professionally led support groups, educational meetings and symposia, and screened physician referral.

Stories about infertility and fast-evolving treatments fill the media, offering great promise but creating the illusion that there is a miraculous solution to every infertility problem. Indeed, developments in the treatment of infertility in recent years have been wondrous, ranging from sophisticated ultrasound equipment that simplified egg retrieval for assisted reproductive technology to the injection of one sperm into the nucleus of an egg to create an embryo. And yet, many of the calls and e-mail messages our national and chapter HelpLine peer counselors receive are still coming from kitchen tables, where individuals and couples are feeling isolated, confused about their options, and anxious to find a way to afford treatment. So, although infertility may be less hidden today, the need for understanding and reliable, accurate information about treatment and options for family building has never been greater.

So much has happened in the world of infertility since RESOLVE was founded. Louise Brown of the United Kingdom, born in 1978 as a result of the first in vitro fertilization procedure, is now an adult. Since her miraculous birth, thousands of families have been created through the use of assisted reproductive technologies. Yet, these techniques remain out of the reach of many. The cost of this and other infertility treatments is high when borne individually by patients but adds minimal burden to the average family premium when included in insurance contracts.

Owing to the very personal and private nature of infertility and the lack of a visible constituency, legislators have often misunderstood or dismissed the issue as one undeserving of legislative attention. RESOLVE has not been easily discouraged, however. In recent years, our advocacy efforts for health care coverage for infertility have accelerated. Tireless chapter leaders and other volunteers have worked since the 1980s with enlightened legislators to help pass mandates for better infertility insurance coverage in thirteen states. In 1992, we established the Government Affairs Program at our national office to support these and other important advocacy efforts.

Some individuals have brought lawsuits successfully against employers who have not provided infertility insurance coverage, and the Supreme Court addressed the issue when it found in 1998 that "reproduction is a major life activity" under the Americans with Disabilities Act. We continue to explore other avenues for establishing equity for infertility patients seeking treatment and to build much-wanted families affordably with adoption and third-party parenting options.

There is much left to do. We see a tremendous need for more infertility research. RESOLVE continues to work to improve both infertility treatment quality and patient access in coalition with the physician community, mental health providers, nurses, embryo laboratory directors, and government agencies. RESOLVE's policies advocate for quality care for consumers and appropriate oversight of the field of infertility.

We have written this book to reach not only those personally coping with the infertility struggle, but also the friends and family members wishing to provide help and support. Today, the disease of infertility affects more than 10 percent of the U.S. reproductive-age population. It strikes diverse groups—cutting across all socioeconomic, racial, ethnic, and religious lines. Thus chances are great that a friend, relative, or neighbor is attempting to cope with the medical and emotional aspects of infertility. In this book, we offer some concrete suggestions for providing sensitive support to individuals struggling with the life crisis of infertility.

*Resolving Infertility* is meant to provide readers with an overview of the medical issues involved in treating infertility and not to serve as a comprehensive guide to treatment or as medical advice. Readers should, of course, consult qualified medical professionals for individual advice. In addition, RESOLVE offers a list of more than 60 detailed fact sheets on infertility issues, including a series on coping and self-help and treatment options. This collection is updated regularly and may be reviewed at the back of the book or at our Web site: **www.resolve.org.**

These days, RESOLVE's national board, staff, and hundreds of volunteers at the chapter level are busier than ever providing the support, information, and advocacy consumers need to resolve infertility issues. As RESOLVE's executive director since 1991, my days have often been filled with travel and administrative work. But it is the letters of appreciation and thanks from our members and correspondents that keep me, and all of us at RESOLVE, happy to come to work each day. Here is a sample of our mail:

*Thank you! We have been to a few RESOLVE meetings, and they are helpful—but your newsletters—national and local, are a big help!*
*—Member from Ohio*

*Although I am a new member, I must take this time to thank your organization for the wonderful support network. My husband and I appreciate learning of all the information we can on infertility.*
*—Member from Michigan*

*Please accept my thanks and gratitude for approving my membership scholarship. It is greatly appreciated. Were it not for your generosity and caring, I would not be able to avail myself of your benefits. Thanks again for a little light in my world that often seems dark and bleak.*
*—Member from California*

*I am sending a letter to my employer's benefits department to protest the
complete lack of coverage for infertility-related diagnosis and treatment.
In my short time as a member of RESOLVE, I have already
found many helpful resources. Thank you.*
—*Member from Missouri*

*Enclosed is a check for RESOLVE in honor of the birth of our
granddaughter. We applaud the work of your fine organization.*
—*Grandparents from Massachusetts*

*Thank you so much for your newsletter and all of your support.
On May 9, our adopted daughter was born. Keep up all you are doing.
You have touched our lives, and for that we are truly grateful.*
—*Member from Washington*

I, too, remember some days of isolation and despair as I journeyed on my
path to resolution. I was grateful then to have found support from RESOLVE
and celebrate now this opportunity as I work each day to assist others who are
striving to build much-wanted families.

We are glad that you, too, have discovered RESOLVE. We hope *Resolving
Infertility* will help you begin the infertility journey, explore its many paths, and
ultimately reach the destination that is right for you.

DIANE D. ARONSON
Former Executive Director
RESOLVE, The National Infertility Association

# PART 1

# UNDERSTANDING INFERTILITY

# 1 Face to Face with Your Options

RESOLVE: "Good morning, RESOLVE HelpLine."
Caller: "Is this RESOLVE . . . if someone is trying to have a baby?"
RESOLVE: "Yes, we help those experiencing infertility with information, referral, support, and advocacy. How can I help you today?"
Caller: "Well, I've had your number in my wallet for over a year. I just kept hoping I wouldn't need it."
RESOLVE: "We're glad you called! How can I help?"

If you are trying to have a baby, it is not unusual to hope, month after month, that a pregnancy will occur and that you will not need a resource such as RESOLVE. Please know that if you are having trouble conceiving a child on your own, or trouble carrying a pregnancy to delivery, *you are not alone*. Millions of men, women, and couples struggle with the very same issues you face today. Indeed, the statistics show that infertility affects 6.1 million people in the United States. According to the 1995 National Survey of Family Growth by the U.S. Department of Health and Human Services, this figure represents 10.2 percent (1 in 10) of couples in which the woman is of reproductive age.

There are very human stories behind these straightforward statistics. Infertility knows no boundaries: Couples and individuals of every race, religious background, and financial stratum face the dilemma you may be confronting right now. More than 1 million people seek medical treatment for infertility every year. In the pages of this book are the stories of many individuals and couples who would recognize how you are feeling, because they too are struggling with infertility or have only recently resolved it.

Sandy and Peter are a couple in their late 30s who had been trying to conceive for about 4 years. Sandy not only had trouble ovulating, but also had poor cervical mucus and a very narrow cervix. (We will explain medical terms and procedures in depth in later chapters.) They went through several cycles of intrauterine insemination (IUI), suffered a miscarriage, and finally had a full term pregnancy last year. Right now, they are enjoying taking care of their healthy baby boy.

Mary Beth, a single, 36-year-old woman, has been trying to get pregnant for about 2 years. She wanted a child but had no male partner in her life, so she chose a donor from a sperm bank and went through more than a year of inseminations without getting pregnant. After visiting several doctors who tried to pinpoint the cause of her infertility, Mary Beth underwent treatment with drugs to help her produce eggs. Although she recently became pregnant, the pregnancy is at high risk, and she is on bed rest through the remainder of her pregnancy.

Jenny and Scott discovered very early in their marriage—she was only 24 and he 26—that Scott had no viable sperm. After discussing their options, they decided to choose treatment with donor sperm, and Jenny underwent several rounds of donor insemination before becoming pregnant. She miscarried in her second month, for no known reason. After grieving for their loss, they tried again; and today Jenny and Scott are raising two healthy children.

Anna and Mike had no reason to suspect an infertility problem, as Anna had given birth to a healthy child years before their marriage. Between then and now, however, Anna's fallopian tubes had somehow become blocked. When she still did not become pregnant after undergoing a tubal surgery, Anna's doctor suggested in vitro fertilization (IVF). They have tried two cycles without success; and although they would be willing to try again, Anna and Mike simply cannot afford to pay for another round of the expensive procedure. For the time being, they have had to put aside their dream of having a child together.

Harry and Lois, a couple in their late 30s, have been trying to get pregnant for 2 years. Lois underwent two surgeries to remove severe endometriosis that had encased her ovaries and fallopian tubes. The couple then spent thousands for three rounds of IVF, without success. Lois's hormone levels now indicate she is approaching perimenopause, and while they would consider attempting a donor egg pregnancy, they feel exhausted from the cycles of hope and lost hope.

As you continue with us through *Resolving Infertility*, you will read about other men and women with various medical conditions who have undergone a variety of procedures and, ultimately, have chosen to explore the alternatives to carrying a pregnancy, such as surrogacy, resolving without children, or adoption. These individuals and couples face a new set of issues as they pursue their wish to create or expand a family, and we are defining *family* as any *constellation of people—related by genetics or not, including a baby or not—that helps sustain others throughout life.*

Whatever path is chosen, some people find the maze of insurance and financial issues among the toughest challenges to face in the journey to resolve infertility. Others are daunted by the emotional ups and downs, still others by the perceived or very real lack of support by, and understanding of, the world around them. You are not alone. As you learn more about the challenge of infertility and the options available to resolve it, listen to the voices of courageous men and women from RESOLVE chapters and support groups nationwide who share with you, in their own words, what this struggle has meant to them.

## INFERTILITY TODAY

Infertility is not a new disease, and rates of infertility have remained relatively stable over the past century. However, an increase in infertility rates apparent in recent decades appears to have several causes. An increase in the age of women wanting to conceive, an increase in the spread of sexually transmitted diseases, and the rise in the level of toxic chemicals in our environment are all factors that could be affecting fertility rates.

### *Meanings*

Infertility is a disease or condition affecting the reproductive system that interferes with the ability of a man or woman to achieve a pregnancy or of a woman to carry a pregnancy to live birth. Generally speaking, doctors use the term *infertile* to describe individuals who try for more than a year to become pregnant without success and those unable to carry a pregnancy to term because of miscarriage. Infertility, however, is *not* sterility, which means conception is not possible under any circumstances. Here are some facts about infertility:

- Infertility, both a disease and a life crisis, is the inability to have a child despite regular sexual intercourse.
- Infertility interferes with one of the most fundamental and highly valued human activities—building a family.
- Infertility affects people of all ages, ethnic backgrounds, and socioeconomic groups, and both sexes.

We hear more about infertility today because medical technology now offers more answers and treatment options to men and women trying to conceive a child. From hormonal treatments to more advanced technologies to surrogacy, diagnostic and treatment options abound for women and men. And now some employers and insurance companies across the country are beginning to cover fertility treatments.

Another advance has occurred in the social realm: First and foremost, it is less taboo to talk about infertility. Individuals and couples have more choices when it comes to building the family that is right for them: Both single individuals and couples pursue adoption and childfree living by choice. Every day, babies conceived with the help of fertility drugs, surgery, and assisted reproductive technologies (ART), such as in vitro fertilization (IVF); through insemination with donor sperm; or through donor egg pregnancy or surrogacy; are welcomed into loving families.

Unfortunately, other aspects of infertility have not changed at all, including the exhausting cycle of emotions experienced by the majority of people confronting this disease. The pain begins with a fundamental belief that conceiving, carrying, and bearing a child is the most natural thing in the world and that the inability to do so quickly and easily feels like a failure. For example, for women who delay child bearing until age 35 or older, it may be a surprising revelation that becoming pregnant may not be as simple as it might have been when they were a younger age. The feeling of having to make up for lost time adds to the determination to "succeed."

Although medical advances offer new hope for millions of people, the process of treatment for infertility itself is not easier or less stressful than it has been in the past. The commitment you make to the treatment process may be a great one—one that can and often does interfere with your regular working, social, and intimate activities and relationships. The good news is that you, like most others in your situation, will find a way to navigate through this process successfully and discover the resolution that is right for you.

With this book, we at RESOLVE offer our help to sort through the options, the way we have for men and women, couples, and families since our founding in 1974. Like you, the people we have helped found themselves immersed in a whole new world—one of physicians and clinics; of medical tests, procedures, and treatments; of unfamiliar adoption terms and regulations—and an experience filled with a mixture of hope, disappointment, joy, and acceptance. Our goal in writing this book is to help you travel through this new experience with as much confidence and knowledge as possible.

## SEPARATING THE MYTHS FROM THE FACTS

Before we outline the medical, personal, social, and financial challenges you face—we want to dispel some of the myths about infertility. These myths place an extra burden on women, men, and couples. So we will do our best to reveal the truth for you and your family. Let's take them one by one.

**Myth:** *Infertility is a female problem.*
**Fact:** In 1780, America's first president, George Washington, wrote a letter to a friend stating his belief that it was the fault of his wife, Martha, that he had no children of his own—despite the fact that Martha had borne two children in a previous marriage. Washington was not the first or only person to hold this erroneous belief; even today, women and society in general seem automatically to blame the woman first for fertility problems.

The truth is, however, that women and men bear nearly equal responsibility when it comes to infertility. Infertility is a female problem in 40 percent of cases, a male problem in 40 percent of cases, and a combined problem of the couple or unexplained in 20 percent of cases. That is why we stress that it is important for both members of the couple to undergo medical evaluation and, as necessary, treatment.

**Myth:** *Everyone* **else** *gets pregnant easily.*
**Fact:**  A normally fertile couple has only about a 20 percent chance of conceiving each month. More than 6 million people of childbearing age in the United States experience infertility every year, and 1 million seek treatment.

**Myth:** *Relax and you'll get pregnant.*
**Fact:** Infertility is a disease of the reproductive system. Although stress can sometimes affect hormone levels and ovulation, emotions are not keeping you from getting pregnant. The stress and intense emotions you feel are the *result* of infertility, not usually its cause. In chapters 11 and 12, "Staying Centered," and "Staying Healthy," some stress-reduction techniques are included that will help improve the quality of your life as you cope with infertility.

**Myth:** *Be patient; you'll get pregnant with time.*
**Fact:** Infertility is a medical problem that usually requires treatment. At least 50 percent of those who complete an infertility evaluation will respond to treatment with a successful pregnancy. Those who do not seek help have a "sponta-

neous cure rate" of only about 5 percent, which means couples have a ten times greater chance of conceiving if they get medical help for their infertility problem.

If you are concerned for any reason about your ability to conceive, make an appointment with a physician for an evaluation as soon as possible—especially if you

As a woman

- are over the age of 35.
- have irregular cycles.
- experience painful menstrual periods.
- have suffered several pregnancy losses.
- have used an intrauterine device (IUD).
- have had a pelvic infection or abdominal surgery.

- If you are a man or a woman and have had exposure through your mother's pregnancy to the synthetic hormone diethylstilbestrol (DES).
- Or, if you are a man and have had a testicular injury or frequent genitourinary infections.

**Myth:** *Just adopt a baby and you'll get pregnant.*
**Fact:** Unfortunately, this persistent myth is one of the most painful for individuals and couples to hear, because it suggests that adoption is a treatment for infertility, not the happy resolution to infertility that it is for millions of families every year. More important, this statement simply is not true: Studies reveal that pregnancy rates for couples after adopting are the same as those for couples who do not adopt. In chapter 15, "Exploring Other Family-Building Options," we offer information about adoption—if, and when, you are ready to explore adopting an infant or child as the solution to resolving infertility that feels right for you.

**Myth:** *You're probably doing "it" wrong.*
**Fact:** Infertility is a medical condition, not a sexual disorder. On the other hand, the timing of sexual intercourse is crucial to the conception process. Chapter 2, "Normal Fertility," includes information about this aspect of fertility.

**Myth:** *Individuals or couples who already have a child (or children) should be satisfied with their situation and should not "push their luck" by pursuing treatment for infertility.*

**Fact:** Having one child does not necessarily diminish the desire to have one or more additional children. The desire to provide a sibling for a child can be a driving need. Secondary infertility, defined as the inability of an individual or couple to achieve and complete a subsequent pregnancy, may be lonely and isolating. Often there is little understanding and support among family, friends, and co-workers—and even within the medical community. For couples and single parents alike, there is the pressure to "leave well enough alone" and "count your blessings" for the child, or children, you already have.

**Myth:** *Your partner will leave you because of your infertility.*
**Fact:** The rewards of an intimate relationship require hard work and diligent effort every day from both partners, regardless of the difficult challenges posed by infertility. Without doubt, infertility represents a major life crisis, one that certainly affects a marriage or partnership. Fortunately, most couples survive the infertility crisis and learn new ways of relating to each other that deepen their relationship. You may hit a few rough patches along the way, but as long as you keep the lines of communication open, there is a good chance you will grow closer through the experience. See chapter 13, "Enhancing Your Relationship: Sexuality, Intimacy, and Infertility," for suggestions on weathering this difficult aspect of the journey.

**Myth:** *Maybe you are just not meant to be a parent.*
**Fact:** You and your partner have made the decision to become parents because you know how much love and support you have to offer a child. Having a medical condition that makes it difficult to conceive and bear a child is not a sign from God, from the universe, from society, or—for that matter—from anywhere else about your suitability to raise children, or whether it is "meant" for you to become a parent.

**Myth:** *Infertility is just nature's way of controlling the population.*
**Fact:** In 1930, there were 2 billion people on planet Earth. According to the United Nations, the world's population reached 6 billion in October 1999, just at the first publication of this book—a tripling of the total population in less than a century. In 1994, however, the world's fertility rate fell to under 50 percent of the average fertility rate of 1950. The truth is that in industrial nations, fertility rates are moving toward the "replacement level"—2 children per woman—required for zero population growth. Many of the developing nations, such as Mexico, have reduced fertility rates from 6 births per woman in 1950 to 3 per

woman in 1994. The challenge remains, however, for developing nations, where almost 1 billion children are about to reach their reproductive years; as of October 1999, 1 in 3 people worldwide was age 15 or younger.

Individuals or couples can certainly choose to be childfree, but the inability to get treatment for infertility may result in childlessness—and not by choice.

**Myth:** *My life will be overwhelmed with infertility and nothing will ever be the same.*

**Fact:** Infertility is a life crisis, and it will probably have an effect on all areas of your life at one time or another. It is perfectly normal to feel overwhelmed, with surges of guilt, anxiety, and sadness. At the same time, the desire to have a child may fill you with single-minded determination, at the expense of other areas of your life—including your most personal relationships. Long-held notions about who you are and how you envision your life may be tested, but you will eventually move through this crisis. Because resolving infertility is a process that may require you to let go of your initial vision of bearing a biological child, it is important to recognize that feelings of loss and grief are common.

Although the emotions and issues surrounding infertility may surface throughout your life in predictable—and unpredictable—times and ways (at menopause, for example), the intense struggle you are facing now will resolve itself as you work through each decision in the infertility process and move along your unique life path. In chapter 3, "Preparing Yourself for the Journey," we introduce a decision tree worksheet you can use to help weigh all the pros and cons along the way.

### Voices

*"Our greatest fear when we started treatment was that we wouldn't know when to stop," recalls Paige, a 35-year-old woman who just adopted her second child with her husband Gary. "We wondered if—no matter what it took—we'd continue with the treatments until we got pregnant, even when there wasn't any real hope left. But when the time came to quit, we knew. And we did the right thing for our family."*

**Myth:** *It is wrong for women over 40 to want children. Mid-life is the time for both men and women to be emerging from the responsibilities of parenting a small child, not beginning them.*

**Fact:** In 1900, at the start of the twentieth century, the average American lived to be 47 years old. Today, as we enter the twenty-first century, that same average American lives to be 76. Even in developing countries, such as India, the human life span showed remarkable progress over the twentieth century, going from 23 years for men in 1900 to 60 years today. According to the MacArthur Foundation Study on Aging in America, anyone who lived to be 100 years old in 1900 was a precious find; now there are about 61,000 centenarians living in America. By 2050, it is projected that more than 600,000 Americans will live past 100 years of age. In industrialized nations where births per woman are consistently dropping, the old pyramid model of aging, where there are more young people than old, is evolving into a pillar. That means that even as a mid-life parent, through adoption, birth or surrogacy, you have the potential to live long enough and remain healthy enough to spoil your grandchildren.

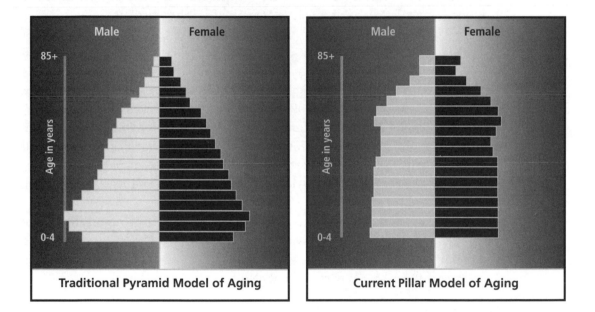

**Traditional Pyramid Model of Aging**

**Current Pillar Model of Aging**

The reality is that fertility declines in women as they age, and markedly for most after the age of 40. Yes, most babies today are born to women in their 20s. Yet in the mid-1990s, more than 1,000 babies a day were born in America to women between the ages of 35 and 44, according to the National Center for Health Statistics, and the trend toward later childbearing is continuing for both married and unmarried women.

### Voices

*Dr. Martha Farnsworth Riche, former director of the U.S. Census Bureau, asserts, "Everyone has been given 20 extra years of fully functional living. . . . Add 20 years to women's lives, however, and women's options shift, even without much change in social conditions. For the first time, women can raise children to maturity and have 20-year careers as well, before confronting care of the elderly. This makes investment in women's education and training more important than ever, along with changes in law and custom that will allow women to reach their full potential."*

There are other myths and misconceptions you may confront while struggling with infertility, so it pays to ask questions of your doctor and to use RESOLVE to help you find the facts. Later in the chapter, we will suggest ways for you to meet the tasks and challenges ahead, including maintaining a journal and using the test result worksheets for women and men located at the back of this book. Now, let's look at the development of fertility medicine.

## THE EVOLUTION OF FERTILITY MEDICINE

In 1978, one of the most remarkable advances in fertility medicine took place when Louise Brown of the United Kingdom—the world's first "test-tube" baby—was born. Three years later, a baby was conceived and born in the United States using the same techniques. Since that time, medical advances and legal precedents have brought fertility medicine to the front pages more than once—for better and for worse—raising medical, social, and legal issues along the way.

These two miracles, and the hundreds of thousands of others that have taken place across the country over the past several decades, are testaments to the importance of family building in our society. This high interest in fertility is hardly new; it has been a part of human culture since time began.

### The Meaning of Fertility

Fertile land, fertile people: Without them, the world as we know it would cease to exist. Adam and Eve were commanded by God to "be fruitful and multiply." "Give me children, or I die!" cried Rachel in the Old Testament. As reported in the Bible, women who were childless often conceived through finding favor with God, forever linking fertility with the ideals of goodness and piety.

But Jewish and Christian communities were not the only ones to revere fertility: The ancient Romans worshiped Venus, the goddess of love, and the Greeks focused on Aphrodite as the symbol of fecundity and procreation. *Fertile* is derived from the Latin word *fertilis*, meaning "fruitful, as in to bear." The mother-goddess was also a symbol of worship in the ancient communities of Asia Minor, Syria, and Libya. In some religious traditions, a woman had to bear children to reach heaven, and in others, a marriage could be annulled if a woman proved infertile.

Secular society has also applied pressure to women and couples to reproduce. For generations, women were denied birth control or safe abortion, both practices considered illegal as well as immoral even today by some sectors of society. How often have couples who have chosen to remain childfree been described as selfish and self-centered?

At the same time, the medical technology that allows women and men to control their fertility was developing. During the colonial period of North America, doctors prescribed herbal elixirs to treat infertility; at the time of the U.S. Civil War, doctors prescribed suspect surgical and other treatments. For example, J. Mann Simms, a prominent New York physician, artificially inseminated a woman with her husband's sperm—but not before surgically enlarging her cervix in the mistaken belief that such a modification was necessary for conception. (To give Simms credit, however, he also developed the Simms speculum, a medical tool that has been adapted and used for gynecologic examinations ever since.)

In 1873, Harvard College physician Edward H. Clarke proposed a theory about infertility that revealed an absurd streak of misguided paternalism. In his widely acclaimed book *Sex Education, or a Fair Chance for Our Girls,* he charged that education was the culprit for "female sterility" by "manufacturing women with monstrous brains and puny bodies." Furthermore, he stated, "the reproductive machinery, to be well made . . . must be carefully managed. Force must be allowed to flow thither in an ample stream . . . and not diverted to the brain by the school."

Fortunately, great strides made in the 1920s put the study of fertility and its obstacles firmly into the scientific arena. In 1920, researcher I. C. Rubin developed the first test for blocked fallopian tubes, a major cause of female infertility. Then, in 1923 and 1925, scientists isolated and identified the two female hormones, estrogen and progesterone (the discovery of testosterone, the male hormone, would not take place for another decade). With this understanding of the anatomy and physiology of women and men, progress was made on both fronts: preventing pregnancy for people who wished to delay parenthood and clearing the path for those who wished to bear children.

Slowly and steadily, the concept of "planned parenthood," of reproductive choices and options, has become firmly entrenched in American society; and it is true that humans have more control over procreation than ever before. There remain, however, higher biological hurdles than even the most advanced medical technology can clear, a fact as frustrating and heartbreaking to modern Americans as it was to their ancestors.

## Today's Challenges

Today, reproduction is an evolving, exciting branch of medicine, offering hundreds of thousands of women and men new hope for experiencing pregnancy and birth. The advance in reproductive techniques comes at a time when several factors have combined to put more women and men at increased risk for reproductive problems. We will discuss these factors—as well as more specific risk factors—at more length in later chapters, but here is a general overview of the pressing issues surrounding fertility today.

*Later Age of First Pregnancy* According to recent statistics, the birthrate for women aged 40 to 44 has increased an astounding 74 percent since 1981, and mothers older than 30 account for more than one out of three new mothers in the United States—more than four times as many as teenage mothers. More and more women and men are choosing to delay starting a family until their 30s and 40s.

As exciting and empowering as the freedom to choose this option may be, it is not always successful. Both men and women suffer a significant decline in their fertility as they age. A woman in her late 30s is about 30 percent less fertile than she was in her early 20s. The clinical term is *subfertile*. As a woman enters her late 30s, her body begins to undergo the changes of *perimenopause*, which may include any or all of the following: rising cycle day 3 follicle-stimulating hormone (FSH) and estradiol levels, irregular periods, decreased ovulation, and more estrogen in relation to progesterone than when she was younger. But perimenopause is not menopause. And subfertile is not the same as infertile. Some women can conceive in their 40s using their own eggs, and researchers continue to look for ways to enhance fertility in older women.

---

### Voices

*Donna waited until she was over 40 to start trying to have children. "I married later than some people do, when I was in my early 30s. Gene and I never felt the pressure to have kids right away, though it was always something we knew we'd want to do someday. Now that* someday *is here. We didn't anticipate that it would be this hard to get pregnant, but we intend to take full advantage of all the recent advances that can help us fulfill our dream of having a child of our own. We're looking for a doctor who can help us try."*

---

*Spread of Sexually Transmitted Diseases*  Every year, according to the National Institute of Allergy and Infectious Diseases (NIAID), 13 million cases of sexually transmitted disease (STDs) are newly diagnosed in the United States, and some of these infections can lead to infertility. If left untreated, they can cause scar tissue and damage to the delicate fallopian tubes. In a man, such infection can also cause scarring and damage to the ducts of the epididymis, vas deferens, and ejaculatory ducts. Sadly, these diseases often work their damage over time and without symptoms.

*Environmental Toxins*  Every day, industry releases roughly 60,000 potentially toxic chemicals into the air we breathe, the water we drink, the food we eat, and the substances we touch, and many of those chemicals may interfere with fertility. Several workplace hazards—lead, chlorinated hydrocarbons, ionizing radiation, kepone, ethylene oxide and ethylene dibromide, PCBs and PBBs, and dibromochloropropane (DBCP)—are known to cause damage to the human reproductive system, but many more may have as yet unproven negative effects. Alcohol, tobacco and nicotine, caffeine, and illicit drugs such as cocaine and marijuana also may impair fertility: A 1985 study published by the *Journal of the American Medical Association* found that smokers were 3.4 times more likely than nonsmokers to take more than a year to conceive. See chapter 12, "Staying Healthy," for more about the environmental hazards and lifestyle risks that may affect fertility.

*Exposure to Diethylstilbestrol (DES)*  During the early to mid-1960s, obstetricians, in a misguided attempt to protect women at high risk of miscarriage, prescribed the drug DES, a synthetic estrogen later banned by the U. S. Food and Drug Administration (FDA). DES may cause a wide range of serious medical problems, including genital cancers and fertility problems, in the people who were exposed to the drug in the womb. DES-related problems may include impaired fertility, endometriosis, ectopic pregnancies, and repeated miscarriages. Some DES daughters were born with malformed fallopian tubes and uteruses, resulting in tubal pregnancies and the inability to maintain a pregnancy.

## Voices

*"My mother told me when I was in my early teens that she'd taken DES when she was pregnant with me, so I always knew I might have trouble getting pregnant," recalls Nancy. At the age of 30, Nancy's doctors discovered that she had an extremely small uterus—a condition common in women whose mothers had taken DES—which was interfering with her ability to become and stay pregnant.*

As you can see, events of the past 30 years have influenced the expectations of men and women and their ability to conceive easily. Perhaps you are among those affected, finding yourself over 35 and not yet pregnant, or coping with the damage from an STD you had years ago. Or perhaps you are among the thousands of people with unexplained infertility, finding yourself searching for a solution to the infertility problem you now confront. And that is where RESOLVE can help.

## MAPPING THE ROAD AHEAD

Without question, you have embarked on a journey into a new world of options, challenges, and emotions that probably feel more than a little overwhelming. One good way to help you make this experience a little more manageable is to keep a journal of your questions and concerns; your hopes and fears; and important names and phone numbers of doctors, clinics, support groups, and other resources. Your journal can become an important record and a therapeutic tool that allows you to vent your feelings of frustration, fear, and hope. You and your partner may want to consider the benefits of keeping separate journals. Throughout this book, we present sidebars called "Perspectives" that give you some ideas for journal writing. You will also want to use the worksheets at the back of this book to help you track your infertility tests and results.

### *Perspectives*

*Tips on Keeping a Journal*  If you choose to keep a journal, and you are a computer buff, create a file (or files) for your journal there. You might enjoy writing in a journal made with high-quality paper covered with an attractive cover; but a plain, old loose-leaf notebook certainly would serve the purpose. Once you have chosen your format, begin, perhaps, by writing down some thoughts about your current situation. Consider your goals, short- and long-term, and don't be afraid to voice your fears as well as your hopes.

In part 1, "Understanding Infertility," you will come face to face with the facts about infertility and learn about the various issues and options. Knowledge is power: Resolving infertility is within your grasp. In the book *The Art of Happiness*, the Dalai Lama counsels readers to face problems and challenges directly: "If you are in a battle, as long as you remain ignorant of the status and combat capability of your enemy, you will be totally unprepared and paralyzed by fear. However, if you know the fighting capability of your opponents, what sort of weapons they have and so on, then you're in a much better position when you engage in the war. In the same way, if you confront your problems rather than avoid them, you will be in a better position." In this book, we provide the knowledge and tools to help you make the decisions to resolve infertility in the way that feels right for you and your family.

## The Medical Process

In part 2, "The Medical Journey," you will find a map through the medical process, from diagnosis to treatment. We outline the way conception *should* work, offer tips on finding a skilled physician and clinic, and describe the techniques and treatments—from low-tech to high-tech—that you may encounter on your journey. Among the many questions we will answer are the following:

- How long should you try to get pregnant before seeing a doctor? And what kind of doctor should you see?
- What are the risk factors for infertility?
- How does having a miscarriage affect future pregnancies?
- If you are over 35, what special challenges could you be facing?
- What are the effects and side effects of hormone treatments for women and for men?
- Is surgery necessary to treat your problem; and if so, what type is best?
- How do the different insemination techniques work and what are the advantages and disadvantages of each?
- Are there successful ways to reverse a vasectomy or tubal ligation?
- If you do get pregnant, what do you need to do to take care of yourself?
- What assisted reproductive technology (ART) techniques might help you become pregnant—from in vitro fertilization to egg or embryo donation?

## The Emotional Roller Coaster

In part 3, "Coping with Infertility," we discuss the myriad of social and emotional issues connected with infertility. Infertility is more than physical; it affects every aspect of an individual's or couple's life. Intense feelings of anger, frustration, determination, loss of control, isolation from family and friends, depression, and grief erupt in unpredictable cycles. To help you cope with the process, we offer tips on:

- Establishing and maintaining a healthy diet and an exercise routine.
- Reducing stress and learning new ways of coping.

- Coping with your family, friends, and co-workers who, though well meaning, may not fully understand or accept your struggle.
- Staying intimate with your partner through this difficult time.

Some couples—despite their commitment and the help of modern medicine—may realize that having a biological child is not an option. In part 3, we also help you sort out your other family-building options—from adoption to donors and surrogacy to resolving without children—and we do so keeping in mind the emotional, financial, and legal considerations of each choice.

We will also explore the special challenges and emotions of individuals and couples experiencing secondary infertility. For those who become pregnant after infertility, we will help to guide you through the experience. And, for any individual or couple who has grappled with infertility, we will take a look at the long-term effects of that experience at each stage along the life path.

## The Financial Maze

Chapter 14, "Creating a Financial Game Plan and Getting Through the Insurance Maze," outlines some important issues that you must consider as soon as possible—your financial responsibilities and your insurance options. Consider this, if your treatment requires ART, a single cycle of IVF may cost between $7,000 and $10,000. Hormone treatments can run from $200 to $3,000 per month, depending on the drug and your needs. An individual or couple may spend $30,000 or more in the quest to have a baby. Unfortunately, insurance coverage is not always available; it is important for you to assess realistically your resources, opportunities, and goals.

The most important things for you to remember right now are that you do not need to absorb this information all at once or to make any final decisions at this time. Take it slowly, ask questions of your doctors and your peers, and allow RESOLVE to help you through this crisis.

## Resolving Infertility

*To every thing there is a season, and a time to every purpose under heaven.* These words from Ecclesiastes have been co-opted by everyone from Shakespeare to the Byrds. And they are still true today. As you and your partner face the challenges and options posed by infertility, you may find within yourselves reservoirs of strength, resilience, and depth of feeling you never knew you had to draw upon. Writer Alice Walker talks often about "honoring the difficult." Martin Luther King Jr., said, "What does not destroy me, makes me stronger." Facing infertility is not easy. But whatever option you choose to resolve infertility—by a pregnancy carried full term, by adopting, by donor egg pregnancy or surrogacy, or by resolving childfree—the decision is yours. And we applaud that decision and all the effort, time, determination, honesty, and emotion you have given to making it.

## POSITIVE STEPS YOU CAN TAKE FROM CHAPTER 1

**Find strength in numbers.** You are not alone in the challenges you face in conceiving and bearing a child. Infertility affects millions of men and women in the United States today, and hundreds of scientists and physicians are working to discover new treatments for infertility in laboratories around the world.

**Dismiss the myths.** Myths about infertility still abound, and it is imperative that you learn the facts. Do not let misconceptions hold you back from thinking logically about your current situation, from accepting the full range of emotions you are feeling, or from considering your future with equal parts hope and realism.

**Commit your experience to paper.** Maintaining a journal may be a key to maintaining your center when things get hectic or seem overwhelming, as they no doubt will from time to time along the way. Writing down your thoughts and keeping written accounts of important medical and financial information may help you feel more in control as you travel on this journey. Be sure to use the decision tree introduced in chapter 3 and the test result worksheets for women and men, found at the back of this book.

# 2  Normal Fertility

As you start to deal with the challenges of infertility, learn as much as you can about the normal reproduction process. Unless you have a good understanding of how conception, pregnancy, and childbirth are *supposed* to occur, taking a proactive and positive role in your own care and treatment will prove especially challenging.

The human body is a miracle of precise and elegant engineering, and in no function is that more apparent than in reproduction. The description of the anatomy and physiology of reproduction that follows shows just how synchronized various systems of the body must be for fertilization and successful implantation of an embryo to take place. We will describe the female and male reproductive systems, identify the important reproductive hormones and discuss their function, and then outline the complicated process of a successful conception and pregnancy.

## Voices

*"I thought I knew at least the basics about the monthly cycle and reproduction," admits Tom, a 35-year-old man who went through 3 years of infertility treatments with his wife, Fran. "But I had to go back to the beginning when my wife and I started infertility treatment. To make sense of and feel comfortable with the treatments, I had to know what they were meant to correct or help. Once I did, a lot of the fear about the whole process went away, and so did the feeling that the doctors knew everything and I knew nothing. I could really participate. Our doctor involved us in the decision-*

*making process concerning diagnostic tests and treatments. That felt good. Fran and I felt more connected to the whole process and more focused about pursuing our options."*

## THE FEMALE REPRODUCTIVE SYSTEM

The female reproductive system includes the following organs and glands:

- *Ovaries:* About the size of walnuts, the ovaries have two important functions: to produce the female hormones, estrogen and progesterone, and to produce one ripened egg (also called an ovum) each menstrual cycle. Each month (or cycle), one of the two ovaries produces an oocyte, or egg. The egg develops within a small, fluid-filled sac called the follicle. When the egg is mature, it is released from the ovary and passes through one of the fallopian tubes.

- *Fallopian tubes:* The fallopian tubes are two muscular, trumpet-shaped, flexible tubes about 2 inches long that are connected to the uterus. Once the egg is released from the ovary, flared projections from the far end of the fallopian tube, called the *fimbriae*, catch the egg and move it into the tube. Then *cilia*, small hairlike structures that line the tube's wall, help move the egg down toward the uterus. It is during this journey that egg and sperm meet. The cilia then transport the newly fertilized egg, or embryo, to the uterus.

- *Uterus:* The uterus is a thick, muscular organ about the size and shape of a pear in its nonpregnant state; when carrying a growing fetus, it is capable of expanding more than forty times this size. The cavity of the uterus is triangular in shape, wide at the top (fundus) and narrow at the bottom (cervical end). Its lining, the endometrium, plays a pivotal role in the process of implantation and nourishment of the embryo.

- *Endometrium:* The endometrium is the mucous membrane that lines the uterus; it thickens and thins under the influence of hormones. This tissue must be in a state of readiness—thickened, spongy, and filled with a web of new blood vessels—when an embryo arrives in order for implantation to occur. If there is no implantation, the thickened endometrium is shed from the body with the menstrual period.

- *Cervix:* A fibrous ring of tissue, the cervix is situated at the top of the vaginal canal. Sperm move up through the vagina to the cervix. The cervix secretes mucus in which sperm collect, later to be released into the uterus. Cervical secretions change in consistency from an impassable plug to

# FEMALE REPRODUCTIVE SYSTEM

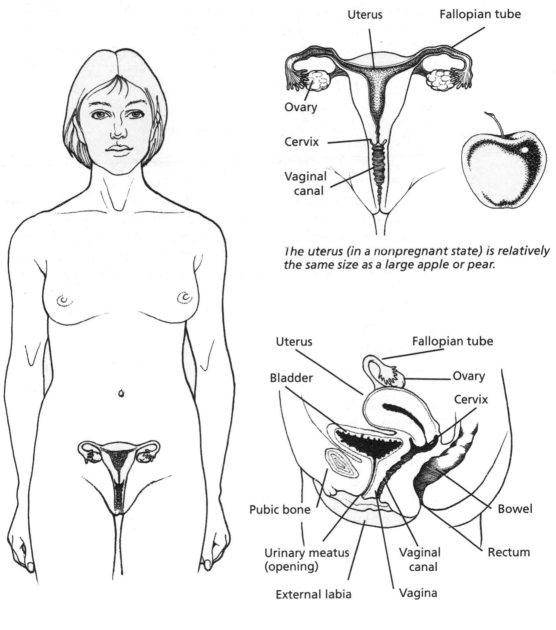

Uterus

Fallopian tube

Ovary

Cervix

Vaginal canal

*The uterus (in a nonpregnant state) is relatively the same size as a large apple or pear.*

Uterus

Fallopian tube

Bladder

Ovary

Cervix

Pubic bone

Bowel

Urinary meatus (opening)

Vaginal canal

Rectum

External labia

Vagina

watery strands during the course of a woman's cycle. Just the right amount and quality of mucus must be present for sperm to pass through the cervix into the uterus. The cervical mucus also serves as a protection against infection; cells produced by the immune system patrol the mucus looking for "enemies," such as bacteria, and viruses.

- *Vagina:* The vagina is the opening to the vaginal canal, a muscular structure 5 to 8 inches long and lined with a mucous membrane. The vaginal canal leads to the cervix. During sexual intercourse, sperm enter the woman's body through the vagina.

## The Reproductive Hormones

The word *hormone* comes from the Greek word meaning "to set in motion, to spur on, to excite." A hormone is a chemical messenger that enables one organ, such as the pituitary gland, to communicate with another, such as the ovary. This chemical signal carries information from the endocrine gland that secretes it to a specific organ or tissue. Humans produce about 50 hormones, which travel through the body, either in the bloodstream or in the fluid around cells, looking for target cells. A target cell is a cell that has the ability to respond to a particular hormone. Once a hormone finds a target cell, it binds to specialized receptors inside or on the surface of the cell and changes the cell's activities in precise ways. The female sex hormone estrogen, for example, binds to target cells primarily in the uterus, bone, and breasts. Target cells often contain receptors for more than one hormone. The uterine, bone, and breast cells that are target cells for estrogen also contain receptors for progesterone and androgens (male sex hormones).

The primary female reproductive hormones—gonadotropin-releasing hormone (GnRH), follicle-stimulating hormone (FSH), luteinizing hormone (LH), estrogen, and progesterone—trigger actions that affect the menstrual cycle and fertility. The endocrine glands that secrete these hormones are the hypothalamus (located in the brain), the pituitary gland (a small, rounded gland attached at the front of the brain), and the ovaries (the female sex glands—also known as gonads).

The female sex hormones and their function in reproduction are outlined below.

- *GnRH:* The hypothalamus releases GnRH, which in turn stimulates the release of FSH and LH, which are also called *gonadotropins*. The hypothalamus releases GnRH in pulses every 60 to 90 minutes. The effects of GnRH

**FEMALE ENDOCRINE SYSTEM**

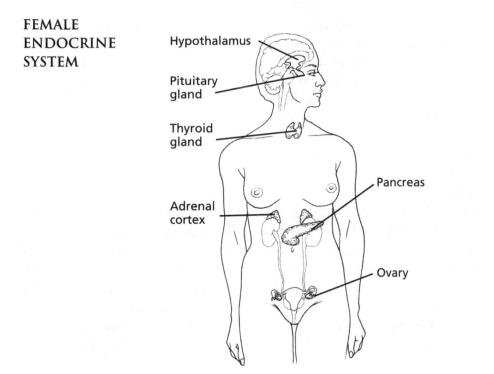

Hypothalamus

Pituitary gland

Thyroid gland

Pancreas

Adrenal cortex

Ovary

are cyclical: In the first half of a woman's menstrual cycle, it stimulates the pituitary gland to release FSH and in the second half of the cycle, when the frequency of GnRH release slows down, it stimulates the release of LH.

- *FSH:* Produced by the pituitary, FSH stimulates the growth of follicles, the structures inside the ovaries that contain eggs.
- *LH:* The pituitary gland also releases LH, which stimulates the ovarian follicle to release the egg.
- *Estrogen:* Estrogen is the primary female sex hormone. The ovaries—specifically the follicles within the ovaries—produce most of the body's supply of estrogen. Estrogen triggers many actions and reactions throughout the body, in addition to its role in the reproductive system. During the menstrual cycle, estrogen stimulates the lining of the uterus, the endometrium, to grow and thicken in preparation for a fertilized egg. The presence of estrogen also causes the cervical mucus to become thin, clear, and watery at the time of ovulation so that sperm can travel through it into the uterine cavity.
- *Progesterone:* Produced by the ovaries, progesterone prepares the uterine lining to receive a fertilized egg. If there is no implantation, progesterone

production falls, triggering the shedding of the endometrium (i.e., a menstrual period) and thus the end of the cycle.

- *Other hormones:* Other hormones, such as *prolactin* and *testosterone*, are also necessary (in small concentrations) for the normal function of the female reproductive system. If produced in excess, they can disturb ovulation and possibly implantation.

## How the Female Organs Respond to the Signals of the Reproductive Hormones

### THE OVARIES

Primarily under the influence of FSH, 10 to 20 (or more) follicles begin to mature. Usually only 1 follicle—known as the *dominant follicle*—develops fully; and as it grows, it secretes estrogen. During ovulation, which occurs about 14 days after a menstrual period begins, the mature follicle opens at the ovary's surface to release the egg. The hormone progesterone is then secreted by the empty follicle, also called the *corpus luteum*. If fertilization and implantation of the embryo occur, the corpus luteum continues to produce progesterone, which helps maintain the pregnancy. If no pregnancy occurs, the corpus luteum stops secreting progesterone.

OVULATION

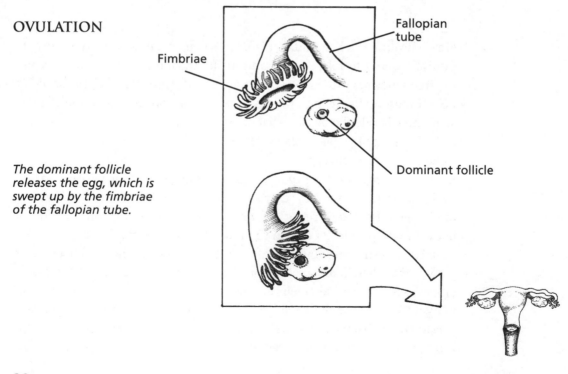

*The dominant follicle releases the egg, which is swept up by the fimbriae of the fallopian tube.*

## *All About the Egg*

The eggs held in each ovary in a female fetus are formed at 14 to 16 weeks after fertilization. The process is called *oogenesis*, and the original cells continue to develop until birth. When a girl is born, she has between 1 and 2 million eggs in her ovaries. At that time, the eggs are called *primary oocytes*. She will begin to lose eggs early in life; by the age of puberty only 300,000 to 500,000 eggs remain in reserve in the ovaries.

As the eggs are formed, thin layers of cells called *granulosa cells* grow around them. The granulosa cells and the oocyte are contained within a follicle. The follicle cells support the egg they enclose for 50 years or more, providing it with nourishment but preventing it from maturing. The great majority of follicles and eggs never grow to maturity and ovulation. Follicles begin to develop, but if conditions for continued growth are not right, the eggs they contain lose nourishment and die. The follicle cells then are absorbed back into the ovary. This process is called *atresia*. Atresia continues throughout a woman's life until all the follicles are gone, and she enters menopause.

During the hours leading up to ovulation when the mature egg is released from the dominant follicle, two important processes begin. A few hours before ovulation, the primary oocyte undergoes a cell division process called *meiosis,* which results in an egg that contains 23 chromosomes—the same number of chromosomes in the sperm that fertilizes it. Once fertilization occurs, the embryonic cell contains all 46 chromosomes that will be necessary for the continued development of the embryo.

The follicle cells surrounding the oocyte secrete mucus, forming a circular barrier (the *cumulus*) around the oocyte. Just beneath the jelly-like cumulus is the tough, glassy-looking membrane called the *zona pellucida*. Sperm must be able to breach the cumulus and the zona pellucida of the egg if fertilization is to take place. Conception usually occurs within 24 to 36 hours after ovulation. If no sperm fertilizes the egg, the egg disintegrates and flows out with the vaginal secretions, before or during menstruation.

### THE CERVIX

Cervical mucus changes in response to the different hormones. During the majority of a woman's cycle, the mucus is a maze of tangled fibers, which makes it difficult for sperm and other cells to penetrate. At ovulation, under the influence of estrogen, the mucus changes, forming long strands that are able to guide the sperm into the uterus. At this time, the mucus is thick enough to coat the vagina and protect the sperm from the acid secretions produced there. After ovulation, as estrogen levels drop and progesterone levels rise with the approach of menstruation, mucus production diminishes and the vagina gradually becomes drier.

### THE ENDOMETRIUM

At the beginning of a menstrual cycle, the secretion of estrogen from the maturing follicle causes the endometrium to grow and thicken. After ovulation, the progesterone secreted by the corpus luteum causes the endometrial lining to thicken. If conception does not occur, the corpus luteum will produce less and less estrogen and progesterone for about 12 days. As the estrogen and progesterone levels drop, the tiny blood vessels that supply the endometrium close off. The endometrial lining is no longer nourished, and the body sheds it.

---

### *The Menstrual Cycle*

*Note: Not every woman experiences the "classic" 28-day cycle. Some women may have shorter or longer cycles and still be fertile.*

**Day 1:** The first day of a woman's menstrual cycle is the first day of blood flow. Some women bleed for 3 to 6 days, others for 2 to 3 days. It is not unusual to have some light spotting just before the menstrual bleed.

**Days 2 to 14:** This is called the follicular phase. During this time, the endometrium starts to grow, the follicles on the ovary become active, and cervical mucus begins to thin.

**Day 14:** Ovulation takes place at midcycle. Rising estrogen levels trigger the pituitary to release LH (the "LH surge"). The climbing level of LH causes the follicle to ovulate, releasing an egg. The timing of ovulation is not precise; it may occur between days 12 and 14, depending on the woman's individual cycle.

**Days 15 to 22:** After releasing the egg, the follicle transforms into the corpus luteum. The corpus luteum produces the hormone progesterone, which thickens the uterine lining for implantation of the fertilized egg (embryo). This stage of the cycle is called the luteal phase.

**Days 23 to 24:** If there is no embryo implantation, estrogen and progesterone levels fall.

**Days 25 to 28:** The falling progesterone levels trigger the shedding of the endometrium.

---

## MENSTRUAL CYCLE

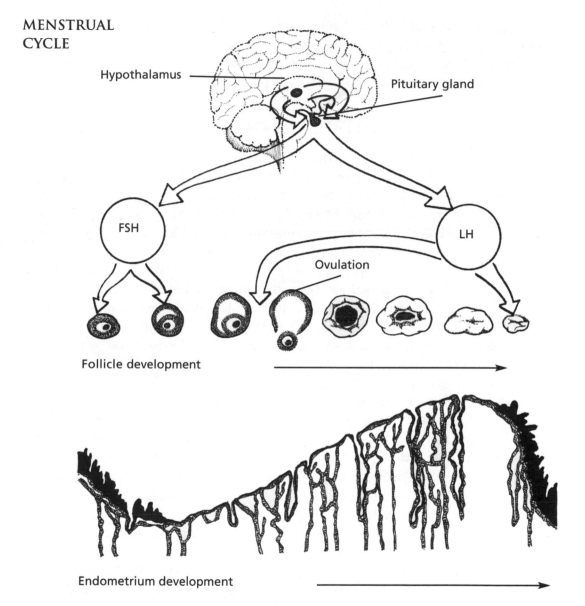

A Voice on Perspectives

"Every month when my period comes," reveals Ilana, a 28-year-old woman with unexplained infertility, "a feeling of such failure comes over me. I have a friend from a support group going through the same treatments as I am, and she's more positive about it. She looks at her period as a kind of starting bell for the next try. I'm trying to look at it that way, too."

*In your journal, write down what getting a monthly period means to you now that you are trying to have a baby and what it has meant to you in the past. Can you communicate these feelings to your partner or significant other? What are your partner's views? How has an awareness of your monthly cycle affected intimacy and sexuality?*

## THE MALE REPRODUCTIVE SYSTEM

Although a man's reproductive system is not controlled by the cyclical rising and falling levels of hormones, it is far more intricate and delicate than might appear at first glance. It consists of the testes and a system of ducts and accessory structures. Its function, like the female reproductive system, depends on the presence and action of hormones, including GnRH, FSH, LH, and testosterone, which act to stimulate certain activities.

In the male, the hypothalamus pulses out constant doses of GnRH in 60- to 90-minute intervals. GnRH triggers the pituitary gland to release FSH and LH. FSH stimulates cells in the testicles to grow, mature, and release male germ cells (*sperm*). At the same time, the LH secretion from the pituitary stimulates the testicles to produce the male hormone testosterone. Testosterone causes development of the normal male sexual characteristics such as facial hair and muscular development, as well as sex drive and ejaculatory function.

As you will note in chapters 5, "The Basic Infertility Work-up for Women and Men," and 8, "The Male: Diagnosis and Treatment," disruptions in the balance of these hormones can interfere with fertility. Only about 5 percent of male factor infertility can be traced to a hormonal imbalance or congenital abnormality of the endocrine system. It is more likely that a problem exists somewhere in the structural and functional anatomy of the male reproductive tract that affects the ability of the sperm to grow or be ejaculated from the man's body.

The male reproductive system includes the following organs and glands:

- *Scrotum:* The scrotum is a pouch of skin that hangs behind the penis. It contains the testes, the sperm-producing organs. The location of the scrotum outside of the body cavity keeps the testes slightly cooler (by about 2 degrees) than body temperature. The temperature difference is vital to normal sperm production. The scrotal muscles contract to bring the testes closer to the body in cold weather and relax to drop the testes away from the body in warm weather.
- *Testes:* A pair of oval glands located within the scrotum, the testes have two major functions: to produce testosterone and to produce sperm cells.

# MALE
# REPRODUCTIVE
# SYSTEM

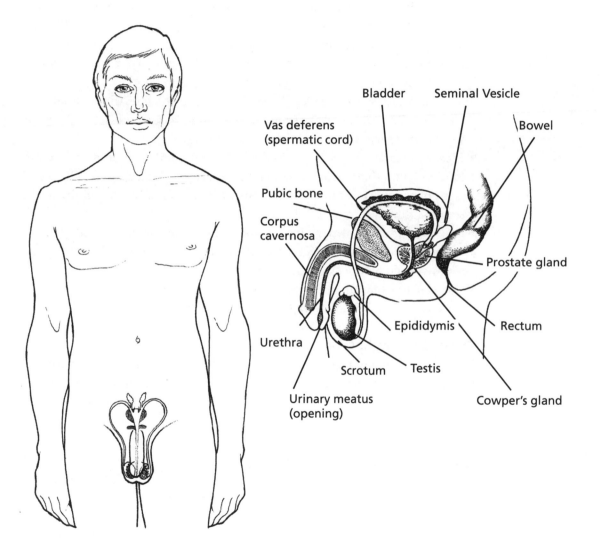

Bladder

Seminal Vesicle

Bowel

Vas deferens
(spermatic cord)

Pubic bone

Corpus
cavernosa

Prostate gland

Epididymis

Rectum

Urethra

Scrotum

Testis

Urinary meatus
(opening)

Cowper's gland

- *Leydig cells* produce the hormone testosterone and *Sertoli cells* produce growth factors that nourish the sperm. The sperm begin to mature and are stored in the seminiferous tubules for about 3 months. To mature fully, the sperm leave the testes and travel to the epididymis.
- *Epididymis:* The epididymis is a long, coiled tube that lies beside and behind the testes. The epididymis helps the sperm mature and transports them to the vas deferens. Sperm remain in the epididymis for 2 to 12 days.
- *Vas deferens:* A long tube with thick walls, the vas deferens (the terminal portion of which is called the ejaculatory duct) runs from the end of the epididymis upward into the pelvis behind the bladder.
- *Seminal vesicles:* Two accessory glands near the prostate, the seminal vesicles contribute most of the seminal fluid and produce the sugar fructose, which the sperm use to fuel their long journey.
- *Prostate gland:* The prostate gland contributes additional fluid and important enzymes that cause the semen to liquefy after ejaculation. The secretions of the prostate are highly alkaline, which neutralize the acidity of the seminal fluid.
- *Cowper's glands:* Cowper's glands, located beyond the prostate at the base of the penile shaft in the urethra, add a small amount of lubricant to the seminal fluid before ejaculation takes place.
- *Penis:* A rod-shaped, muscular organ, the penis allows the man to deposit the seminal fluid into the vagina of the woman.

## The Physiology of Healthy Sperm

Sperm development begins in the Sertoli cells of the testes. Over a period of 72 hours, a single sperm cell (spermatozoon) develops a head that contains 23 chromosomes, a middle piece that contains fuel for movement, and a tail to pro-

HEALTHY SPERM

Head

Tail

Midsection

pel it forward. Once the sperm cell separates from the Sertoli cell, it moves into the lumen (center) of the seminiferus tubules within the testes—and then on into the epididymis. There, over a period of days, the sperm mature and begin to move through the actions of their tails. It takes 90 to 108 days for the sperm to traverse the tubules leading from the testicle to the penis. During that time, the sperm continue to mature and develop the ability to swim.

The fully mature sperm remain within the vasa deferentia until ejaculation occurs. The process necessary for sexual stimulation and ejaculation begins in the brain. Signals transmitted from the brain travel down the spinal cord to the penis. These messages tell the corpora cavernosa, two rod-shaped bundles of muscles on either side of the penis, to relax and fill with blood. As they fill, the corpora cavernosa expand and press against the veins that would normally drain blood from the penis, which causes the penis to become firm and erect. In this state, the penis can penetrate the female vagina during sexual intercourse.

During intercourse, nerve impulses from the penis are carried back to the brain. The sexual stimulation gradually builds in intensity until the brain senses the threshold and sends other messages to trigger ejaculation. Rhythmic contraction of the smooth muscles of the testicles causes them to expel their contents—0.5 milliliters of fluid, which normally contain 20 to 150 million active sperm. The seminal vesicles, prostate, and Cowper's glands all add their secretions to the sperm, thus forming semen, or seminal fluid, before ejaculation through the urethra and out of the body. Healthy sperm can live up to 48 hours in the cervical mucus, more than enough time to make the journey to the fallopian tube and a waiting egg. Ejaculation should take place approximately every other day around the time of ovulation. This ensures motile sperm are present in the cervical mucus at the time the egg may be fertilized (egg viability).

Reaching the egg is only part of the process. To breech the egg's outer layers, the sperm must undergo a change (become *capacitated*) that will allow it to penetrate the egg. Changes in the sperm membrane, called the *acrosome membrane*, facilitate their binding to and penetrating through the egg, in a process called the *acrosome reaction*. This reaction releases enzymes from the sperm head, which help make a tiny opening in the egg's outermost layer to allow one sperm, from the thousands surrounding the egg, to penetrate it. Thousands more sperm attack the next layers, the zona pellucida and the vitelline membrane. When one sperm finally gets through all the egg's layers, fertilization occurs and the potential for a new life begins.

## FERTILIZATION

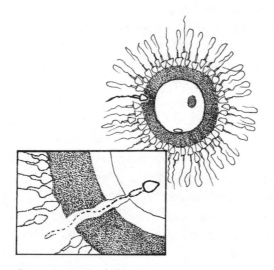

*Sperm surround the egg.*

### Conception

An incredible confluence of events must occur for successful conception. Here is a summary:

1. The woman must release a healthy, mature ovum, which must be picked up by a healthy, functional fallopian tube.
2. The man must produce healthy sperm and deposit it in the vagina, near the cervical opening. (Once deposited into the vagina, only about 10 percent of the sperm will survive to penetrate the cervical mucus and begin the long swim toward the oocyte.)
3. Because sperm live for only about 48 hours in cervical mucus, a couple must have intercourse about every other day around the time of ovulation (for example, days 10, 12, 14, and 16 of the woman's menstrual cycle, if the cycle is a total of 28 days).
4. Sperm must make it through the cervix and then swim through the uterus into the fallopian tube.
5. One healthy sperm must successfully breach the egg's protective layers, including the cumulus layer and the zona pellucida.

## FROM FERTILIZATION TO EMBRYO IMPLANTATION

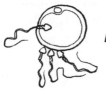

*Egg and sperm meet.*

*Sperm has fertilized this egg to produce a 2-celled embryo.*

*Cells continue to divide as the embryo moves through the fallopian tube.*

*About 3 to 4 days after fertilization, the embryo enters the uterus.*

*As the embryo reaches the blastocyst stage, it is ready to hatch and implant in the woman's endometrium.*

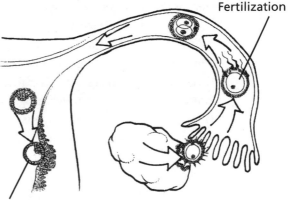

Fertilization

Implantation

# THE EMBRYO, IMPLANTATION, AND GESTATION

When the sperm combines with the egg, a completely new and unique cell forms. Within about 12 hours, the head of the sperm disintegrates, and the 23 chromosomes from the man and the 23 chromosomes from the woman combine to create a single cell. The fertilized egg then divides into an embryo with 2 cells. A total of 46 chromosomes are held in each one of the embryo's 2 cells. (This is one point at which some genetic disorders can occur, especially in older women whose eggs are unable to replicate their chromosomes as consistently as are those of younger women.) The embryo divides again in approximate 16-hour cycles, from 2 cells to 4 to 8 to 16, continuously, as it grows. The chromosomes double too during each cell division so that each new cell contains the full complement of 46 chromosomes.

When the embryo arrives in the uterus, it floats for several days; then the implantation process begins. First is the step called hatching, during which the zona pellucida opens, allowing the embryo—which has now developed into a blastocyst—to attach to the endometrium. After implantation is well established, the cells that will form the placenta begin to surround the embryo. The placenta connects with the uterine blood vessels, allowing the exchange of oxygen, nutrition, and waste products between the woman's circulatory system and that of the developing embryo.

Implantation triggers a series of remarkable changes. Estrogen and progesterone levels begin to rise rapidly, which ironically leads to premenstrual-like symptoms in some women: breast tenderness, fluid retention, and sometimes a little vaginal spotting. At this point, a new hormone enters the picture. The placenta, acting as an endocrine gland, secretes human chorionic gonadotropin (hCG), which signals the corpus luteum in the ovary to continue its secretion of progesterone to nourish the growing embryo. hCG is called the *pregnancy hormone* because its levels are what pregnancy tests are designed to measure. The hormone's level generally doubles every 2 to 3 days during the first 6 weeks of pregnancy and every 3 to 4 days during the following 2 to 4 weeks.

The woman's immune system must also cooperate for the implantation process to succeed. The immune system functions as the first line of defense against disease, or any cells that it views as foreign to the body. Immune system cells could prevent fertilization at the start of the process by killing sperm that enter the vagina, and they may also prevent the embryo from properly implanting in the uterus, resulting in miscarriage. Doctors believe that immune system problems play a role in some cases of recurrent miscarriage, as you will read in chapter 10, "Pregnancy Loss."

If all goes well, the embryo will continue to grow and develop for the next 9 months or so. As you can see, getting to a developing, growing, healthy embryo involves a long and intricate series of steps and processes that can be interrupted by a number of problems, leading to infertility. Learning about the physical process of reproduction helps you understand the factors that may be affecting you and your partner. This knowledge may allow you to feel more in control and to make informed decisions.

In chapter 3, "Preparing Yourself for the Journey," we explore some of the emotions individuals and couples encounter when experiencing infertility and introduce the infertility decision tree as a tool for working through the tough challenges and choices.

## POSITIVE STEPS YOU CAN TAKE FROM CHAPTER 2

**Keep perspective:** It is important always to keep in mind that even the healthiest, youngest couple has only a 20 percent chance of becoming pregnant in any given menstrual cycle. Conception and childbirth remain, in part, miracles that medical science attempts to replicate.

**Gain confidence:** The more you know about the anatomy and physiology of reproduction—about what is *supposed* to happen for a successful conception and pregnancy—the better able you will be to participate in medical decision making through the infertility process.

**Protect your reproductive health:** Eating a well-balanced diet, maintaining your proper weight, and avoiding toxic substances can only improve your chances of conceiving and bearing a healthy child. For more information, see chapters 11, "Staying Centered," and 12, "Staying Healthy."

# 3 Preparing Yourself for the Journey

The world of infertility is filled with challenges, hopes, frustrations, and occasionally despair. The hope the new technologies provide to individuals and couples who otherwise would be unable to bear children is wondrous. But this hope comes at a price. Pursuing infertility treatments may mean confronting feelings about self-image, about intimate relationships, and about a person's place in the world with or without children. This pursuit may also require serious, life-altering decisions.

## INFERTILITY: A LIFE CRISIS

The drive to have a child is a basic one—some say even a primal one—with deep psychological and sociological roots. Psychologists and anthropologists have developed a variety of theories about the roles of childbirth and parenting within the structure of society. Being unable to participate in either or both puts infertile couples out of synch with their peers and may leave them feeling they are failures. Infertility does not just affect the couple; it impacts on extended family, such as potential grandparents or aunts and uncles.

---

### Voices

*Infertility is an intergenerational family developmental crisis in that it prevents not only the couple themselves but also their parents and siblings from proceeding through appropriate life cycle stages. "My husband Eric had a younger sister who*

---

*was born with birth defects, and she died when she was 5 or 6 years old," says Denise. "His mother was very, very supportive of our situation, but she was definitely eager to become a grandmother. Because she'd lost her daughter, Eric was now the end of the family line."*

The desire to experience a pregnancy and have a baby is intensely personal. For various reasons—such as lack of effective birth control, childhood diseases, and shorter life expectancies—delaying a family did not become a viable option until well past the middle of the twentieth century. Today, most men and women assume they can postpone starting a family, then become parents when they feel the time is right. For individuals or couples to discover that this dimension of the American dream—building a family—is closed to them is an extraordinarily harsh shock.

## THE CYCLE OF GRIEF AND ACCEPTANCE

Infertility poses such enormous challenges for individuals and couples that mental health professionals consider it a life crisis. Coping with infertility requires the same kind of psychological and physical strength as does coping with the death of a parent, a divorce, or a life-threatening disease. According to Barbara Eck Menning, RESOLVE's founder, the crisis of infertility is so intense it results in people experiencing a cycle of emotions similar to that associated with the stages of grief related to death and dying set forth by pioneer therapist Elizabeth Kübler-Ross. These stages may follow the same order, although the length of time it takes an individual to work through them varies. You may pass through some stages quickly, then seem to get stuck in one for a long time. Eventually, however, most people complete the cycle, which Kübler-Ross identified as essential for healing to take place.

### *Voices on the Kübler-Ross Stages*

1. **Shock or numbness.** As you begin your struggle with infertility and at various other points in your journey, you may not feel emotional. "It was still shocking," says Trish, "even after 2 years, that Bob and I didn't have a baby and nobody could tell us why." You will not feel sad, or angry; you may feel numb. Many psychologists believe that this kind of shock helps protect a person from being overwhelmed by too many emotions at once.

2. **Denial.** Denial emerges as the numbness and shock begin to wear off. You begin looking for mistakes—*the lab reported the wrong results, the doctor got you*

*confused with another patient, of course your cervix is fine because you've been having periods since you were 12....* Denial shelters you from reality a little longer, allowing your emotional core to process the intellectual information your brain has received. Denial eventually succumbs to increasingly strong signals from reality, preparing you for your transition to the next stage in the cycle. "During the first intrauterine insemination (IUI)," says Jill, "I took David's sperm sample to the lab. The doctor then found that the sperm count was lower than normal. We thought it was a fluke. We did another IUI; the sperm count was low again. Then we realized we had a male factor involved that we hadn't considered originally."

3. **Anger.** The anger stage of the infertility response is often triggered by the feelings of unfairness and injustice that accompany month after month of disappointment. After all, there has to be a reason this is happening to you. "It was so painful at times," says Madeline. "I couldn't talk about it without crying, and I didn't want to cry at work or with my family. My husband reacted with a sullen withdrawal. We were so angry and upset." In this stage, you begin to realize there has been no mistake, this is really happening to *you*. Now the inequity of this reality strikes you. *It isn't fair, you have done nothing to deserve this, how can it be that so many people can get pregnant right away while you, the potentially ideal parent who has so much to offer to a child or children, can't conceive.* As long as you do not let anger consume you, it can help you mobilize and focus your energy to get the medical information and support you need.

4. **Bargaining/guilt.** "Many times I railed and cursed God for not hearing my pleas," says Roxanne. "Then I would bargain and make promises if my goal could be met." During this stage, you often look back on your life and see what you perceive as reasons for your current situation. Guilt feelings are not uncommon. "I had three unplanned pregnancies, and I had three abortions," says Althea. "I went from being 'fertile Myrtle' to the depths of despair in dealing with the ordeal of infertility. I started to regret the last abortion, to think about how old that child would be if I had allowed the pregnancy to continue. I could not stand the emotional impact it was having on my psyche." This stage helps you to examine your feelings of responsibility—realistic or not—and deal with them, so you can move beyond blaming and toward resolution.

5. **Acceptance.** At some point, you will have to accept that you are experiencing infertility and may need medical help to get pregnant and have a baby or that you may need to consider other family-building options. Although you may still have periods of despair, anger, and depression, you will begin gradually to manage your emotions better and to notice that infertility is not dominating your life as much. Says Ron, who with his wife Lydia resolved as childfree, "Eventually,

there were more days when it felt great. I think once in a while about what we've lost—and this is a loss, this wasn't Plan A. It's a great Plan B."

The Kübler-Ross model, although originally created to define and understand the stages of psychological healing for people coping with death or the prospect of dying, works well for people facing infertility because they, too, must cope with loss. In addition to losing the dream pregnancy, birth, and child you thought you could have easily and naturally, you have also lost the image of yourself as a healthy person. At times, you may feel as if you have lost parts of your personality. Your sense of humor may disappear, resentment and jealousy may replace your sense of closeness with friends and family, and you may feel you have lost your capacity for optimism and joy. Feelings of sadness will be more intense after a late period, a failed in vitro fertilization (IVF) cycle, or a miscarriage.

## DECISIONS, DECISIONS

Knowing what to do and when to do it are significant challenges in infertility diagnosis and treatment. Most couples who seek treatment for infertility require only low-tech medical solutions to their problems. For others, infertility treatment may involve more complex procedures and many decisions. Certain options, particularly those involving assisted reproductive technologies (ART) or donor sperm/egg, may bring up questions of morality and ethics. You may have to consider the short- and long-term impact that infertility treatments will have on your financial situation, and the physical and emotional toll repeated testing and treatment will take on your relationship.

### Voices

*"We've gone from one doctor who says it's all me to another who says it's all my husband," says Chloe. "How do we make a decision?"*

Many who struggle with infertility would feel more comfortable if there were an established sequence of testing and corresponding treatment options. Unfortunately, this is not the case. Infertility care, like infertility itself, is individual. The physician determines what tests and treatments are appropriate for you on the basis of your individual circumstances and your medical history. For a woman who conceives but continually miscarries, for example, it makes sense to start the testing procedure with her by looking for hormonal irregularities and uterine abnormalities. For couples who can not conceive, it makes more sense to start by examining the woman's ovulatory cycle and the man's sperm. If the woman ovulates and the sperm analysis is normal, the next step might be testing for tubal patency and uterine structure in the woman, or postcoital examination to determine what happens when sperm are in the cervical mucus, or. . . . All those "ors" cause so much frustration. There are more mysteries surrounding infertility than there are answers in many situations. And technology can change the answers seemingly overnight. Although there has never been a better time to deal with infertility, there also have never been so many choices.

## CREATING YOUR INFERTILITY DECISION TREE

Despite the uncertainty that envelops infertility treatment, there is a fairly simple way you can assess your options and make decisions that are best for you. The infertility decision tree is a series of circles and lines on a piece of paper to help you visualize your journey. Not all options will be choices for you. For example, your finances, or your core belief system or religious beliefs, may make IVF or gamete intrafallopian transfer (GIFT) choices that are not right for you. The decision tree process is also a progressive decision-making tool. You can use it to examine your overall situation, and then to take a closer look at each "branch" decision you face.

To create your decision tree, start with a plain piece of paper. Draw a circle in the top left-hand corner, and write your primary goal inside it—for example, "Start a Family." Draw a line coming away from this circle, and draw another circle. Inside, write one option about which you need to make a decision—for example, "Continue Trying on Our Own." Beneath this circle, make a list of the pros (positives) and cons (negatives) of this option. When you are done with that, draw another line from your main circle and create another subcircle. Write in another option, for example, "Seek Medical Testing," and below it a list of pros and cons. Even if you feel you have already eliminated an option, go through the process of putting it in your decision tree.

For each option you are considering, start a new decision tree on a fresh piece of paper, with that option as the main topic. For example, perhaps your doctor is recommending surgery to remove a uterine fibroid. Write "Surgery to Remove Uterine Fibroid" as your main topic circle in the top left-hand corner. If you had a lot of pros and cons, do one branch decision tree for pros and one for cons, so you have plenty of room to work everything through. Draw a line with a circle at the end for each pro and con. Your pros under "Surgery to Remove

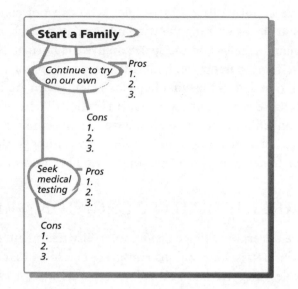

Uterine Fibroid" might include "Remove obstacle to conception" and "Less painful periods." Under cons, you might have "Possible risks of surgery" and "Might not be cause of infertility." Think through each of these pros and cons, and continue your tree by writing down your thoughts about each.

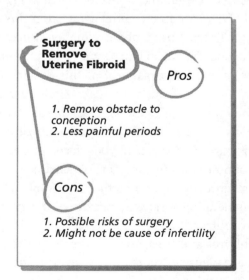

> ### *A Voice on Perspectives*
>
> *Use the decision trees in combination with your journal to help you work out the decisions you need to make and how you and your partner feel about them. Writing things down can help you plan more clearly, working toward a balanced perspective and the decisions that are right for you as an individual and/or as a couple. You may find that the tough challenges you face may lead you to explore and discover new things about yourself, your partner, and your relationship. Thirty-three-year-old Rebecca, now the mother of two, says, "My husband, Frank, was right there with me, which was an interesting development as it had taken us some time, years, to agree to start a family. And then to have difficulty created a new strain and tension between us. I had to manage my anger at him for making me wait longer than I had wanted to, and he felt guilty about making me wait that long—it all added to our baggage. You really are thrown into a life crisis, faced with many issues that you never thought would pop up about what you want in life, about what you want from each other. You can be married 5 or 10 years, and still be getting to know each other. During treatment, plenty of decisions—opportunities—presented themselves that needed to be worked on and thought through. We can say we're better off for having dealt with each one."*

## A Sample Decision Tree

To give you an example of how a decision tree might unfold, we created Patrick and Elizabeth, a fictional couple with fertility problems. In their late 30s, Patrick and Elizabeth have been trying to get pregnant for 3 years. They know that Elizabeth is a diethylstilbestrol (DES) baby and has cervical stenosis (a narrowing of her cervix) that may or may not be interfering with her ability to get pregnant. Her physician thinks that once that problem is corrected with surgery, Elizabeth and Patrick should be able to conceive on their own. On the other hand, she also has poor cervical mucus (cervical mucus serves as the transport for the sperm). So another option is for the couple to go straight to IUI, a procedure that allows them to avoid the cervical mucus problem by placing the sperm directly in the uterine cavity. Unfortunately, that procedure is not covered by their insurance and would require them to pay out of pocket. To increase their chance for the IUI to work, the physician also suggests that Elizabeth take medication to stimulate the production of eggs. Not only does this option increase the cost, but also Elizabeth is terrified of needles (the medication must be injected) and worries about the side effects of medication. Here is their decision tree.

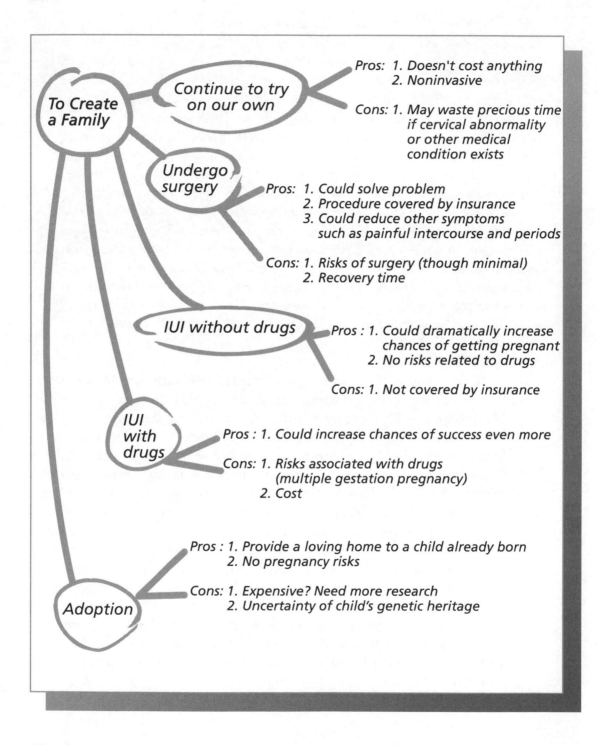

To Create a Family

**Continue to try on our own**

Pros: 1. Doesn't cost anything
2. Noninvasive

Cons: 1. May waste precious time if cervical abnormality or other medical condition exists

**Undergo surgery**

Pros: 1. Could solve problem
2. Procedure covered by insurance
3. Could reduce other symptoms such as painful intercourse and periods

Cons: 1. Risks of surgery (though minimal)
2. Recovery time

**IUI without drugs**

Pros : 1. Could dramatically increase chances of getting pregnant
2. No risks related to drugs

Cons: 1. Not covered by insurance

**IUI with drugs**

Pros : 1. Could increase chances of success even more

Cons: 1. Risks associated with drugs (multiple gestation pregnancy)
2. Cost

Pros : 1. Provide a loving home to a child already born
2. No pregnancy risks

Cons: 1. Expensive? Need more research
2. Uncertainty of child's genetic heritage

**Adoption**

As a result of their decision tree, our fictitious couple, Elizabeth and Patrick, decided Elizabeth should have surgery. Even though this might not solve the problem, they knew the cervical stenosis was undoubtedly a serious barrier to conception. Going forward with surgery did not rule out other options, yet would eliminate one potential problem. And it could provide relief from occasionally painful intercourse and periods for Elizabeth. The couple also decided that they would try conceiving on their own for 6 months, then revisit their decision tree if they did not get pregnant.

## As You Make Your Decisions

What decisions are you, as an individual and/or as a couple, facing? What options remain open, and which ones are closed because of medical, personal, or financial considerations? Here are some points to consider when you begin to construct your decision tree(s).

Be sure you understand all your medical and other family-building options.

- Talk with your physician about the medical treatments that are possible for you.
- Read all you can about treatments, and talk with others who have been through the treatments or selected alternative options.
- Attend a seminar on an option you may not be considering now, like donor egg pregnancy, adoption, or childfree living. You do not have to commit yourself, and you may learn something that will help in your decision-making process.
- Consider short-term counseling with a therapist who can help you explore paths to family building and your own feelings about it.

Consider your emotional resources.

- How have you done with the roller-coaster aspect of treatment, the highs of hope and the lows of disappointment?
- What emotional reserves do you have for the various options ahead?

Analyze what is important to you about family building.

- Is a pregnancy extremely important?
- Is genetic connection to one or both of you paramount?
- Is your picture of family one of similarity, or do you ever imagine a multicultural family?

What are your financial resources, and what compromises are you willing to make?

- Have you reviewed your health insurance policy thoroughly for all the treatment it provides? (See chapter 14, "Creating a Financial Game Plan and Getting Through the Insurance Maze," for help with this exercise.)
- Are you willing to borrow, and have you reviewed the consequences to your monthly expenses?
- Are you willing, or do you have the time, to wait to save money to attempt to reach your primary goal?
- Are there lifestyle changes you are willing to make to save money for further treatment, surrogacy, or adoption, for example?

Remember that there are no perfect decisions. Thoughts about the path not taken are familiar to anyone who has made difficult choices. Learning all your options and making rational choices will help you make peace with your ultimate decisions and may reveal some interesting trails you hadn't originally considered exploring on this journey.

## POSITIVE STEPS YOU CAN TAKE FROM CHAPTER 3

**Consider every option.** Use the decision tree to explore fully each of the options available to you and your partner. Seeing the pros and cons on paper can help put each option into a perspective that moves you toward the best decision for your situation. Without writing it all down, you might overlook an important detail that could be one of the keys to your choice.

**Value your feelings.** You will be making many tough decisions throughout your journey of infertility treatment. Give your feelings, and your partner's feelings, a legitimate role in the decision-making process. Suppressing emotions may hinder, not help, your search for the right solution.

**From crisis comes opportunity.** It may be hard to imagine that you can come through this experience stronger—as an individual or as a couple—but you can. You may learn new coping skills to help you get through this crisis. You can learn to manage your stress and to keep lines of communication open with your partner, family, friends, and co-workers. And you may improve your decision-making skills.

# PART 2
# THE
# MEDICAL JOURNEY

# 4 Choosing Your Medical Team

Whether you are just getting started or you have already had a consultation or started treatment for a possible infertility problem, the most positive thing you can do is to select the best medical care possible. By taking a proactive role in your medical care and finding the right group of healthcare professionals, you can regain some control over your situation and perhaps expand the options available to you and your partner. No matter the outcome, it is important to know that you sought out the best medical resources for your needs.

Many of your decisions about what physicians to see and what treatment to pursue may depend on your insurance coverage, especially if you belong to a health maintenance organization (HMO) or managed care plan. Financial issues also may play a central part in your care (see chapter 14, "Creating a Financial Game Plan and Getting Through the Insurance Maze").

## YOUR MEDICAL TEAM

If you are like most individuals and couples who suspect they have an infertility problem, you will start addressing the issue by asking your primary care physician or obstetrician-gynecologist (OB-Gyn) this question: "How long should we try before starting tests or treatments for infertility?" The standard answer is "1 year," and it is an appropriate response for couples in which the woman is younger than 35 years of age with no history of reproductive problems or risk factors for infertility. Remember that 80 to 90 percent of couples will get pregnant within a year of unprotected intercourse. However, if you are a woman older than 35 years, or you have known reproductive problems or risk factors, your physician may recommend starting an infertility work-up sooner. Your primary care physician or OB-Gyn may refer you to an infertility subspecialist for evaluation and to discuss treatment options.

### *Voices*

*Jorie, a woman with blocked fallopian tubes who suffered ectopic pregnancies and went through three in vitro fertilization (IVF) cycles before having a baby boy, recalls, "I can only imagine how much time would have been lost if my OB-Gyn had tried to play infertility expert. As much as I adore my doctor, I was glad for the referral to an infertility subspecialist. I hated to leave my OB-Gyn, but I needed more help to get pregnant. What a joy it was to return to her care when I got pregnant!"*

All physicians with MD (medical doctor) after their names have completed 4 years of medical school and an internship, either in a specified field or in a so-called rotating internship providing exposure to many areas of medicine. If a physician decides to specialize in a specific field such as OB-Gyn, a residency program in that area must be completed. In general, infertility training in an OB-Gyn internship and residency is limited, and does not provide physicians with a thorough understanding of reproductive medicine or insight into the emotional component of infertility. That is why it is important for individuals and couples experiencing infertility to consider consulting a physician trained and experienced in infertility as a subspecialty.

The following is an overview of the medical professionals who may be a part of your infertility healthcare team.

## Primary Care Physician

Many couples find it more comfortable to start exploring their infertility problems with their family or primary care physicians. Primary care physicians may be certified in Family Medicine or in Internal Medicine. Primary care physicians can assess your general health and investigate the potential effects that your medical history, environment, and medications might have on your fertility. They can document ovulation, order a semen analysis, and do the basic blood tests needed (see chapter 5, "The Basic Infertility Work-up for Women and Men," for a description of the diagnostic tests you and your partner may undergo). Some infertility problems can be treated at this level. For example, your primary care physician may change medications that could interfere with your fer-

tility or advise you to avoid using sperm-kill⏑ ⏑ ever,
if your infertility problem is more complex, ⏑ ⏑ specializes in infertility or another qualified s ⏑

## Obstetrician-Gynecologist (OB-Gyn)

OB-Gyns specialize in the diagnosis ⏑ ⏑ roductive
diseases, including genitourinary proble ⏑ ⏑ pregnancy
and childbirth. OB-Gyns often can star ⏑ ⏑ ess, including the semen analysis, hysterosalping ⏑ ⏑ (see chapter
5, "The Basic Infertility Work-up fc ⏑ ⏑ OB-Gyns are
surgeons and can perform diagnosti ⏑

Ask your OB-Gyn about his o⏑ ⏑ perience. Many
OB-Gyns are able to treat ovulation proble⏑⏑ citrate (Clomid
or Serophene), and some can perform intrauterine inse⏑⏑⏑s (IUI). However,
if a high percentage of your physician's practice is obstetrics (the treatment of
pregnant women and the delivery of babies), effort and time will be diverted to
those patients. This could mean that this physician is not as current with infertility diagnostic and treatment protocols as OB-Gyns who take a special interest
in infertility. You may also find it difficult to be in the office with pregnant
women as you struggle with infertility. You may decide to start treatment with
an OB-Gyn, but choose to continue treatment with a physician specializing in
infertility, and, if you become pregnant, return to your OB-Gyn to be followed
during your pregnancy.

### When to See an Infertility Specialist

You and your partner may want to consider seeing a physician board-certified in
the medical subspecialty of Reproductive Endocrinology and Infertility if you are
a woman:

- experiencing irregular menstrual cycles or evidence of irregular ovulation; or
- who has a history of three or more miscarriages; or
- older than 35 years of age; or
- with a history of pelvic infection or previous pelvic surgery.

In addition, consider transferring care to a specialist if, after undergoing the
initial round of diagnostic tests described in chapter 5, "The Basic Infertility
Work-up for Women and Men," you find that you:

- have unexplained infertility—your basic tests came back normal, but after 2 years of treatment, you have not yet succeeded in conceiving; or
- are a woman who needs microsurgery for endometriosis or for tubal damage; or
- are a man who has a poor semen analysis showing low count, motility, or appearance (morphology), or who may require microsurgery; or
- need more advanced treatment, such as injectable ovulation-induction medications or assisted reproductive technology (ART).

## Reproductive Endocrinologist (RE) and Other Infertility Specialists

A board-certified RE is an OB-Gyn who has completed additional training in reproductive medicine. In addition to completing requirements for board-certification in obstetrics-gynecology, an RE must complete a 2- or 3-year fellowship in reproductive endocrinology; pass a written board examination in reproductive medicine; complete a 2-year practice experience in reproductive endocrinology and infertility; and then pass a 3-hour oral examination. Some physicians have passed the written examination and are still completing practice experience in reproductive endocrinology and infertility before taking the oral examination. These physicians are "board-eligible to become certified" in this field. REs are trained in advanced procedures, such as difficult reproductive surgeries and treating hormonal imbalances, and in the use and monitoring of injectable fertility drugs, IUI, and ART procedures, such as IVF. REs may be in private practices, but often are affiliated with ART programs or large university-based infertility clinics.

Currently, about 500 physicians certified in reproductive endocrinology practice in the United States. Another 800 or more are board-eligible to become certified. Many REs are engaged in research in reproductive medicine and teach medical students and residents, as well.

## Reproductive Immunologists

Reproductive immunologists are scientists (usually MDs) with advanced training in the study of the immune system as it affects the reproductive tract. They are able to diagnose immunologic barriers to achieving pregnancy, such as autoimmune conditions that cause recurrent miscarriage and antisperm antibodies. There is no training program for reproductive immunology; it is not a medical specialty or subspecialty, but rather an area of interest.

## Urologists

Urologists are medical doctors who specialize primarily in the genitourinary tract. They can perform semen analyses and diagnose varicocele, endocrine problems, genetic defects, or other physical abnormalities that may cause fertility problems in men. In addition, urologists may be trained to perform testicular biopsies, surgical varicocele repair, and vasectomy reversal (see chapter 8, "The Male: Diagnosis and Treatment"). A reproductive urologist is an MD with additional training in treating urinary tract disorders, plus 2 years of general surgical training and microsurgical training in repairing obstructions, varicoceles, and other anatomic disorders of the male reproductive tract.

## Andrologists

Clinical andrologists specialize in treating the male reproductive tract. Some are urologists, some are PhDs in technical areas such as microbiology, biochemistry, or andrology. Many andrologists are affiliated with fertility treatment centers and play a key role in performing ART cycles. The andrologist's focus is on hormonal issues and sperm quality. Andrologists develop and direct procedures for handling sperm in larger clinics, where they work closely with embryologists to prepare sperm for the fertilization procedure.

## Embryologists

Every ART clinic should employ a professional with expertise in the handling of embryos. The following criteria for the embryologist are drawn from Society for Assisted Reproductive Technology (SART) guidelines. The embryologist should be an MD, or have a doctorate degree in a chemical, physical, or biological science. An embryologist should have a minimum of 2 years of documented experience in a program performing at least 100 IVF-related procedures per year. Each embryologist should perform at least 20 complete ART procedures annually. An embryo laboratory technologist should have a bachelor's or master's degree and documented experience in tissue culture, sperm-egg interaction, and sterile technique, and have completed at least 30 IVF procedures.

## Geneticists and Genetic Counselors

A clinic should be able to refer couples to a geneticist when they may have genetic abnormalities that affect fertility, who have recurrent pregnancy losses, or who may need prenatal screening tests.

## Nurses and Physician Assistants

Nurses and physician assistants perform—and often educate patients about—tests, procedures, and treatments. They often cover the telephone during call-in hours to answer patients' questions and concerns. If it is a large infertility clinic or practice, you may have a designated nurse who works with your physician and will be your contact person.

## Mental Health Professionals

Psychiatrists, psychologists, therapists, and counselors are trained to offer support in dealing with life crisis issues, options, and decisions. Infertility counselors can help you deal with the emotional aspects of the infertility experience. Many clinics require psychological counseling for individuals and couples considering ART procedures, donor sperm, or donor egg options (see chapter 11, "Staying Centered," for more information on choosing a therapist).

## The Most Important Members of the Healthcare Team: You and Your Partner

Consider you and your partner to be equal participants with the healthcare professionals providing your care. During the infertility experience, being proactive may help you feel more in control of your options and decisions. You may find that you will wear many hats:

- *Diligent medical researcher.* Learn about your medical condition and appropriate treatments. Collect information from your physician(s), other medical professionals, RESOLVE resources (see the appendix at the back of this book), books, reliable Internet resources, and medical journals. Join a support group: hearing other couples' experiences with infertility treatments can help you gain perspectives that may be valuable to your own decision-making process.

### Voices

*"I learned early on that the best thing I can do to help myself is to be an intelligent, aware, and optimistic person," notes Margaret, a 32-year-old woman now in her third year of infertility treatment. "That way, I can participate in my own care and not hinder it. I constantly seek information and try to improve my odds by choosing the best protocols and the best physicians. And I always have a backup plan, which may be the key to solving my problems if the first plan fails."*

- *Savvy medical consumer.* Remember, *you* choose your healthcare team.

Choosing the best physician depends on your treatment needs as well as your personal compatibility. Be prepared to be your own advocate, to search for the best, appropriate care—and to deal with any financial or insurance concerns that may affect access to that care.

- *Solid financial and insurance manager.* You will need to budget and manage the costs of treatment and keep track of insurance claims and approvals.
- *Medical record keeper.* Although the physician has a medical chart on you, keep your own record of each appointment, medications you take, and every question you have for your physician and the answer given. The longer you continue treatment or the more complex your case is, the more important your role as record keeper becomes. Request written records of laboratory reports and test results. Use the test result worksheets for women and men and the clinic information sheets that appear at the back of this book. A complete record of treatment becomes especially valuable should you decide to change physicians or seek a second opinion.
- *Personal trainer.* Keep yourself healthy, focused, and positive. See chapter 11, "Staying Centered," and chapter 12, "Staying Healthy," for information on diet, exercise, and stress-management techniques.

## CHOOSING A PHYSICIAN

A good place to start your search for an infertility specialist may be with a referral from your primary care physician or OB-Gyn. Suggestions from satisfied patients should not be your only criteria, but they certainly can help you narrow your search. A word of caution: A treatment that works for a friend or relative may not be appropriate for you. The more you learn about infertility and your own specific problem, the better able you will be to choose your care wisely. Other sources to help you locate qualified physicians and clinics in your area include the following:

- *RESOLVE.* Contact your local RESOLVE chapter or the national RESOLVE office for a referral. Physicians on this referral list have to meet specific criteria and standards regarding education, training, and concentration in the practice of infertility medicine. When you contact RESOLVE, we will provide you with several physician referrals in your area. As a RESOLVE member, you can request a regional list of specialists.
- *The American Society for Reproductive Medicine (ASRM) and local county medical societies.* These organizations can provide you with a list of physi-

cians who have an interest in infertility treatment. Membership in these organizations does not indicate additional training or certification in infertility medicine.

- *Fertility clinics.* There are more than 300 fertility clinics in the United States. Some are for-profit; others are nonprofit, research-based clinics, usually associated with universities. Many clinics can perform a basic infertility work-up and provide treatment, from simple intervention through ART.

When evaluating an RE or infertility clinic, consider the following criteria:

- *The training and background of your physician and his or her staff.* Before your first appointment, inquire whether the physician is board-certified in reproductive endocrinology and infertility or has other infertility training.
- *The experience the physician and clinic staff has with infertility treatments, including ART.* The U.S. Centers for Disease Control and Prevention (CDC) requires that infertility clinics publish ART pregnancy success rates (for information on ordering the CDC report, see chapter 9, "Assisted Reproductive Technology [ART]," and the Resource Guide at the end of this book). In July 1999, the CDC also released guidelines that states may use to develop programs for certification and inspection of embryo laboratories. ASRM supports the federal guidelines and is in the process of accrediting clinics through its own certification process.
- *Availability of staff and technicians 7 days a week.*

### Voices

*"My wife and I were lucky because our physician and staff really went out of their way to help us get pregnant," 39-year-old Hunter reveals. "At our first clinic, we were all geared up to start our first IVF treatment, but—wouldn't you know it—the perfect day to retrieve the eggs would have been on Thanksgiving, which is the only day besides Christmas and New Year's that the clinic wasn't open. We had to wait a month, and that was hard."*

- *Experience with and routine use of transvaginal ultrasound equipment.* You should not undergo treatment with injectable fertility medications unless the ultrasound equipment and skilled staff are available for routine monitoring through ultrasound supplemented by laboratory blood testing.
- *A qualified, competent, on-site laboratory.* The clinic should have a labora-

tory for blood analysis, semen analysis, and preparation of sperm for IUI.

- *Access to facilities for freezing and storing sperm and embryos.* Donated sperm are usually stored at a sperm bank and then shipped to the physician's office, and it is best to have storage and thawing facilities at the site where the donor insemination (DI) will take place. If you are undergoing ART, your clinic should be able to cryopreserve additional embryos that are not transferred during a "fresh embryo" treatment cycle.
- *If you are doing ART, experience with micromanipulation procedures.* The success of these procedures, which include the microscopic injection of one sperm into an egg, depends on the skill of the embryologist or technician performing the micromanipulation technique.

## WORKING WITH YOUR PHYSICIAN

To get the most out of your relationship with your physician and the practice, you should do the following:

- *Formulate a clear-cut treatment plan.* After your first conference, your physician should be able to outline the initial phases of your infertility work-up. After the basic work-up (described in chapter 5, "The Basic Infertility Work-up for Women and Men"), your physician should be able to outline a treatment plan. You should feel confident that your physician is using specific step-by-step procedures—explained to you in clear and understandable terms—to identify and then try to solve your particular problem.
- *Feel free to speak openly and honestly with your physician.* If you find it difficult to talk freely to your physician, you are faced with a serious obstacle. Although physicians are usually very busy, you should always feel comfortable enough to ask questions and express your concerns. Your physician should take the time to address each in full detail and with full respect for you and your partner. A recent Tufts University study reveals that patients who request medical records and discuss their treatment plan and options with their physicians have better outcomes than those who do not have access to records or do not discuss the details and options of treatment with their physicians. Here are a few tips that might help you facilitate communication with your healthcare team:

- Write down your questions before your appointment.
- Consider requesting permission to record the consultation with the physi-

cian so that you can listen to the physician's comments later at home. Or, designate one partner to take notes during the conference so that details are not missed or forgotten.

- Telephone after the appointment with any further questions you may have.

• *Make sure you feel comfortable about the way your physician and other healthcare team members treat you.* You should feel comfortable about the physician's approach to treating infertility, and you should have adequate time to talk about any concerns you have about the treatment options. If the physician is unwilling to discuss treatment philosophy or answer specific treatment-related questions, you may want to consider changing physicians or seeking a second opinion.

• *Realize that your physician cannot act as your personal support system.* Create a support network by joining RESOLVE and by seeking emotional comfort from your partner, your family, and friends. Ask your physician for a referral to a therapist who offers infertility counseling if you feel that the emotional aspects of the experience are becoming more intense and difficult to handle.

## *Signing Consent Forms or Contracts*

Informed consent is a medical term. It means that the patient gives permission for a test or invasive procedure to be performed, after having been informed by the physician in clear language of what the test or procedure involves. When you are asked to sign a consent form or contract, consider the following:

- Ask for clarification if you have questions about wording used on the form.
- When possible, have a third party (spouse, friend, lawyer, etc.) review any forms before you sign them.
- Ask how long a period of time the signed consent document will be applicable.
- Use a pen, not a pencil, to complete and sign forms.
- Answer all relevant questions; do not leave any questions blank. If a question is not relevant to your situation, write "NA" (not applicable).
- Write your initials beside any changes made, for example, if you delete a word or phrase in the original document.
- Always date the form when you sign it.
- Ask for a copy of the consent form for your own records.

- If you are signing a consent form for an ART procedure, request in writing what the clinic agrees to do financially if the cycle is cancelled.
- Ask if the clinic has a policy regarding storage and transfer of sperm or embryos to other facilities either in or out of state. Sign and date any statements relating to this policy.

## GETTING A SECOND OPINION

At some point along the infertility journey, you may decide to get a second opinion or change physicians. Here are just a few of the reasons you might do so:

- The physician does not seem to have an organized treatment plan for you or wants to continue the same treatment that has failed for four or more cycles.
- The physician seems confused about your case. You have to remind the physician of your treatment plan and progress.
- You receive treatment without a diagnosis, for example, the physician prescribes fertility drugs before completing an infertility work-up. (Please note, however, that your diagnosis and treatment needs may change over time.)
- The physician fails to monitor cycles using injectable fertility medications with ultrasound and blood tests.
- Communication between you and the physician is poor. You feel reluctant to ask questions and feel as if your concerns are quickly dismissed.
- The obstetrical part of a practice seems to diminish the amount of quality time the physician can spend with you and other infertility patients.
- You are at a decision-making point in your treatment, for example, considering stopping treatment or undergoing major surgery, and may be in need of a second opinion.

Knowing that you want to change physicians and feeling comfortable about doing so are two different things. If at all possible, talk to your physician about your concerns before you leave the practice. If you decide to move on to another physician for any reason, ask in writing for a complete copy of your medical records. Remember that most physicians are not offended that a patient might want a second opinion before undergoing major surgery, making major decisions about treatment options, or ending medical treatment.

## POSITIVE STEPS YOU CAN TAKE FROM CHAPTER 4

**Find the best care possible.** Begin your search for the right physician or clinic with your primary care physician or OB-Gyn; also consult your local RESOLVE chapter or the national RESOLVE office. RESOLVE maintains one of the most accurate, up-to-date lists of screened physician referrals.

**Do your research.** Look to legitimate sources of information, such as your physician, RESOLVE, the Web sites of established legitimate organizations such as ASRM or the CDC, and medical journals and references to learn about your condition, your options for treatment, and their success rates for couples in your situation. The better informed and educated you are, the better you will be able to discuss your situation with the members of your healthcare team.

**Advocate, advocate, advocate—for yourself!** Getting the best care often means being assertive with your physician and healthcare team. Stay on top of your care by keeping well informed, asking questions, and maintaining good records.

# 5 The Basic Infertility Work-up for Women and Men

Despite its profound personal implications, infertility is really a medical disease. In most cases, either the woman's or the man's reproductive system is not working properly, causing difficulty with getting pregnant and giving birth. In many cases, a physician can diagnose and treat the infertility, and patients go on to conceive and have a baby. Conception and birth can sometimes occur without pinpointing a cause for infertility, with or without medical treatment. Occasionally, all efforts to find a problem or correct a problem fail. In the end—despite remarkable advances in medicine—science has not uncovered all of the mysteries surrounding conception and childbirth.

As you learned in chapter 1, "Face to Face with Your Options," statistically, female problems and male problems are equally accountable for infertility—and one in four couples has multiple problems.

## For Your Information

The likelihood that infertility treatment will result in a pregnancy depends on numerous variables. Some of the most important include the following:

- The experience of the clinic or health care provider.
- The nature, complexity, and number of identified problems.
- The age of the woman (and, to a lesser extent, the age of the man). **If you are a woman older than 35 years and you are having trouble getting pregnant,** ask your primary care physician or OB-Gyn for an immediate referral

to an infertility specialist or board-certified reproductive endocrinologist (RE), who will perform your basic infertility work-up.

Here is a more specific breakdown of what causes infertility:

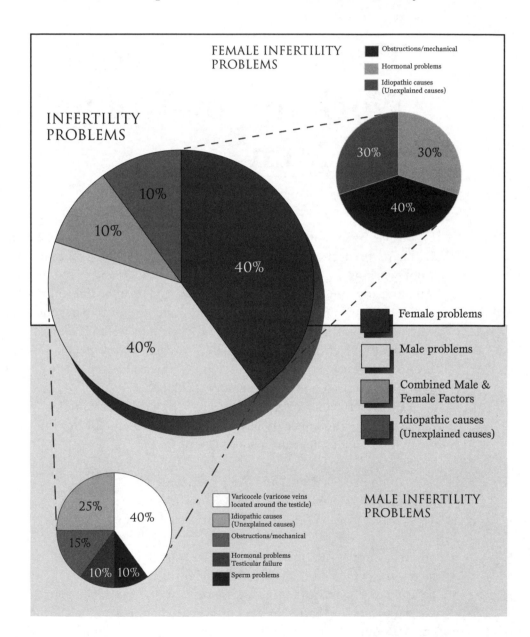

If you suspect that you may have an infertility problem, you have probably started doing research and have made an appointment with either your primary care physician or OB-Gyn. Or, your physician has referred you to the specialized care of an infertility clinic. As you consider starting to have the diagnostic tests to identify the reason you are having trouble getting, or staying, pregnant, you and your partner should know what to expect. This chapter provides you with an overview of the basic infertility evaluation for women and men. For women, the work-up is the same whether you are experiencing primary or secondary infertility (trouble getting pregnant or carrying a baby to term after having given birth). For more information on the special emotional concerns of women experiencing secondary infertility, see chapter 16, "Surviving Infertility."

Be sure to take your health records to your first office visit, or send them to the physician or clinic in advance of your appointment. Your physician will want to see which, if any, medical tests you have already had and what the results were. After reviewing your medical histories, your physician will perform a complete physical work-up, including laboratory tests (whether retests or original testing), on both you and your partner, to determine whether your reproductive systems are functioning normally. Couples seeking infertility treatment should go to the first appointment together.

You should be aware, though, that finding the cause of the infertility problem may be a difficult process in itself, and is usually necessary before deciding what treatment(s) may be needed. In many cases treatment for infertility is a *progression*, one that may take unexpected twists and turns.

---

### *Voices*

*Lisa is a 34-year-old mother of a 1-year-old boy she gave birth to after IVF treatment, and after several years of unexplained infertility. "It's important to understand as you wend your way through this process that you may never have a complete diagnosis. For years, the only diagnosis I had was that I was a poor responder to fertility medications. Then it became clear that I had an autoimmune problem that caused me to lose several pregnancies. Later my husband developed a low sperm count—and we now had a male factor to deal with as well."*

*Josh, who's experiencing secondary infertility with his wife, Emily, notes, "I wish there were some kind of a checklist that doctors could run down so that they could say you do hysterosalpingogram (HSG) before you do laparoscopy and then do this and that. . . . But everyone's different, so I guess that will never happen."*

*It is important to work with a medical team you trust and to be as flexible and patient as possible during the infertility treatment process.*

This is the perfect time to take a look at the test result worksheets for women and men, which you will find at the back of this book. Completing the worksheets will help you and your partner to remember important clinical details and to have a way to track the process of infertility treatment.

# THE BASIC WORK-UP FOR WOMEN

## Medical History and Lifestyle

At your first appointment, the physician will take a medical history and ask questions about your lifestyle that may seem very personal. Answer each question as openly and honestly as possible. Without accurate information, your medical team may not be able to assess and treat an infertility problem quickly and successfully. Do not intentionally hold back information, or assume that a detail will not be important to your health care team.

The topics covered include the following:

- *Menstrual history:* The physician will need to know the age that you began to menstruate, how regular your periods are, what the flow is like, and what, if any, discomfort you feel during your cycle. Irregular or painful periods may indicate a problem with ovulation, the presence of endometriosis and/or scar tissue, or structural problems that may be interfering with your ability to get pregnant.
- *Pregnancy history:* The physician will ask you for details about any previous pregnancies, miscarriages, or abortions you may have had.
- *Birth control history:* The physician will need to know what birth control methods you have used. Some intrauterine devices (IUDs) have been linked to increased risk of pelvic infection and damage to the fallopian tubes. Recent use of birth control pills may contribute to irregular ovulation and menstrual cycles.
- *History of sexually transmitted disease:* The physician will inquire about any vaginal, cervical, or pelvic infections you have had. Sexually transmitted diseases (STDs) can interfere with fertility by causing scarring of the reproductive tract. In many cases, these infections may be nearly symptom-free, which is why your physician may take a cervical swab to culture for infection or a blood test to check indications in your blood that you had certain STDS in the past.

- *Current sexual patterns:* Your physician will ask how often you have sexual intercourse and whether you use any lubricants.
- *Medications:* The physician will ask you about any medications, prescription or over-the-counter, you are taking. If you take vitamins, herbal remedies, or supplements, you will want to mention those, too.
- *Surgical history:* Any kind of abdominal or gynecological surgery may leave scars or adhesions on the reproductive organs. The presence of scar tissue can interfere with the ovary's release of an egg, block the egg from reaching the fallopian tube, or keep a fertilized egg from moving through the fallopian tube to the uterus.
- *Other significant health problems:* The physician will want as complete a history about major health problems you and your immediate family members may have had.
- *Lifestyle and work environment:* Your physician may ask whether you smoke cigarettes, drink alcohol or caffeine-containing beverages, or use recreational drugs. Questions will be asked about your diet, weight loss or gain, and whether you exercise vigorously. All these factors may contribute to diminished fertility. Tell your physician about environmental hazards at home or in the workplace (see chapter 12, "Staying Healthy").

### Perspectives

Undergoing the basic work-up for infertility can leave you feeling vulnerable and embarrassed. Consider writing in your infertility journal about your feelings. Pinpoint any overwhelming emotions that surface as you are writing, such as fear, remorse for past actions or habits, or confusion about what it all means. Taking the time to express and then identify the nature and source of your feelings will help you manage the sometimes overwhelming experience of infertility treatment.

## The Physical Examination

Chances are, you have been through more than one physical examination in your life, so the routine will probably be familiar to you. Although you may feel uncomfortable emotionally, the physical examination and the pelvic examination should not be painful.

- *Thyroid:* Your physician will palpate (or gently press) the base of the front of your neck, looking for signs of abnormality in your thyroid gland. The thyroid secretes thyroxine and regulates the body's metabolism. Both hyperthyroidism (overproduction of thyroxine) and hypothyroidism (underproduction of thyroxine) may interfere with fertility. In particular, hypothyroidism can interfere with ovulation, either making it irregular or stopping it altogether.

- *Hair distribution:* Unusual or excessive hair distribution patterns on the face or body may be evidence of increased male hormone levels. The pubic hair pattern, which is normally triangular, may be diamond-shaped, extending upward toward the navel, which is also a clue that male hormone levels may be high.

- *Breast examination:* Your physician will look at the size and shape of your breasts during the examination, and may also gently squeeze behind the nipples to see whether any discharge or milk can be expressed. If it can, you may be overproducing a hormone called prolactin. Prolactin stimulates milk production in nursing mothers and prevents them from ovulating or getting pregnant. If your prolactin level is elevated, it may explain why you are having trouble conceiving.

## The Pelvic Examination

The pelvic examination may be uncomfortable, but it is essential in evaluating the internal female reproductive tract. In preparation for a pelvic examination, you lie on your back with knees bent and feet placed in stirrups. A speculum will be inserted to hold open the vaginal canal so that the physician can inspect the cervix, looking for signs of unusual growths, sores, discharge, or infection. Often a Pap smear to check for cervical cancer is taken, which involves scraping a bit of tissue from the cervix (it may sting and cause a bit of cramping and spotting, but it should not be painful) to be sent to a laboratory for evaluation. In addition, the physician may want to culture the cervical mucus for possible infections such as gonorrhea or chlamydia. The physician may do a bimanual examination (an examination that requires two hands) by placing one or two fingers in the vaginal canal and placing the other hand on the abdomen to palpate the uterus, ovaries, and pelvic cavity for signs of abnormalities. A rectal examination may be performed, particularly if you have reported experiencing pain with your menstrual cycle or with bowel movements, or a problem with constipation and diarrhea around the time of your period.

If your medical history, physical examination, or pelvic examination results in information that explains your difficulty in conceiving, specific treatments will be started. Otherwise, tests designed to investigate these other areas of your reproductive system will be ordered:

- Your ovulatory pattern and the quality of your uterine lining.
- The quality of your cervical mucus and its ability to support sperm.
- The size and shape of your uterus and whether your fallopian tubes are patent (open).

These tests are done at specific times in your menstrual cycle.

## BIMANUAL PELVIC EXAMINATION

Uterus

Cervical opening

Vaginal canal

Rectum

## PELVIC EXAMINATION USING SPECULUM

Vaginal canal

Speculum

Uterus

Cervical opening

Rectum

## Ovulation Evaluation

In about 30 percent of cases, women experiencing infertility have some type of ovulation disorder. The problem with ovulation can exist at any stage of a cycle—in the stimulation of the follicles (the follicular phase), the release of the egg (ovulation), or the preparation of the uterus for a fertilized egg (the luteal phase). We explore the diagnoses and treatment of specific ovulation disorders in Chapter 6, "The Female: Hormonal Disorders and Treatment." For now, we will show you how your physician might evaluate your ovulatory cycle.

There are five objectives to ovulation tests:

1. To confirm that you have been ovulating in the past.
2. To predict when you will be ovulating next.
3. To evaluate ovarian function or reserve (the ability of the ovaries to produce eggs).
4. To test whether or not you did ovulate in the current cycle.
5. To measure how receptive your uterus is to pregnancy during the second half (the luteal phase) of your cycle.

## Preliminary Step to Evaluate Ovulatory Patterns

A test that helps document past patterns of ovulation is the basal body temperature chart.

*Basal body temperature (BBT) charts:* Keeping track of your BBT (your body temperature at rest, typically when you first wake up) is a way to document whether you have ovulated. A specific hormonal change during your cycle—the secretion of progesterone after the follicle releases the egg at the time of ovulation—triggers a rise in BBT, so if you are taking your temperature every day, you will see that temperature rise if you have ovulated. The BBT chart will not *predict* when you are going to ovulate, but can serve as a record of your cyclical patterns.

To create a BBT chart, take your temperature at the same time every morning. At the time of ovulation, or just after, you will notice an increase of about 0.6 or 0.8 degrees. As you chart your temperature on a graph, you will see whether there is a rise in temperature, and then you will know whether you ovulated during that particular cycle. Here is what you need to do:

1. Purchase at the pharmacy a special BBT thermometer, which is designed to make reading small temperature increments easier. Both oral and rectal thermometers are available; oral thermometers may be more convenient to use.
2. Before you go to bed, shake down the thermometer to below 95 degrees, and leave it on a bedside table.

BASAL BODY TEMPERATURE (BBT) CHART

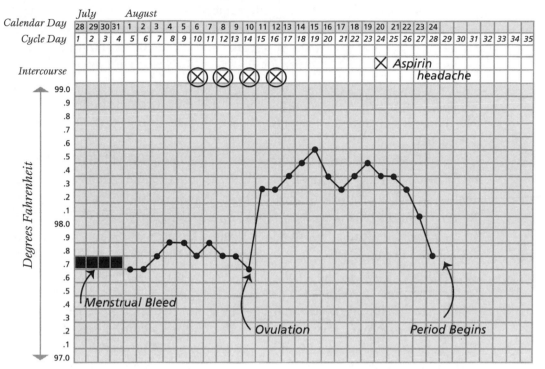

3. Upon waking, before getting out of bed or drinking anything, place the oral thermometer under your tongue and leave it there for about 3 minutes, or follow the package instructions. Do not get up until you complete the 3-minute test.

4. Record the temperature every day for several months, or according to your physician's instructions. Annotate the chart to mark days on which you have sexual intercourse. You may also want to note days when you take any kind of medication, stay up late at night, feel like you are ill with a cold, etc.

## To Predict When You Are Going to Ovulate

*Urine test kits to monitor luteinizing hormone (LH):* Ovulation predictor kits are designed to help you *predict* the time you will ovulate, so that you may maximize the timing of sexual intercourse or intrauterine insemination (IUI) to help ensure that sperm will be present when the egg is present. You will perform a simple urine test with the kit to document the surge in LH released by the pituitary just before ovulation—usually 24 to 38 hours before the follicle ruptures to release the mature egg. Remember to continue having sexual intercourse for 2 days after the LH surge (through day 16, more or less, of your menstrual cycle); do not stop with the surge! There are many ovulation kits on the market, each with its set of directions. Most kits offer a toll-free number for patients to call if they have questions about test results or are on certain fertility medications, such as clomiphene citrate (see chapter 6, "The Female: Hormonal Disorders and Treatment"), which may require testing of urine for LH earlier.

*Blood tests and ultrasound:* Other tests used to predict ovulation include frequent blood tests that measure levels of estrogen and LH, and frequent ultrasounds that track follicular growth. These tests are expensive and are usually reserved for cycles in which the woman is taking superovulatory drugs. Transvaginal ultrasound, if performed on the day of your LH surge, will confirm whether a follicle has begun to swell in preparation for release of an egg. Transvaginal ultrasound is painless and involves no radiation; the physician will insert an ultrasound probe into the vagina to produce images of the uterus, ovaries, and fallopian tubes for diagnostic analysis. In the hundreds of studies performed on the procedure since its invention in the mid-1970s, no abnormalities of soft tissue have been reported as a result of its use. Transvaginal ultrasound is a different procedure from the abdominal ultrasound procedure, which requires that you drink large amounts of liquid before the test. During abdominal ultrasound, no vaginal probe is used; the transducer is used on the skin of the abdomen only.

## To Evaluate Ovarian Function

To evaluate ovarian function, your physician may use several tests. Normal values for these tests vary from laboratory to laboratory. Therefore, your physician will have to interpret your results for you. Refer to the test result worksheet at the back of this book. The tests of ovarian reserve, as they are called, include the following:

*Day 3 FSH:* This blood test, taken on day 3 of your menstrual cycle, measures the level of the hormone FSH, or follicle-stimulating hormone. As cycle day 3 FSH levels rise, the ability of the ovary to produce good quality eggs and embryos is decreased. FSH levels often rise as women grow older, but occasionally younger women, even in their 20s and 30s, may have elevated FSH levels. A normal range for day 3 FSH may be either less than 20 mIU/mL (milli-International Units per milliliter), or less than 10 mIU/mL depending on the type of laboratory procedure used. Make sure you ask your physician to interpret the test results for you. Ask what is considered normal or abnormal ranges for the laboratory used by your physician or clinic.

*Day 3 estradiol test:* At the same time that your physician measures your day 3 FSH level, the amount of estradiol (the main type of estrogen) in your blood may also be measured. A high level of estradiol at this point in your cycle may also indicate poor egg quality or quantity. Normal range for day 3 estradiol is less than 50 pg/mL (picograms per milliliter).

*Clomiphene challenge test:* The clomiphene challenge test may be performed if the physician wants more information on how your ovaries function after stimulation with an oral medication, clomiphene citrate (Clomid or Serophene). The test involves the following series of steps:

1. A cycle day 3 FSH blood level will be taken.
2. You will be instructed to take 100 mg of clomiphene citrate on days 5 through 9 of your cycle.
3. FSH levels will be retested on cycle day 10.

A normal clomiphene challenge test would show a low FSH and a low estradiol on cycle day 3 and also a low FSH level on day 10. Your physician will explain your values to you and what they may mean to your fertility. Some physicians will also perform an ultrasound to evaluate follicular growth during the clomiphene challenge test.

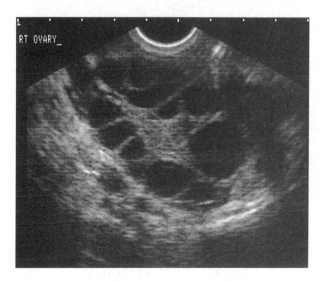

*Ultrasound of an ovary under the influence of fertility medication; multiple follicles are developing.*

## To Determine Whether You Have Ovulated and the State of Your Uterus in the Luteal Phase

- *Plasma progesterone level:* A plasma progesterone level (blood test) can be drawn in the last part of your cycle; high levels indicate that you have ovulated.
- *Ultrasound:* Transvaginal ultrasound may also be used several days *after* the LH surge to detect whether the follicle has ruptured and collapsed, which usually indicates that ovulation has occurred. An exception is a rare condition called luteinized unruptured follicle syndrome (LUF).
- *Other hormone tests:* Your physician may take a blood test to measure the amount of prolactin—a pituitary hormone that stimulates milk production. High prolactin levels in a woman who is not pregnant or nursing may disrupt ovulation and may indicate a benign pituitary tumor. Blood tests may also be performed to evaluate androgen (male hormones) levels. Androgen testing helps the physician diagnose a common condition called polycystic ovarian syndrome (PCOS), as well as hypothalamic and pituitary dysfunction.
- *Endometrial biopsy:* An endometrial biopsy can reveal how well your uterine lining is prepared for the potential implantation of a fertilized egg. An endometrial biopsy is not surgery and does not require anesthesia, but it is an invasive procedure.

### Voices

*Most women find the endometrial biopsy painful. "Everyone told me it would be a breeze," recalls Adrienne, a 37-year-old woman who went through 2 years of treatment before getting pregnant with her now 2-year-old son. "But I thought it hurt a lot, and I experienced some bleeding and severe cramping afterward. Before my second biopsy, my doctor gave me some Valium, which really helped."*

The endometrial biopsy is performed in the office, usually after day 21 in the cycle. The physician places a speculum in the vagina and then threads a small instrument through the cervix to "biopsy" a small area of the lining of the uterus. Cramping, especially during the small tissue biopsy, is common. Relaxation techniques, such as taking deep abdominal breaths, can help. Also, taking medication, such as Valium or pain medications, just before the test will lessen the discomfort. Many physicians suggest that you take antiprostaglandin medications, like Advil or Motrin, one half hour before the test.

After an endometrial biopsy, you may notice some spotting, either bright red or dark brown. If you start to have a heavy blood flow or develop a fever greater than 100 degrees Fahrenheit, or have a vaginal discharge that has an odor, contact your physician. The results of a biopsy will be available to your physician in 1 to 2 weeks; if the results show a lag of more than 2 days in endometrial development, a diagnosis of luteal phase defect (see chapter 6, "The Female: Hormonal Disorders and Treatment") will be made.

If the results of any of these tests point clearly to a hormonal imbalance affecting ovulation or endometrium development, your physician may proceed to treatment, or order additional tests on other areas of your reproductive system.

## Evaluation of the Cervical Mucus

*Postcoital test (PCT):* The PCT, also known as the Sims Huhner test, is performed at midcycle, as close to ovulation as possible. This test serves two purposes: to evaluate the quality and quantity of cervical mucus and to document that live, motile sperm are present in the mucus. You will be instructed to monitor ovulation, and when you detect an LH surge on your urine test kit, you should have intercourse, making sure not to use a lubricant. The physician's office will instruct you not to douche and to come to the office within a certain number of hours after intercourse. The nurse or physician will take a swab of your cervical mucus and check under the microscope for specific patterns, such as "ferning" (a pattern that looks very like a plant fern and indicates fertile mucus), and that there are at least 5 to 15 sperm alive and moving in the mucus. *A PCT should never serve as a substitute for a semen analysis.*

### Voices

*"Before you know it, you find yourself being able to undergo all kinds of tests and procedures that you thought would embarrass you when you first got started," admits Cherilynn, a veteran of infertility treatments. "As long I just kept my mind on my end goal—a successful pregnancy and a healthy baby—I could get through anything and know it would be worth it."*

## Evaluating Your Reproductive Organs

For successful fertilization, pregnancy, and birth to take place, each one of your reproductive organs must work normally. The tests we describe below help your physician evaluate them.

*Hysterosalpingogram (HSG):* An HSG is an x-ray procedure performed in the first half of the cycle, using a water- or oil-based dye to identify any structural abnormalities in your uterus and fallopian tubes, such as an unusually shaped uterus, fibroid tumors, scar tissue, or blockages in the fallopian tubes. Most women report cramping and mild to moderate discomfort with this procedure.

### Voices

*Some women, especially those who do have blockages, report intense pain during the HSG procedure. "It felt like someone lit my uterus on fire," is how Rachel describes it. "And I didn't even have a blockage."*

Ask your physician about giving you a pain medication 30 minutes before the procedure, which can help alleviate discomfort. Your physician may also prescribe Valium to help relax your uterine and tubal muscles. Finally, many physicians order a few days of a broad-spectrum antibiotic to be taken at the time of the HSG to prevent infection that could be caused by the procedure.

## HYSTEROSALPINGOGRAM (HSG)

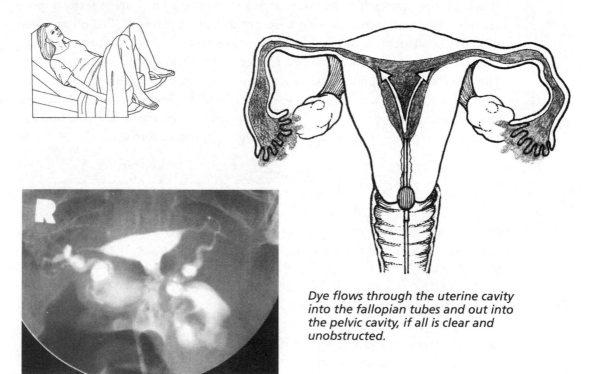

Dye flows through the uterine cavity into the fallopian tubes and out into the pelvic cavity, if all is clear and unobstructed.

*Normal HSG*

The HSG is usually conducted in the radiology department. The test is performed in the first part of your cycle, before ovulation. The gynecologist or radiologist will insert a speculum into the vagina, then thread a small catheter through the cervix and into the uterus. The physician then injects radiographic contrast material (dye) into the uterine cavity, which reveals blockages and other abnormalities on x-ray film.

The test can take 15 to 30 minutes, during which time a series of x-ray pictures will be taken. Recent studies report that women who have the oil-based dye have a slight increase in pregnancy rates after the HSG if their fallopian tubes are open. When the test is completed, you may feel tired and groggy if medication was given. It is a good idea to have a friend or family member be available to drive you home. You should not have any pain, discharge, or fever after the test. If you do, call your physician.

### *Breakthroughs*

Two new procedures are available to assess the uterine cavity or the fallopian tubes. Sonohysterography (hystogram) is an ultrasound-monitoring procedure using saline solution instead of the radio-opaque dye; this procedure can be performed in a physician's office instead of a radiology facility. In addition, no x-rays are needed. Falloposcopy is the visual examination of the inside of the fallopian tube through the use of a fiber-optic endoscope that takes pictures of the inside of the uterus and fallopian tubes. Ask your physician whether one or both of these procedures are performed at their facility.

## SONOHYSTEROGRAPHY

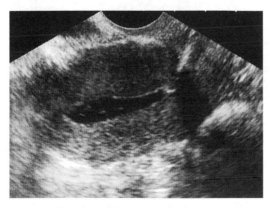

*Normal, side view of uterus.*

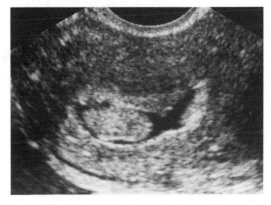

*Abnormal, showing uterine polyp.*

*Hysteroscopy:* If the results of your HSG indicate that you have a uterine abnormality, your physician may want to examine the inside of your uterus with a hysteroscope, a tiny telescope mounted with a fiber-optic light. When used for diagnostic purposes, hysteroscopy can be performed in the office under local anesthesia. After giving you medication to relax you, the hysteroscope is inserted through the cervix into the uterus. The physician will be able to see any uterine abnormalities or growths, such as polyps. Photographs are taken for future reference. This test is usually performed in the first half of your cycle so that the build-up of the endometrium does not obscure the examination of the uterine wall and endometrium. Small polyps or scar tissue can be removed at that time. Hysteroscopy is also performed in combination with diagnostic laparoscopy.

## HYSTEROSCOPY

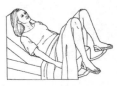

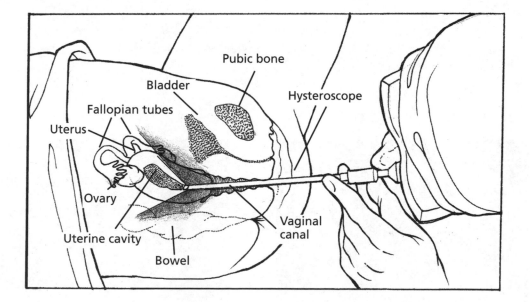

*Laparoscopy:* A laparoscopy is a surgical procedure performed under general anesthesia. Most laparoscopies are conducted in a hospital as an outpatient

## LAPAROSCOPY

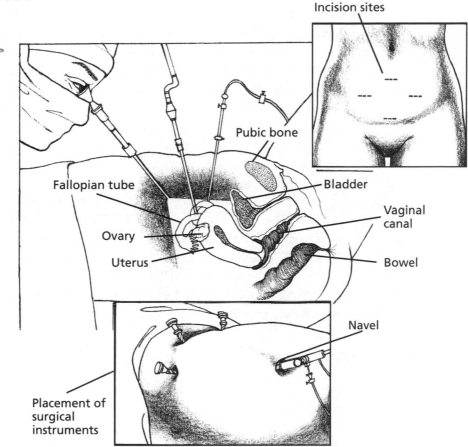

Incision sites

Pubic bone

Fallopian tube

Bladder

Ovary

Vaginal canal

Uterus

Bowel

Navel

Placement of surgical instruments

procedure. The laparoscopy is performed around or before ovulation. If it is going to be combined with a hysteroscopy, it may be performed even earlier in the cycle.

You will be instructed not to eat or drink anything after midnight on the day of the procedure. You may meet with the anesthesiologist before the procedure and will need to have a series of preoperative blood tests, chest x-ray films, and possibly an electrocardiogram. The operation consent form that you will be requested to sign can be frightening, because it lists all possible complications. Laparoscopy is one of the safest surgical procedures, however, and it has a very low complication rate.

During the laparoscopy, a telescope-like instrument is inserted through a tiny incision made just below your navel. Small incisions may be made in the groin area as well. These incisions allow the physician to insert instruments to move and position the pelvic organs. Carbon dioxide is introduced through a catheter to inflate the abdomen and push the abdominal wall and bowel away from the other pelvic organs. With such a clear view, your physician can examine your ovaries, fallopian tubes, and other pelvic organs. If endometriosis or adhesions are found, a surgical instrument, such as a laser, can be used to remove them. Dye can be injected through the cervix into the uterus, and the physician can observe through the laparoscope whether the dye spills out from each tube, indicating open fallopian tubes. At the end of the procedure, the abdomen is deflated, and several stitches are used to close the small incisions. Most women are discharged from the hospital's day surgery unit once they can urinate, take fluids without being nauseated, and stand and walk.

It is not uncommon to experience shoulder and neck pain for several days after laparoscopy. This is because any carbon dioxide still remaining in the abdomen pushes against the diaphragm and causes referred pain to the upper chest and shoulder area. The physician will give you a prescription for pain medication and instruct you to take it easy for 1 to 2 days. If you develop fever or increased pain or have vaginal bleeding or discharge, redness, and swelling at the site of the incision, call your physician.

## THE BASIC WORK-UP FOR MEN

The basic work-up for men begins with an appointment with the physician to discuss medical history and current medical, sexual, and lifestyle factors. Past medical problems that may affect fertility include having had mumps after puberty, hernia repairs, athletic injuries to the groin, or a history of undescended testicles. The physician will also ask about sexual history, especially details about possible STDs, urinary tract infections, or prostatitis. The physician will also ask about any impotence or ejaculatory problems (premature or delayed ejaculation), which make it difficult to release the sperm during sexual intercourse necessary to fertilize the egg. (Treatment for male factor infertility problems is discussed in chapter 8, "The Male: Diagnosis and Treatment.")

### The Physical Examination

The male reproductive tract is largely external, including the penis and the scrotal sac, which contains the testes. The physician will check the man's hair growth pattern in the genital area, which should be diamond-shaped, extending upward toward the navel. After examining the penis for abnormalities, the physician will examine the scrotum, using his fingers to distinguish each testicle, the epididymis coiled on top and behind it, and the vas deferens, which runs like a cord up the back of each testicle and upwards through the scrotal sac. Careful attention is paid to the size and firmness of the testes. Small, very soft, or hard and irregular-shaped testes may be indicators of compromised fertility.

One of the most common anatomic defects that could interfere with male fertility is the varicocele, a dilated vein (also called a varicose vein) found around and on top of the testicle and often occurring on the left testicle. Physicians may suspect that a varicocele could be causing an infertility problem after a semen analysis (described below) reveals a low sperm count and/or poor sperm motility. Abnormally shaped sperm are often found. Usually, the physician diagnoses varicocele by palpation (touch) during the physical examination. The physician will ask the man to stand up and bear down or cough, which pushes blood into the vein, making it easier to detect a varicose vein. The physician may also use ultrasound to measure the enlarged veins and identify abnormal blood flow in the vessels (more about varicocele diagnosis and treatment in chapter 8, "The Male: Diagnosis and Treatment").

- *Prostate examination:* This part of the physical examination is not painful, but it is invasive. The man will be asked to stand and bend over the examination table, and the physician will insert one finger into his rectum to feel the seminal vesicles and the prostate gland. If the gland is tender or swollen, the physician will massage the prostate gland to trigger the release of a little fluid through the penis that can be cultured and evaluated for the presence of white blood cells and bacteria.

The next step in evaluating the male's fertility is the semen analysis.

## The Semen Analysis

The single most important test of male fertility is the semen analysis, which evaluates the following:

- sperm count (how many millions of sperm per milliliter)
- ability of the sperm to swim (motility)
- velocity or forward progression of the sperm
- size and shape of the sperm (morphology)
- total semen volume
- the liquefaction of the semen (the ability to go from the normal gel-like state at ejaculation to a liquid state)

- viscosity of the ejaculate (how sticky it is)
- presence of fructose in the ejaculate (fructose, a type of sugar, is its source of energy)
- presence of white blood cells

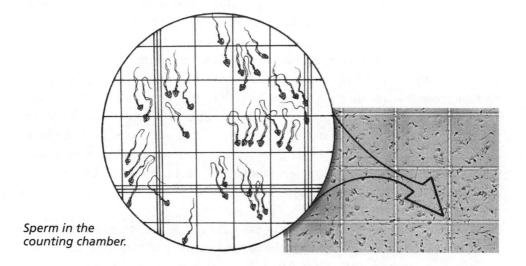

*Sperm in the counting chamber.*

The laboratory can evaluate all of these factors with one semen specimen. Most physicians recommend that you abstain from ejaculating for 2 to 3 days before collecting a semen sample. The man masturbates and collects the total ejaculate into a cup; for best results, the semen should be examined within a few hours of ejaculation. The total volume of the ejaculate is usually 2 to 3 teaspoons. The specimen can be collected at the laboratory or physician's office. If the specimen is collected at home, however, it must be kept at body temperature and should be delivered to the laboratory within about an hour of collection. Because sperm counts and quality can vary, at least two or three samples may be necessary to establish a baseline.

### *Voices*

*"We did some very odd things to get pregnant," says Walter, a 34-year-old man who went through 5 years of infertility treatments—and many semen analyses—before he and his wife got pregnant this year. "It's all surreal. You have to dissociate a little bit from what's going on to get through giving a sperm sample. One time I went in to give a specimen, the nurse was a big male guy who proceeded to talk to other nurses right*

*outside the door while I was supposed to get things done. You're supposed to be doing what is normally very private. All your life you are told you're not supposed to masturbate—especially me because of my strict religious upbringing—and now it is necessary."*

Two methods are used in the laboratory to evaluate the specimen. In some laboratories, technicians examine the sperm by placing it on a slide, looking at it under a microscope, and making calculations and evaluations themselves. Other laboratories and clinics use the CASA (computer-assisted semen analysis) method, which uses a computer-programmed instrument to count the sperm cells and evaluate their motility, velocity, and morphology. Either method is acceptable if done correctly.

These are the factors that are reported in a semen analysis (also refer to the test result worksheet for men located at the back of this book):

- *Total volume:* Two to five milliliters is normal volume. A very low volume indicates that the seminal vesicles may not be making enough fluid or that these ducts may be blocked. It may also indicate a problem with the prostate gland, which contributes about 30 percent of the seminal fluid.
- *Sperm count:* The normal range for the number of million sperm per milliliter is between 40 million and 300 million. Counts of 80 million are average. However, you certainly do not need this high a count to establish fertilization and a pregnancy. Counts below 10 million are considered poor; counts of 20 million or more might be just fine if motility and morphology are normal. Generally speaking, the higher the sperm count, the better. On the other hand, if it is too high, chances are that the sperm may have poor motility or morphology and thus hinder fertility.
- *Motility and velocity:* Motility and forward progression—how fast and well the sperm swim in a forward direction—are important factors when it comes to male fertility. Your physician will evaluate two aspects of motility: the number of active cells as a percentage of the total number of cells, and the quality of the movement of the sperm. The motility is measured in a percentage from 0 to 100. Two or three hours after ejaculation, 50 percent of the sperm cells should be active (motile); more is even better. The progression of sperm cells in a straight line across a grid is rated from 0 (no progression) to 4 (excellent progression). A score of 2 or more is satisfactory.
- *Morphology:* All sperm cells are not alike. Some are immature and others may be of abnormal shape. At least 30 percent of cells should be of normal

shape (World Health Organization [WHO] criteria). Normal sperm heads are oval-shaped without irregularities. The midsection and the tail should not be too narrow or thin (called tapered). If the heads are large and round, the sperm may be missing the acrosome, the packet of enzymes that allows sperm to bore through the coating of the egg. Evidence of a large number of immature cells, called spermatids, may indicate the presence of a varicocele or possible testicular dysfunction.

## ABNORMAL SPERM

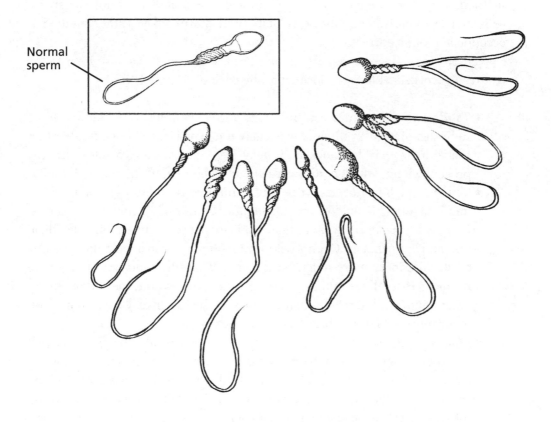

Normal sperm

- *Kruger (strict) morphology test.* Another test done on sperm cells during a semen analysis of sperm morphology focuses only on an examination of the shape and size of the sperm head. In this test, normal results are when 14 percent or more of sperm have normal-shaped heads; men with less than 4 percent normal-shaped sperm may have a significant infertility problem.

- *Liquefaction:* At ejaculation, liquid semen immediately coagulates into a pearly gel that liquefies within 20 minutes. Failure to coagulate and then liquefy may be a sign that the seminal vesicles are malfunctioning. Increased viscosity (thickness) of the semen may indicate a problem with the seminal vesicles, or the presence of white blood cells resulting from infection or inflammation.
- *Seminal fructose:* If no sperm are present, the physician will test the semen for seminal fructose, which the seminal vesicles normally produce. If no fructose is present, congenital absence of the vas deferens or seminal vesicles or obstruction of the ejaculatory duct are possibilities.
- *Cultures:* The physician may culture the semen and/or the urethra for the presence of chlamydia, gonorrhea, and other bacteria.

### Normal Semen Analysis Results

On at least two occasions:

| | |
|---|---|
| Volume | 2.0 to 5.0 mL or more |
| Sperm number | 20 million/mL or more |
| Motility | 50 percent or more |
| Forward Progression | at least 2 + forward progression |
| Morphology | WHO > 30 percent; or, Kruger, at least 4 percent normal forms |

and

No significant sperm clumping or agglutination

No significant white blood cells or red blood cells

No hyperviscosity (increased thickening of the seminal fluid)

Other tests done on semen include the following:

- *Sperm antibodies:* If the sperm agglutinate, or do not move well, the physician may order tests that can localize and quantify specific antibodies in the blood and on the sperm's surface. Depending on where the antibodies attach to the sperm, different problems with fertility can result. If they stick to the head of the sperm, the sperm may not be able to penetrate the egg for fertilization. If the tail becomes covered, the sperm may not be able to swim fast enough or in the right direction.
- *Sperm penetration:* The sperm penetration assay (SPA), also called the *ham-*

*ster egg test*, is a specific test to evaluate the sperm's ability to capacitate and complete the acrosome reaction. This reaction allows the sperm to break through the outer membrane of an egg and then fuse with the egg cytoplasm. The SPA involves mixing sperm with hamster eggs (the hamster produces eggs that are capable of being penetrated by human sperm). The eggs have been stripped of their outer layer (the zona pellucida). If the sperm successfully fuse with hamster eggs, it is assumed that they will do so when they come into contact with human eggs.

Another test, the hemizona assay test, evaluates the sperm's ability to fuse with a previously frozen but no longer viable human egg with an intact zona pellucida. The hemizona assay test is rarely done now with the advent of the assisted reproductive technology (ART) procedure, intracytoplasmic sperm injection (ICSI) (see chapter 9). With both the SPA and hemizona assay test, the number of eggs should be divided into two groups. Healthy donor sperm (the control sperm) should be placed with one half of the eggs, while the sperm of the man being examined (the test sperm) should be placed with the other half.

The cervical mucus penetration test (Pentrak) is a laboratory test that uses cow mucus to simulate the sperm's ability to move through the woman's cervical mucus. A normal result is 30 mm (millimeters) or more.

## Hormone Levels

Hormone levels or concentrations in the male are very important in defining normal fertility. FSH and LH levels are usually in the normal range if sperm production is relatively normal; for FSH, this is 4 to 10 mIU/mL. Androgen levels, testosterone specifically, should be in the normal range of 300 to 1,111 ng/dL (nanograms per deciliter). If the level is too high, it can result in testicular disturbances. The hormone prolactin should be less than 20 ng/mL. High levels may be indicative of a small benign tumor in the pituitary gland. These men may have a milky discharge from their breast nipples, decreased sex drive, low volume ejaculate (a small amount of semen on ejaculation), and some changes in their vision.

In some cases of severe male factor infertility, a testicular biopsy may be needed to assess sperm production in the testicles. This surgical procedure is performed in an outpatient hospital setting; a small biopsy of testicular tissue will be taken and evaluated. If the results of the testicular biopsy reveal that sperm are present in the testes, but no sperm is found in the ejaculate, an obstruction of the vas deferens or ejaculatory ducts may be suspected.

Vasography is usually done at the time surgery for microsurgical reconstruction is planned (see chapter 8, "The Male: Diagnosis and Treatment," for more information about testicular biopsy).

Together, the basic infertility work-ups for women and men described in this chapter will uncover the vast majority of fertility problems and lead you to a next stage of treatment. The 10 percent of cases that remain unexplained may require more testing, or your physician may try treatment to enhance one or more phases of the reproductive process.

After your evaluation is complete, meet with your physician to review the results and discuss treatment options. At this point, you might want to create a decision tree that can help you put what you have learned from the basic infertility work-ups into context and explore what steps you may want to take next.

**Basic Infertility Work-up**

*Male Work-up:*
*Tests Performed and Results*

1.

2.

3.

*Female Work-up:*
*Tests Performed and Results*

1.

2.

3.

*What's next?*

## POSITIVE STEPS YOU CAN TAKE FROM CHAPTER 5

**Understand that the diagnostic work-up is part of a process.** You may come away from the basic work-up without a definitive diagnosis. Some of the tests may be inconclusive; some may need to be repeated. Your fertility status, and treatment plan, may change as you go through treatment.

**Control what you can.** You and your partner are the ultimate decision makers at this stage, as in all stages, of the infertility journey. Your physician will identify fertility roadblocks and help map a reasonable course for you, but you will decide what, if any, treatment you wish to pursue and for how long. Infertility touches many areas of your life, and the experience makes most people feel a loss of control and privacy, even a sense of betrayal by their bodies. This is normal, and to some degree unavoidable. We will give you information in part 3, "Coping with Infertility," to help you restore control wherever you can.

**Use the test result worksheets.** Record your test results in the worksheets provided at the back of this book. Remember to enter in retest results, if necessary.

# 6 The Female: Hormonal Disorders and Treatment

This chapter covers ovulatory and hormonal disorders, and the methods of diagnosis, treatments, and medications used to help resolve them. "Fertility drugs" generally refer to those hormonal preparations used by women to help stimulate ovulation and/or support the development of the uterine lining. We will discuss each drug, including the benefits, risks, and potential side effects. Some of these drugs are also used to treat male factor infertility hormonal problems (see chapter 8, "The Male: Diagnosis and Treatment").

## OVULATORY DISORDERS

About 30 percent of female infertility problems result from ovulation disorders. This is a broad category under which we include discussions of hypothalamic anovulation, polycystic ovarian syndrome (PCOS), premature ovarian failure (POF), and luteal phase defect (LPD). Some important terms used to describe ovulatory problems include the following:

- *Amenorrhea*: a term used if a woman has not had a period for 3 or more consecutive months.
- *Oligomenorrhea*: a term used to describe irregular periods.
- *Anovulation*: a term used to describe the absence of ovulation, with or without a menstrual bleed.

## *Evaluating Ovulation with Hormonal Blood Tests*

- **Follicle-stimulating hormone (FSH) and luteinizing hormone (LH):** If the cycle day 3 FSH level is elevated, a woman's ovaries may be unable to produce a good quality egg each month because of age or other problems. If FSH and LH levels or their ratio (FSH/LH) are low, there may be an abnormality in the hypothalamus-pituitary circuit.
- **Estradiol:** On cycle day 3, the estradiol level should be normal. Otherwise, it can indicate that the ovary is not capable of creating good quality eggs.
- **Prolactin:** Excess levels of prolactin can affect normal ovulation and endometrial (uterine lining) growth.
- **Thyroid-stimulating hormone (TSH):** The thyroid gland controls the metabolism in the body and is important in maintaining the hormonal balance between the pituitary and ovary. Both hyperthyroidism (an overactive thyroid) and hypothyroidism (an underactive thyroid) can interfere with normal ovulation.
- **Androgens:** Excess levels of testosterone or dehydroepiandrosterone sulfate (DHEAS)—hormones made by the ovaries and the adrenal glands that have male hormonal effects—can affect ovulation. Elevated male hormones may also trigger excessive body hair, oily skin, or acne.
- **Progesterone:** This hormone is produced by the ovary and rises after ovulation. One test of ovulation is to measure the progesterone level during the midluteal phase, approximately 1 week before expected menses.

## *Normal Results for Female Hormone Levels*

This chart indicates the normal results for hormone levels. The cycle day column indicates the day of your menstrual cycle when the blood test will be taken. Refer to the test result worksheet for women at the back of this book to keep a log of your test results.

| TEST | CYCLE DAY | NORMAL RANGE |
|---|---|---|
| FSH | 3 | < 10 mIU/mL |
| | | < 20 mIU/mL depending on laboratory |
| Estradiol | 3 | < 50 pg/mL |
| Progesterone | Midluteal: 7 days after LH surge | > 10 ng/mL |
| Prolactin | Any cycle day | < 25 ng/mL |

| TEST | CYCLE DAY | NORMAL RANGE |
|---|---|---|
| Thyroid-stimulating hormone (TSH) | Any cycle day | 0.5–3.8 IU/mL |
| Total testosterone | Any cycle day | 6.0–8.6 ng/dL |
| Dehydroepiandrosterone sulfate (DHEAS) | Any cycle day | 35–350 mcg/dL |

*Code: IU = international units; mL = milliliters; mIU = milli-International Units; ng = nanograms; dL = deciliters; pg = picograms; mcg = micrograms

## Primary Amenorrhea and Ovarian Failure

Today in the United States the median age for menarche (the age at one's first period) is about 12 years. If a girl is older than 16 and has not menstruated, she has primary amenorrhea, an unusual condition affecting less than 2.5 percent of all women. Women who have primary ovarian failure, amenorrhea, will not ovulate or have periods. This is not to be confused with *premature ovarian failure* (POF), which is the loss of ovarian function before 40 years of age but after having had at least one period. Women with primary ovarian failure have abnormal ovaries, as seen in women with Turner's syndrome and other gonadal dysgenesis (failure of organs to develop or form properly).

The main causes of primary ovarian failure include congenital abnormalities due to chromosome problems. The sex of the embryo is determined at the moment of fertilization, when the father's 23 chromosomes join with the mother's 23 chromosomes. If a girl is conceived, both the mother and father contribute an X chromosome (women contribute only X chromosomes). During the conception of a male, the woman contributes an X chromosome and the man contributes a Y chromosome. When a defect occurs in either the X or the Y chromosome, problems can result. If the X chromosome from either the mother or the father has a defect in one of its genes, development of a full range of female characteristics may be impossible. Such defects may result in abnormal sexual development and a woman's inability to ovulate. Among the most common of these rare defects are the following:

• *Turner's syndrome* is the most common congenital cause of primary amenorrhea and primary ovarian failure. Women with Turner's syndrome are born with a missing second X chromosome, which makes it impossible for normal sexual development to take place. Women with Turner's syndrome do not have normal ovaries and are unable to ovulate, even with medication—but they do have a uterus.

• *Ovarian dysgenesis* results when a woman has a normal female chromosomal pattern but has a defect in one of the X chromosomes. Women with this condition are born with a uterus but without eggs in their ovaries. They do not produce follicles or estrogen, and can never have biological children. Because they have a uterus, however, they may be able to carry a fertilized donor egg—as long as they receive hormonal treatment to support the lining of the uterus, and as long as the uterus is of adequate size and normal shape (as can women with Turner's syndrome).

• *Androgen insensitivity* is a rare genetic disorder in which an individual is born with a male chromosomal pattern but with an abnormal gene on the X chromosome. Someone born with this defect appears to be female, but has a shortened vaginal canal, no uterus, and, instead of ovaries, tissue that produces both estrogen and male hormones. Although individuals with this problem have normal secondary sex characteristics, such as breasts, and appear female, they are genetically male. These individuals cannot have biological children.

Several other conditions may cause primary ovarian failure, including severe malnutrition or extreme weight loss in childhood, which also delay the onset of puberty. If a young girl does not reach a certain weight—and this level varies significantly from person to person—she may not menstruate.

## Hypothalamic Anovulation

In hypothalamic anovulation, lifestyle factors may contribute to a cessation of ovulation. Stress, extreme weight loss, and excessive exercise can reduce the output of gonadotropin-releasing hormone (GnRH) from the hypothalamus, which in turn causes the pituitary to reduce its production of FSH and LH. No ovulation occurs because FSH and LH are necessary for follicles and eggs to mature and be released from the ovary.

• *Stress.* One of the myths about infertility dispelled earlier was "just relax and you'll get pregnant." In part, stress may play a role in the disease of infertility; but more often, it is the infertility that causes stress. Stress that can impair fertility usually results from a crisis situation, such as a family health emergency or a traumatic event. You may know how it feels: Your heart beats faster, your palms sweat, your breath comes in shallow and rapid measure. This is the so-called "fight or flight" response. The same endocrine glands largely responsible for regulating the menstrual cycle—particularly the hypothalamus and the pituitary—are also involved in these physiological reactions. Severe stress and even chronic low-level stress can disturb ovulation patterns. Perhaps you have experienced this yourself: Have you noticed that your periods change in length or come late or early when you have been faced with a stressful situation?

• *Infertility itself is a life crisis.* Every month a pregnancy does not happen, every time you get an invitation to yet another baby shower, every time you hear "just relax and you'll get pregnant" may contribute to the chronic stress of infertility and may trigger a hormonal imbalance and ovulatory disturbance. In part 3, "Coping with Infertility," we offer stress-management techniques that may help.

• *Extreme weight loss or obesity.* A woman's body weight should not fall below or go above a certain set point to maintain a regular pattern of ovulation and menstruation. Fat tissue is important in estrogen storage and metabolism. If a woman is extremely underweight, her body may not have the estrogen it needs to keep the cycle going. Being grossly overweight, or obese, on the other hand, may cause high estrogen levels, which could interfere with regular ovulation. Regaining weight, or losing it, through proper diet and exercise programs may restore fertility in a few women. However, cases of extreme obesity caused by endocrine problems such as hypothyroidism need to be medically treated.

• *Excessive exercise.* Excessive exercise interferes with fertility in three ways: First, it can cause substantial weight loss and the loss of estrogen-storing body fat, which can disrupt hormonal balance. Second, strenuous exercise may alter brain signals to the hypothalamus, which then fails to emit its regular pulses of GnRH every 60 to 90 minutes as a message to the pituitary to release LH and FSH. As a result, the pituitary releases less than normal amounts of the reproductive hormones, LH and FSH, which interferes with the ovaries' ability to produce estrogen and progesterone. Third, endorphins—the opiate-like chemicals that the brain releases during strenuous exercise that cause the so-called runner's high—may also hinder the normal production of GnRH and other hormones.

Your physician may ask questions about your exercise patterns, weight, and stress levels during your infertility work-up. Remember, losing or gaining a little weight (if you are overweight or underweight) or exercising on a regular basis will not interfere with your fertility. A healthy lifestyle that involves a balanced diet and regular exercise may help you cope with the stress of the infertility experience (see chapter 12, "Staying Healthy").

## Polycystic Ovarian Syndrome

Polycystic ovarian syndrome (PCOS), also known as *polycystic ovarian dis-*

*ease, Stein-Leventhal syndrome,* and *hyperandrogenic chronic anovulation,* occurs in a small percentage of the female population. It is a complex disorder of ovulation involving the hypothalamus, pituitary gland, adrenal gland, and ovaries. With this disorder, ovulation may be irregular, and tiny cysts—which are actually tiny follicles—accumulate in the ovaries. These follicles contain eggs, but instead of the follicles maturing, very small cysts develop.

## PCOS

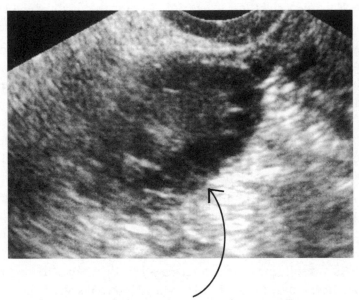

*Ultrasound image of an ovary showing PCOS.*

### SYMPTOMS

The primary symptom of PCOS is irregular or absent periods, and this menstrual dysfunction usually dates back to the onset of menses. Some women with PCOS have symptoms related to the excess levels of male hormones in the blood, including hirsutism (excess facial and body hair), a tendency to develop acne, high lipid levels that can lead to future cardiovascular disease, and possible disturbances of sugar metabolism. Many (about 50 percent), but not all, women with PCOS are overweight. It is important to note that some women with polycystic-appearing ovaries have *none* of the symptoms described above. Women with PCOS often experience infertility that may be related to their irregular ovulation patterns.

**Voices**

*Carolyn, a 29-year-old woman who recently gave birth to twin boys after 6 years of infertility treatment, said: "I always thought I had irregular periods because I was a gymnast. I competed in gymnastics all through my teens into my early 20s. And my doctor thought that, too. But when I stopped competing, my periods got worse, not better. My doctor, still convinced it was my exercise patterns that threw my cycles off, put me on the birth control pill to regulate my cycle—I wasn't trying to get pregnant yet—and I felt normal for the first time. But when we started trying to get pregnant when I was 23 and couldn't after a year and a half of trying on our own, we went to a specialist. Right away, he told me my problem had nothing to do with my past as a gymnast, that what I really had was a medical condition called polycystic ovarian syndrome, or PCOS. I was relieved. I thought 'Good. Now we can fix it and everything will be all right.' I didn't realize how much of a journey I had ahead of me." After a few years of treatment, including an in vitro fertilization (IVF) attempt that ended in a heartbreaking miscarriage at 20 weeks, Carolyn and her husband Larry had twins.*

## DIAGNOSIS

An ultrasound examination on a woman with PCOS often reveals ovaries that contain small, immature follicles just beneath the ovarian cortex (lining). Because healthy women without PCOS may also have immature follicles, however, an ultrasound examination alone is not enough to make the diagnosis.

After a careful physical examination and obtaining a history of menstrual cycle patterns, the physician should take blood tests to evaluate FSH, LH, estradiol, prolactin, progesterone, testosterone, and DHEAS levels. The LH to FSH ratio may be abnormal in women with PCOS: LH levels are often two to three times as high as FSH levels. Prolactin, testosterone, and DHEAS levels are also often elevated.

Some women with PCOS have abnormal insulin and glucose (sugar) interaction. If the physician suspects this problem, a glucose tolerance test may be done. This involves drinking a thick, sweet drink and having several blood samples drawn at intervals afterward to see whether the body can respond to this sugar load.

## TREATMENT

Women with PCOS who are trying to conceive and who have ovulation problems have several options. The first treatment for ovulation induction is an oral medication, clomiphene citrate, which is successful for many women with this condition. About 80 percent of infertile women with PCOS ovulate after taking clomiphene citrate, and if no other infertility factors are present, they should have increased pregnancy rates. For those patients with PCOS who do not respond to clomiphene citrate alone, physicians may add human chorionic gonadotropin (hCG)—one shot of hCG at the time of expected ovulation. Finally, therapy with human menopausal gonadotropin (hMG) (or purified FSH) may help women who fail to ovulate or to conceive with clomiphene citrate and hCG. Read more about each of these medications later in this chapter.

Women with PCOS who undergo ovulation induction are at greatly higher risk for ovarian hyperstimulation syndrome (OHSS). OHSS is overstimulation of the ovaries, and it results in painful enlargement of the ovaries, fluid retention in the abdominal cavity, and other symptoms. Physicians who treat patients with PCOS are particularly vigilant about monitoring the effects of ovulation-induction drugs. Many physicians recommend a low starting dose of hMG or FSH, followed by small incremental increases in amount to control the number of maturing follicles.

A surgical approach called *ovarian drilling* may be successful in producing ovulatory cycles in women with PCOS. During laparoscopy, the surgeon uses a laser or electrosurgical instruments (the newest is the harmonic scalpel) to puncture the tiny cysts. The potential risks of anesthesia and surgery, as well as the increased risk of the development of ovarian adhesions (scar tissue), make this option less appealing than drug therapy as an initial option for women with PCOS.

### Voices

*Gail is 28. Her husband, Paul, is 33. Gail recalls, "During the surgery, the doctor did something called ovarian drilling. The thought is that the ovaries will function normally for about 6 to 9 months—you'll ovulate normally—until the cysts come back. Later, the doctor saw that I ovulated, but I didn't get pregnant, even though everything seemed to be working normally. I did two more cycles with clomiphene citrate and intrauterine insemination (IUI), and then went on to IVF. The third IVF cycle took, but I miscarried. After the fourth IVF, I'm pregnant with twins. It's been years of persistent effort. We're hoping I'll be able to carry the pregnancy full term."*

If a woman with PCOS has elevated DHEAS levels, dexamethasone, a type of oral steroid, may be administered. This medication may be used at low dosage for 2 weeks each cycle or until pregnancy occurs, but should be used cautiously, because when used long term, it can have potentially serious side effects, such as bone changes in the hip joint.

Several new drugs are being studied that help trigger ovulation by correcting the abnormal insulin and glucose interaction that some PCOS patients have.

## Premature Ovarian Failure

Premature ovarian failure (POF) is defined as the loss of ovarian function in women younger than 40 years. It occurs in 1 in 1,000 women between the ages of 15 and 29 and in 1 in 100 women between the ages of 30 and 39. The average age of onset is 27 years. A family history of POF is found in about 4 percent of women experiencing the condition.

A woman is born with all the eggs she will ever have—usually about 1 to 2 million. By puberty, she has just 400,000 left, and by menopause, very few. This loss of eggs is a normal process that occurs steadily throughout a woman's natural reproductive life, which usually lasts until about the age of 51 or 52. In women with POF, however, the process of egg loss is greatly accelerated and may lead to infertility at a very early age. Some women with this disorder have infrequent or irregular menstruation. It is important to note that a woman can have a menstrual period but may not have ovulated.

Usually, if a woman has POF, irregular periods eventually stop. Either her cycle day 3 FSH or her estrogen levels may be elevated. She may experience symptoms of menopause such as hot flashes, no menses, and vaginal dryness. These symptoms may appear suddenly over 1 to 2 months, or more gradually over several years.

In most cases of POF, no cause is ever identified. Pelvic surgery, chemotherapy, and radiation therapy can cause POF, as can, uncommonly, severe pelvic inflammatory disease (PID). There are two theories about other causes:

- *Chromosomal abnormalities.* Certain inherited disorders can trigger premature loss of eggs. Other conditions cause ovaries to become resistant to the hormones necessary for ovulation and menses. A rare cause of POF is associated with a defect in the enzyme 17-hydroxylase, which affects the formation of hormones necessary for ovulation.
- *Autoimmune oophoritis.* In autoimmune diseases the body's immune system attacks the body's own tissues, and in this theoretical case, the ovaries. Rheumatoid arthritis is an example of an autoimmune disease. Several studies show that some women with POF also tend to have other autoimmune disorders, such as Graves' disease (an autoimmune disease that involves the thyroid gland) and Addison's disease (an autoimmune disease of the adrenal glands). Some scientists suspect that autoimmune oophoritis is responsible for certain cases of POF.

DIAGNOSIS

The following tests are used to diagnose POF:

*FSH,* and *estrogen levels.* Elevated cycle day 3 hormone levels should trigger investigation. It is important to ask your physician what the clinic considers a normal range for cycle day 3 FSH levels. Depending on the type of test used, some clinics consider 12 mIU/mL or above to be abnormal; others use 25 mIU/mL or above as the abnormal reading. Unfortunately, researchers have found that even though these levels may fluctuate from cycle to cycle, once an FSH or an estradiol level is confirmed as elevated, it has a negative effect on future cycles in terms of ovarian response and egg quality.

- *TSH level:* This blood hormone level should be checked to rule out severe hypothyroidism.
- *Chromosome study:* Karyotyping involves a blood test that will reveal any chromosomal abnormalities that could explain the loss of eggs.

---

### *Questions to Ask*

**If You Suspect You Have Premature Ovarian Failure**

If your physician suspects that your ovaries are failing and that you are going into early menopause, ask the following questions:

- Have thyroid tests been done, including tests to detect thyroid antibodies?
- Have repeat day 3 FSH and estradiol blood serum levels been drawn?
- Has a clomiphene challenge test been done? (This is not usually done if the initial day 3 FSH and estradiol blood levels are extremely elevated.)

---

TREATMENT

Unfortunately, there is no effective way of stimulating ovaries if POF is diagnosed. However, if you have untreated hypothyroidism, your physician will place you on thyroid medication. If ovarian antibodies are present, treatment with high doses of steroid medications may be able to restore ovarian function in a few rare cases. However, side effects of steroid therapy can be severe, and this treatment is not usually recommended for women with POF. In a small number of cases, women with POF have been able to get pregnant after being treated with estrogen replacement therapy or birth control pills, followed by high-dose hMG or FSH therapy.

Most physicians recommend estrogen replacement therapy for POF patients because this will lessen side effects of estrogen loss, such as osteoporosis (a condition characterized by reduction in bone mass and density) and cardiovascular disease. Progesterone is also administered to prevent the endometrial lining from becoming too thick.

A diagnosis of POF can be devastating and means putting an end to a woman's dreams of conceiving and bearing a genetically related child. However, if the uterus is intact, it is possible for a woman to attempt pregnancy using a donor egg, a process described in chapter 15, "Exploring Other Family-Building Options."

## Luteal Phase Defect

The luteal phase of the menstrual cycle derives its name from the *corpus luteum*, the structure on the ovary that forms and remains after the follicle releases the egg at ovulation. Before ovulation, the endometrium, or uterine lining, thickens under the influence of estrogen. After ovulation, the endometrium continues to mature as the corpus luteum secretes progesterone. The luteal phase is normally the 12 to 14 days of the cycle occurring after ovulation and before the next menstruation. Continued secretion of progesterone by the corpus luteum is essential for maintenance of pregnancy through week 8 or 10. At that time, the placenta takes over the primary responsibility for providing progesterone.

In luteal phase defect (LPD), either the corpus luteum fails to secrete adequate progesterone or the endometrium does not respond to the progesterone to grow and develop sufficiently. If the endometrium is not prepared for implantation of the fertilized egg at the right time—about 4 to 8 days after ovulation—no pregnancy will result. The incidence of LPD in infertile women is estimated to range from 3 to 4 percent, although women who suffer recurrent miscarriages may have an incidence as high as 25 percent.

This condition may be associated with hyperprolactinemia (excess amounts of the hormone prolactin, which can interfere with normal ovulation), vigorous exercise or low body weight, PCOS, and endometriosis (see chapter 7, "The Female: Structural Problems, Age-Related Factors, and Treatment," for more about endometriosis). Furthermore, a higher incidence of LPD occurs in some women treated with the fertility drug, clomiphene citrate.

### Diagnosis

One test used to document LPD is the endometrial biopsy, often performed 1 to 2 days before the onset of menses. A tiny sample of endometrial tissue is examined for thickness as well as cellular changes that should have occurred at this stage of the cycle. If the development of the endometrium shows a lag of more than 2 days from the point at which it should be, an LPD may exist. To avoid disturbing a pregnancy, the physician may order a sensitive blood serum pregnancy test to detect an early pregnancy before performing the biopsy, or ask the couple to abstain from sexual intercourse during the cycle of testing.

Serum progesterone levels may be taken during the luteal phase, but these levels only indicate whether ovulation has occurred and are not precise enough to diagnose LPD. A normal mid-luteal range would be 10 ng/mL (nanograms per milliliter) or more.

Vaginal ultrasound can also document different textures and patterns of endometrial development before ovulation. In the early preovulatory phase of the cycle, the endometrium appears as a single line on the sonogram. As it continues to grow and develop, this single line is replaced by a triple-line effect. The endometrium should be at least 6 mm (millimeters), but optimally 8 mm or more, in thickness at the time of ovulation.

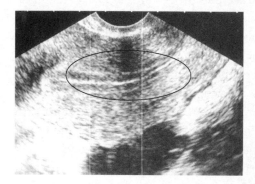

*At left, triple-line effect of a normal endometrial lining on ultrasound.*

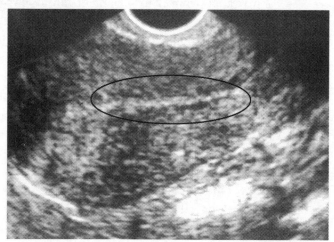

*At right, a thin endometrial lining on ultrasound.*

## Questions to Ask

**About Luteal Phase Defect**

The following questions may be important if you have, or suspect, an LPD:

- Is my luteal phase less than 12 days long?
- Do I have vaginal spotting before the onset of menstruation?
- Do I have a slow or low rise on my basal body temperature chart (BBT) after ovulation?
- Have I had a vaginal ultrasound just before ovulation to document an adequately thick endometrium?
- Has the physician taken a blood test to evaluate progesterone levels midway between ovulation and my menstrual cycle?
- Was my endometrial biopsy done near onset of my next flow?
- If the endometrial biopsy showed a lag and I am being treated for LPD, will another biopsy be done in the future to evaluate results?

### TREATMENT

Treatment of LPD may include using medications to stimulate follicular growth and the corpus luteum, or medications that act directly on the endometrium. Clomiphene citrate and FSH or hMG can be used to stimulate follicle growth. hCG given in a series of injections after ovulation can also help support the corpus luteum and uterine lining. Progesterone treatment is used to mature the uterine lining and is started 2 to 3 days after ovulation. It can be given in pill form, by vaginal suppository or gel, or by intramuscular injection. However, it appears that oral progesterone may not be absorbed as well by the body as the other forms of progesterone.

## The Role of Female Hormones

Some fertility drugs are derived from naturally occurring hormones extracted from human urine; others are synthetic versions created in a laboratory. The following is a brief recap of how reproductive hormones work normally in a woman's body.

A woman's reproductive hormones are released primarily by the hypothalamus, the pituitary gland, and the ovaries. The hypothalamus produces gonadotropin-releasing hormone (GnRH), which stimulates the pituitary gland to release follicle-stimulating hormone (FSH) and luteinizing hormone (LH). FSH stimulates the growth of follicles in the ovaries. About halfway through the cycle, a sudden surge of LH and FSH causes the rupture of one dominant follicle and the release of a mature egg, the process of ovulation.

The other two important hormones, which are produced by the ovary, are estrogen and progesterone. Estrogen supports the growth of the follicles and the development of the endometrium, which is shed if pregnancy does not occur. Progesterone, which the corpus luteum releases after the release of the egg at ovulation, prepares and nourishes the endometrium for implantation and pregnancy.

## UNDERSTANDING HORMONAL MEDICATIONS

In this section, the facts about the most common fertility drugs are outlined: how each is supposed to work, what it is meant to treat, and its potential side effects and contraindications. The drugs discussed are the following:

- Clomiphene citrate
    (Clomid, Serophene)
- Follicle-stimulating hormone (FSH)
    (Gonal F, Fertinex, Follistim, Metrodin)
- Human menopausal gonadotropin (hMG)
    (Humegon, Pergonal, Repronex)
- Human chorionic gonadotropin (hCG)
    (Novarel, Pregnyl, Profasi)
- Gonadotropin-releasing hormone agonist (GnRH agonist)
    (Lupron, Synarel)
- Gonadotropin-releasing hormone antagonist (GnRH antagonist)
    (Antagon)
- Bromocriptine, Cabergoline
    (Parlodel, Dostinex)

Be sure to store all medications properly to ensure their potency. Follow package and pharmacy instructions. Keep medications out of direct sunlight, and avoid excessively hot or cold storage temperatures. The cost of each drug varies among pharmacies, so shop around for the best price you can find. We have included a cost range for each drug to give you a general idea of what to expect.

### *About Generics*

You can ask for generic versions of some fertility drugs—to save some money—but check with your physician on this before switching to a generic substitute. Some physicians prefer that patients not use generic drugs.

## Clomiphene Citrate (Clomid, Serophene)

If your basic infertility work-up indicates that you are not ovulating regularly or if you are ovulating very late or early in the cycle, your physician may suggest clomiphene citrate. This drug, sold under the brand names Clomid and Serophene, is an oral, synthetic drug structurally related to estrogen. Clomiphene is an example of a group of drugs called selective estrogen receptor modulators (SERMs). It attaches to the so-called receptor normally used by estrogen. When given early in the menstrual cycle (typically on days 3 to 7 or days 5 to 9), clomiphene acts as an anti-estrogen and tricks the pituitary into producing more FSH and LH, which in turn stimulate the ovary to develop follicles and eggs. It binds to the sites in the brain—called estrogen receptors—where estrogen normally attaches. The brain then determines that the amount of estrogen in the blood is too low, which triggers the release of more GnRH and FSH. The increased levels of FSH cause a follicle to grow, which produces more estrogen and triggers egg maturation. Clomiphene can also trigger higher progesterone production, which can improve the quality of the uterine lining and/or lengthen the luteal phase of the cycle.

- *Indications for use:* In women, clomiphene is used to induce ovulation, to correct irregular ovulation, to help increase egg production, and to correct luteal phase deficiency.
- *Dosage:* Clomiphene comes in 50-mg tablets. The usual starting dose is one tablet on day 3, 4, or 5 of your cycle, and for 5 days afterward. Ovulation usually occurs on cycle day 13 to 18. If you do not ovulate, your physician may increase the dose in increments in future cycles; the maximum dose is usually 200 mg daily. The American Society for Reproductive Medicine (ASRM) recommends that clomiphene be prescribed for three to six cycles only.
- *Monitoring:* LH urine test kits can be used to document ovulation. Check the instructions in the kit to see when you should start testing your urine if you are taking clomiphene. Some physicians also draw a blood progesterone level after ovulation. If levels are more than 10 ng/mL (nanograms per milliliter), ovulation has probably occurred. Occasionally, a physician will do a series of ultrasound images to document follicular development and egg release. Your physician may have you come to the office to check for ovarian cysts or enlargement before starting your next cycle of clomiphene. Because clomiphene can dry up cervical mucus, the transport and nourishment medium for sperm, a postcoital test may be suggested while a woman is on this drug to be certain that sperm are surviving in the mucus. If the mucus is very thick, low-dose oral estrogen may

be suggested for use at the time of ovulation. If intrauterine insemination (IUI) is being used, a postcoital test is not necessary. Clomiphene may also thin the thickness of the endometrium, which can be documented on ultrasound exams. One approach to combat this problem is to add progesterone. Very rarely, low-dose estrogen is added to clomiphene to improve uterine lining quality.

- *Potential side effects:* Mood swings, hot flashes, breast tenderness, thick cervical mucus, and thinning of the uterine lining may occur. Women often feel bloated and notice sensations in their ovaries at the time of ovulation when taking this drug. Multiple gestation pregnancy occurs in about 8 to 10 percent of women who get pregnant using clomiphene. Discuss the potential outcome with your physician before you start taking clomiphene.

- *Contraindications:* You should not take clomiphene if you are pregnant or if you have a history of liver disease. Careful assessment before starting clomiphene is needed if you have irregular bleeding or ovarian cysts to rule out any other medical or gynecologic problems. Clomiphene can cause large follicular cysts, which may persist into the next cycle. Cysts may be a direct result of clomiphene or may result from hyperstimulation of the ovary.

- *Drugs used in combination:* Drugs combined with clomiphene citrate may include hCG to help release the ripened egg, hMG and FSH, and progesterone, which is started after ovulation has occurred.

- *Cost:* Five 50-mg tablets: $15 to $50; generic is available.

---

### *Voices*

*"I want to start a support group for men called "Husbands of Clomiphene,"" jokes Joe, husband to Grace, a 34-year-old woman with polycystic ovarian syndrome (PCOS). Their treatment consisted of four cycles of IUI with clomiphene citrate, resulting in a pregnancy that ended in miscarriage after 11 weeks, another six rounds of IUI with clomiphene citrate, and then four rounds of hMG until they got pregnant with their son, now 14 months.*

*Albert agrees; his wife Muriel has been through more than 12 cycles of ovulation-induction drugs in one form or another, but so far without a successful pregnancy. "I'd like to suggest a 'safe house' for men. A place where guys could go so they don't have to worry about looking at the wives the wrong way, or sitting the wrong way, or saying the wrong thing, or saying the right thing but at the wrong time. We could call it the 'Hormone Free Zone.'"*

## Follicle-Stimulating Hormone (FSH)

(Urofollitropins: Fertinex, Metrodin)

(Follitropins: Follistim and Gonal F)

Two different types of drugs are available that contain pure FSH. One type, called urofollitropins, is made from the purified urine of postmenopausal women; brand names are Fertinex and Metrodin. The other type, called follitropins, is made synthetically using recombinant DNA technology. Gonal F and Follistim are the two brands currently available. The primary difference between the urofollitropins and the follitropins is purity and consistency. Because the follitropins are created by recombinant DNA technology, they do not contain protein contaminants that may cause allergic reactions or other health problems. They also tend to be more consistent than urofollitropins because the latter preparations vary from batch to batch, depending on the proteins present in the urine at the time it was collected.

All FSH preparations require injections: Fertinex, Gonal F, and Follistim are all injected just beneath the skin (subcutaneous injections), whereas Metrodin requires injection into deep muscle tissue (intramuscular injections).

Both types of drugs are designed to deliver purified FSH to stimulate follicular development and oocyte maturation. Unlike hMG, these drugs contain only FSH, and no LH, and can be helpful to women who produce too much LH in relation to the amount of FSH they produce, such as women with polycystic ovary syndrome (PCOS). All of these medications require careful monitoring to avoid ovarian hyperstimulation syndrome (OHSS) or multiple gestation pregnancy.

• *Indications for use:* These drugs are used for the treatment of ovulation disorders, and to stimulate follicle and egg production for intrauterine insemination (IUI), in vitro fertilization (IVF), or other assisted reproductive technology (ART) procedures.

• *Dosage:* Injections start on day 2, 3, or 4 at 75 IU (international units) to 225 IU or more per day. Dosage may be adjusted as the cycle progresses and as indicated through blood and ultrasound monitoring. One shot of hCG is given just before ovulation to trigger the release and final maturation of the eggs.

• *Monitoring:* After 4 to 8 days of injections, your physician will monitor your response by measuring estrogen (estradiol) levels in your blood and follicular growth with vaginal ultrasound. When estradiol levels reach an appropriate level, and one or more follicles are between 16mm and 18 mm (millimeters) in size on ultrasound, the trigger shot of hCG will be ordered. *In any women using these drugs, careful monitoring is essential.* If estradiol levels are very elevated, or too many follicles are mature at one time, the physician may withhold the hCG shot because of concerns about the development of OHSS or the possibility of multiple gestation pregnancy, particularly in cycles of intrauterine insemination (IUI) or sexual intercourse. Physicians usually let the estradiol levels go higher and want more follicles to develop in ART cycles, however.

• *Potential side effects:* Ovarian hyperstimulation is the most serious side effect of FSH preparations. Signs of hyperstimulation usually do not peak until 7 to 9 days after the hCG trigger shot is given. Multiple gestation pregnancy occurs in about 25 percent of women who get pregnant while taking FSH preparations.

• *Contraindications:* No one with a known allergy to any of the preparations should use these medications. Before starting treatment, your physician should rule out a pituitary tumor by checking prolactin hormone levels and ovarian tumors by ordering a baseline ultrasound. Pituitary tumors can be treated in other ways. Pure FSH can promote the growth of ovarian tumors.

• *Drugs used in combination:* Drugs used with FSH may include clomiphene citrate, GnRH agonists, GnRH antagonist, hMG, hCG (required for release of eggs), and progesterone, which is started after ovulation.

• *Cost:* One ampule: $50 to $60.

---

### Signs of Ovarian Hyperstimulation Syndrome (OHSS)

If a woman notices the following signs of OHSS, she should contact her physician immediately.

• Weight gain of more than 1 pound a day.
• Decreased urine output.
• Shortness of breath.
• Abdominal or pelvic pain, nausea.
• Significant bloating and swelling of the abdominal area.

## Human Menopausal Gonadotropin (hMG) (Humegon, Pergonal, Repronex)

Human menopausal gonadotropin (hMG) (brand names Humegon, Pergonal, Repronex) is a mixture of FSH and LH that is purified from the urine of postmenopausal women. hMG acts directly on the ovaries to stimulate follicle development. To allow for the release of the mature eggs, an injection of hCG must be taken with hMG. hMG is used to induce ovulation in anovulatory patients or to stimulate increased production of follicles and eggs in women who are ovulating but undergoing intrauterine insemination (IUI), in vitro fertilization (IVF), and other assisted reproductive technology (ART) procedures.

hMG carries a risk of ovarian hyperstimulation syndrome (OHSS) and multiple gestation pregnancy, and therefore requires careful monitoring.

• *Indications for use:* hMG is used to stimulate the development of follicles in women who do not ovulate regularly and to stimulate ovulation for intrauterine insemination (IUI), IVF, and other ART procedures.

• *Dosage:* hMG comes in ampules of 75 IU (international units) or 150 IU of FSH and LH and is given by intramuscular injection once or twice a day. Preliminary research suggests that it may be possible to administer low doses of these drugs by subcutaneous injection. Dosages vary depending on patient response and type of treatment cycle.

• *Monitoring:* Your physician will carefully monitor estradiol levels and perform vaginal ultrasounds to monitor follicular development.

• *Potential side effects:* Mood swings (not as intense as with clomiphene) and ovarian hyperstimulation are the most common side effects. Other side effects include abdominal pain, nausea, vomiting, diarrhea, bloating, rashes, and swelling or irritation at the injection site. Multiple gestation pregnancy occurs in approximately 25 percent of women who get pregnant using hMG, and this potentiality should be discussed with a physician before treatment begins.

• *Contraindications:* hMG should not be used by anyone with a known allergy to the preparation.

• *Drugs used in combination:* hMG may be used in combination with clomiphene citrate, FSH, GnRH agonists, GnRH antagonist, hCG (required for triggering egg release), and progesterone, which is started after ovulation.

• *Costs:* One ampule: $30 to $40.

## Human Chorionic Gonadotropin (hCG) (Novarel, Pregnyl, Profasi)

Human chorionic gonadotropin (hCG) (brand names Novarel, Pregnyl, Profasi) is a hormone produced by the human placenta. Commercial hCG is made from the purified urine of pregnant women.

• *Indications for use:* hCG is used for two reasons. First, hCG mimics LH, resulting in the release of matured eggs after controlled ovarian hyperstimulation (COH), with FSH or hMG, for example. Second, after ovulation has occurred, either naturally or in conjunction with intrauterine insemination (IUI) or an assisted reproductive technology (ART) cycle, hCG may be used to support the corpus luteum and to enhance the quality of the uterine lining and the potential for implantation of the embryo(s).

• *Dosage:* hCG comes in vials in dosages of 5,000 IU (international units), and 10,000 IU for intramuscular injection. Dosages vary depending on the purpose of treatment. A new drug made with recombinant DNA technology will soon be available, which can be administered subcutaneously.

• *Monitoring:* None required.

• *Potential side effects:* Other than irritation at the injection site, there seem to be no side effects.

• *Contraindications:* hCG should not be used by anyone who has had a prior allergic reaction to this medication. It should not be given if estradiol levels are extremely elevated or, in IUI patients, if many mature follicles are present on ultrasound. It should be used with caution in the luteal phase support role as this may aggravate ovarian hyperstimulation syndrome (OHSS).

• *Drugs used in combination:* hCG may be used in combination with hMG, FSH, and clomiphene citrate.

• *Costs:* One vial: $25 to $50.

---

### Voices

*"If I could eliminate one sentence from my wife's vocabulary," admits Andy, husband to Hanna, a woman who recently underwent her third IVF cycle, "it would be 'Get away from me with that needle!'"*

---

## Gonadotropin-Releasing Hormone Agonists (GnRH agonist) (Lupron, Synarel)

Gonadotropin-releasing hormone (GnRH) agonists (brand names Lupron, Synarel) are synthetic drugs that bind tightly to GnRH receptors in the pituitary and initially cause the release of FSH and LH from the pituitary. With continued use, however, GnRH agonists quickly suppress these hormones. The body goes into a pseudomenopause that provides a "clean slate" on which to create a controlled ovarian hyperstimulation (COH) cycle with other drugs for an in vitro fertilization (IVF) or other assisted reproductive technology (ART) procedure. The GnRH agonists reduce the risk of premature ovulation in stimulated cycles. Longer-acting GnRH agonists are used in treating endometriosis and fibroids (see chapter 7, "The Female: Structural Problems, Age-Related Factors, and Treatment").

• *Indications for use:* GnRH agonists are used to prevent premature release of eggs in IVF or gamete intrafallopian transfer (GIFT) or to treat endometriosis or shrink fibroids.

• *Dosage:* Short-acting GnRH agonists come in two forms: Lupron, a drug taken by subcutaneous injection daily, and Synarel, a nasal spray taken twice a day. Length of treatment depends on the purpose for which the drug is being used. GnRH agonists may be given under several protocols as part of COH regimens. The drugs may be given in various doses initiated during the midluteal or early follicular phases. The long-acting form is taken by injection once a month.

• *Monitoring:* Effectiveness of these drugs is usually assessed by measuring suppression of serum estradiol levels.

• *Potential side effects:* GnRH agonists put women into a pseudomenopause, which means that side effects usually involve hot flashes, night sweats, headaches, vaginal dryness, and reduced sexual drive. In long-term treatment for endometriosis or fibroids, the use of GnRH agonists, which reduces estrogen, can cause a depletion of calcium in a woman's bones and reduce bone density. Fortunately, bone density returns after the end of therapy. These symptoms are extremely rare in women undergoing the short course therapy used in COH regimens.

• *Contraindications:* You should not use GnRH agonists if you are pregnant, or if you have a known allergy to the preparations. Therefore, patients should avoid conception on the month of the long (luteal phase) GnRH protocol.

• *Drugs used in combination:* GnRH agonists may be used in combination with hMG, FSH, and hCG for COH in an IVF cycle.

• *Costs:* Kit: $250 to $350; generic is available.

## Gonadotropin-Releasing Hormone Antagonist (GnRH antagonist, ganirelix acetate) (Antagon)

This class of drug (brand name Antagon) recently has been introduced to inhibit premature surge of luteinizing hormone (LH).

• *Indications for use:* The drug is used in controlled ovarian hyperstimulation (COH) cycles for in vitro fertilization (IVF) or other assisted reproductive technology (ART) procedures.

• *Dosage:* The drug is given by subcutaneous injection, usually starting on cycle day 8, and continued for 5 days. It is given in combination with ovulatory-stimulating drugs.

• *Monitoring:* The physician will determine monitoring case by case.

• *Potential Side Effects:* Possible irritation at the injection site.

• *Contraindications:* This drug should not be taken if you are pregnant or have a known allergy to the preparation.

• *Drugs used in combination:* GnRH antagonist may be used with hMG, FSH, and hCG for COH in ART cycles.

• *Costs:* Similar to GnRH agonist.

---

### *For Your Information*

• Be aware that it is illegal to import fertility drugs from outside the United States. Medications made or purchased outside the United States for lower prices may not have approval from the U.S. Food and Drug Administration (FDA). In addition, if there is a problem with a particular batch of a drug, the FDA has no way to recall the drug. Consumers with questions about importation of drugs for personal use should consult with their local FDA office or the FDA Imports Operations Branch in Rockville, Maryland.

• If you are considering giving unused, unopened vials or ampules of medication to a friend, consider the liability issues if the medication caused an adverse reaction. It is better to give any unopened medications to your infertility clinic; they can take full responsibility for dispensing it.

---

## Bromocriptine Mesylate and Cabergoline (Parlodel, Dostinex)

In both men and women, hyperprolactinemia (overproduction of the hormone prolactin) can cause fertility problems by interfering with the normal production of FSH and LH. In women, the condition can disrupt ovulation and impact the quality of the luteal phase and endometrial lining. Hyperprolactinemia can be caused by benign tumors of the pituitary gland and disorders of the hypothalamus. In some cases, a woman may be able to express breast milk with pressure applied to the nipples. Bromocriptine (Parlodel) and cabergoline (Dostinex), two oral medications, effectively suppress prolactin secretion by the pituitary gland. They do so because they mimic the action of dopamine, the neurotransmitter released by the brain that normally blocks prolactin production.

• *Indications for use:* Bromocriptine and cabergoline correct abnormal prolactin levels.

• *Dosage:* Bromocriptine, an oral medication, comes in 2.5-mg (milligram) tablets. Because bromocriptine may cause gastrointestinal discomfort and dizziness (see side effects below), most physicians suggest taking one-half tablet per day at first, then slowly increasing it to 2.5 mg per day.

• *Monitoring:* Your physician will order blood tests to monitor prolactin levels and the effect of the medication.

• *Potential side effects:* The most common side effects include nausea, headache, dizziness (particularly when moving from a lying down to a standing position or vice versa), fatigue, vomiting, abdominal cramps, nasal congestion, constipation, diarrhea, and drowsiness.

• *Contraindications:* Women should ask their physician whether to continue bromocriptine or cabergoline if they get pregnant. No one with uncontrolled high blood pressure or with an allergy to any ergot alkaloids should take these drugs. (Ergot alkaloids are drugs that cause the uterus to contract and are used to control hemorrhage of the uterus after delivery, as they cause blood vessels to contract.)

• *Drugs used in combination:* Bromocriptine mesylate and cabergoline may be used with any of the ovulation-stimulating drugs.

• *Costs:* Twenty 2.5-mg tablets: $35 to $50.

## THE FINE ART OF GIVING AND RECEIVING INJECTIONS

If you decide to use injectable fertility medications, in most cases you will have to give them to yourself, or your partner will give them to you. For many people, this is one of the most difficult aspects of infertility treatment. In a recent national survey conducted by the independent polling firm of Louis Harris and Associates, 79 percent of women and their partners found intramuscular injections stressful, and 68 percent found them difficult to administer. In addition, even though 70 percent of patients reported they are more fearful of self-administering an intramuscular injection than being injected by their partner or physician, 57 percent said their partners were not always available to administer all the necessary injections. More than half of those who responded said that they were concerned that they were not performing the injections correctly.

***Voices***

*For Connie and Warren, as for most couples experiencing treatment for infertility, the injectable medication proved to be a difficult challenge. "I did one cycle of clomiphene," recalls Connie, "and then a cycle of FSH and clomiphene. Warren gave me some injections, but he travels a lot, so I had to learn how to do it myself. Sometimes I'd practice on an orange. Often when trying to give myself an injection— I know this is silly—I'd just sit there, almost stick the needle in, and then not be able to go through with it. I hated it. One night, I just waited for Warren to come home and I told him I couldn't make myself do it. He was a good sport about it; he did well with it. Neither of us enjoyed it."*

The following are directions for administering subcutaneous (just below the skin) and intramuscular (into muscle tissue) injections. For more advice, talk to your physician.

## INJECTION SITES FOR FERTILITY MEDICATIONS

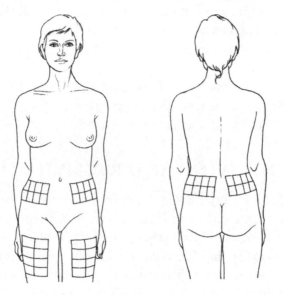

## Subcutaneous Injections

1. Wash your hands thoroughly with soap and warm water and dry them with a clean towel.
2. Assemble supplies: two alcohol wipes, one facial tissue, one syringe, medication.
3. Cleanse the ampule with an alcohol wipe before breaking off the top. If your medication comes in a vial with a rubber top, clean the rubber top with an alcohol wipe.
4. Remove the cap from the syringe, exposing the needle.
5. Insert the needle straight and firmly into the rubber center of the vial and turn the vial upside down, or insert the needle into the ampule opening.
6. Pull the syringe plunger back, filling the medication to the line of the correct dose as directed by your physician.
7. Hold the syringe needle up and flick with finger to remove any air bubbles.

8. Hold the syringe and new alcohol wipe in one hand.

9. Choose injection site (your physician will tell you where, and probably suggest that you rotate the site daily) and clean the area with an alcohol wipe. You may find that putting an ice pack on the area before the injection helps to make it less painful.

10. Grasp the skin and gently pinch it with your other hand.

11. Holding the syringe like a dart, briskly insert the small needle into the pinched area of skin.

12. Pull the needle back gently. If blood appears in the syringe, do not administer the medication. Withdraw the needle and apply pressure at the injection site. Select another site and repeat the sequence beginning with step 10. If no blood appears in the syringe, then push the plunger down gently and slowly until all the medication is emptied from the syringe.

13. Pull the needle straight out of the skin and gently apply pressure with a clean piece of gauze or facial tissue if any bleeding occurs.

14. To dispose of needles properly, remove the used needle from the syringe and put it in a glass jar with a screw top.  Never reuse a syringe.

15. Rub the injection area for 15 to 20 seconds.

### *Reducing the Stress of Injections*

To make injection time less stressful, take a few deep breaths before getting the shot—concentrate on the exhale. Make an audible sigh as you release the air.

## Intramuscular Injections

Follow the directions for subcutaneous injections through step 9. Then, proceed as follows:

10. Do not pinch the skin before giving the injection. Instead, use two fingers to push down gently on the skin. Then, move the fingers apart, spreading the skin between them.

11. After inserting the needle into the skin, check that it did not enter a blood vessel by pulling the plunger back slightly to see if blood comes into the syringe. If it does, remove the needle and try another site.

12. Some people find that applying a warm moist cloth to the area after the injection prevents painful lumps from developing.

Return to steps 12 through 15 above, under the instructions for subcutaneous injections.

> **When You Travel**
>
> If you are traveling, keep your medications at the proper temperature. If you are going out of the country, get a note from your clinic explaining why you are carrying needles and syringes.

# THE RISKS OF FERTILITY MEDICATION

Generally, side effects from fertility drugs are minor and short-term, if the medications are taken as directed and you are monitored appropriately. Here is more complete information on side effects of fertility medications.

## Ovarian Hyperstimulation Syndrome

In a medicated cycle, when the ovaries are stimulated to produce more follicles, estrogen levels rise and all the symptoms that accompany natural ovulation—bloating, spotting, pain (mittleschmerz), irritability, and mood swings—may be increased. The side effect that poses the most potential danger in medicated cycles is ovarian hyperstimulation, which results in fluid accumulation in the abdomen. It is normal for the ovary to produce fluid in the abdomen, but when excessive stimulation occurs—a condition known as ovarian hyperstimulation syndrome (OHSS)—fluid accumulation can cause pressure on surrounding organs, including the lungs and the heart. Breathing difficulties, dehydration, and severe nausea can result; occasionally, hospitalization may be required.

Ovarian hyperstimulation occurs in about 1 to 5 percent of cycles. The clinical symptoms usually occur 7 to 9 days after an injection of hCG. You should always report the following symptoms, if they occur after ovulation: abdominal pain, significant swelling, bloating, weight gain of more than 1 pound a day, nausea, shortness of breath, or decreased urine output. These symptoms could mean OHSS.

When a woman develops OHSS, certain types of substances are produced from the ovaries that affect the tiny blood vessels, or capillaries. Fluid and protein leak out of the capillaries and accumulate in the abdominal cavity. One theory suggests that some women produce proteins that may make the capillaries more permeable—and more prone to leaking fluid into the pelvic cavity. Although a particular woman's susceptibility to hyperstimulation is not well understood, we do know that the chance of ovarian hyperstimulation increases in women with polycystic ovarian syndrome (PCOS).

If a physician suspects that you may be at risk for hyperstimulation because a blood test prior to the hCG shot indicates high levels of estrogen in the blood—more than 1,500 pg/mL or 2,000 pg/mL (picograms per milliliter) for an ovulation induction cycle or more than 3,500 pg/mL for an IVF cycle—the cycle may be canceled. In the alternative, stimulating drugs may be stopped until estrogen levels return to normal, a technique known as "coasting." Physicians also can retrieve all the mature eggs, fertilize them, and freeze the embryos for transfer in a future cycle—in other words, perform in vitro fertilization (IVF) with cryopreservation of the resulting embryos.

### Voices

*Remembers Jessie, "Early on, I had a night of excruciating pain and vomiting. Ray and I called the doctor, who ruled out ectopic pregnancy. At 1 AM, we went to the emergency room, and luckily, the doctor on call had experience with infertility patients. I was diagnosed as being hyperstimulated. I took it easy for a few days and it seemed to subside. That was my only scare."*

OHSS is a serious condition; its symptoms require attention and should never be ignored. If OHSS does occur, your physician will ask you to monitor your urine output, take a daily weight measurement, and record changes in abdominal girth. A physician may order bed rest for OHHS patients, or in serious cases, hospitalization, where fluids and electrolytes may be ordered.

## Multiple Gestation Pregnancy

Up to 25 percent of pregnancies resulting from taking ovulation-induction drugs result in multiple gestation, in contrast to a rate of 1 to 2 percent in the general population. Although twins are the most common outcome of multiple gestation pregnancy, a significant percentage of triplets or more can occur. However, with careful monitoring, multiple gestation pregnancy is largely a preventable complication of fertility drug therapy.

It is not hard to understand how multiple gestation pregnancy can occur with the use of fertility drugs. After all, their purpose is to increase a woman's ability to ovulate more eggs by either indirectly or directly stimulating the ovaries. Once that has been accomplished, a woman can try to become pregnant through sexual intercourse, or through insemination procedures such as intrauterine insemination (IUI), or through assisted reproductive technology (ART). In the cases of intercourse and insemination, it is difficult to ensure that the sperm only fertilizes one egg, as the physician is not able to calculate with precision how many follicles will release eggs at ovulation. On the other hand, when the physician removes multiple eggs from the ovaries for an IVF or gamete intrafallopian transfer (GIFT) cycle, the number of fertilized eggs returned to the uterus can be controlled.

Many of the multiple births you may have read about in the press are from poorly monitored IUI cycles. If cycles are carefully monitored and the physician believes there is a high risk for multiple gestation pregnancy, the cycle can be canceled. The physician will tell the patient not to try to conceive, and the hCG shot which triggers the release of mature eggs will not be given. It is important to understand that you may ovulate and be able to conceive regardless. The physician may decide to lower the dose of the ovulatory drug for the next cycle, in the hope that fewer eggs will be produced.

Unfortunately, because of the expense of fertility drugs and some treatments, many couples will risk a multiple gestation pregnancy to increase their chances of success in any given cycle. However, multiple gestation pregnancy is associated with several serious risks, including pregnancy loss, premature delivery, infant abnormalities, pregnancy-induced hypertension, hemorrhage, and other significant maternal complications (see chapter 16, "Surviving Infertility and Moving Forward"). Add to that the emotional, physical, and financial strain of caring for several infants at a time, and you can see why it is important to reduce the risk of multiple gestation pregnancy whenever possible.

## Ectopic Pregnancy

Taking ovulation-induction drugs has been shown to increase slightly the risk of having an ectopic pregnancy in which the egg fails to leave the fallopian tube to implant within the uterus. Careful monitoring of blood levels of hCG, which should double every 2 to 3 days, and reporting of pain during early pregnancy are vital. Classic symptoms of ectopic pregnancy may include vaginal bleeding, fainting, and rectal, abdominal, or shoulder discomfort. For more about this condition, see chapter 10, "Pregnancy Loss."

## Ovarian and Other Reproductive Cancers

The risk of cancer—particularly ovarian cancer—from fertility drugs continues to be a subject of debate. Some researchers believe that the increased ovulation caused by these medications subjects the ovaries to increased trauma, which raises the likelihood of cancerous changes in an ovary's surface.

A study published in 1994 in the *New England Journal of Medicine* found a possible link between ovarian cancer and the extended regimens (12 or more cycles) of clomiphene citrate taken by 3,837 women participating in the study. Eleven cases of ovarian cancer were reported in this study. The American

Society for Reproductive Medicine (ASRM) currently recommends a maximum treatment of 6 cycles of clomiphene citrate.

A Danish study reported in *Fertility and Sterility* in 1997 indicated that women who took fertility drugs were not at higher risk of ovarian cancer. In this study, 684 women with invasive ovarian cancer were compared with 1,721 age-matched population controls. The researchers compared infertile women who took infertility drugs with infertile women who did not, and compared cancer rates for women who gave birth and for those who never gave birth. They found that the women who took fertility drugs, whether or not they ever had a successful pregnancy, did not develop ovarian cancer more than women experiencing infertility who did *not* take the medications. Moreover, there were no significant differences in risk among the various drug regimens reported, which included clomiphene citrate, clomiphene citrate plus hCG or hMG, or hMG plus hCG. The highest risk for ovarian cancer was in infertile women who did not take fertility drugs and who never had a successful pregnancy. (Fortunately, the overall incidence of ovarian cancer among all women in the United States, regardless of pregnancy history, is relatively low).

Although the news of this Danish study is good, there is still need for more research in this area through carefully controlled long-term studies.

If you have a history of breast cancer or have a suspicious breast lump, you should be thoroughly evaluated before attempting pregnancy or receiving fertility drugs. Researchers continue to study the relationship between breast cancers and pregnancy, and you should keep up-to-date on new information as it becomes available through RESOLVE and other advocacy organizations. Talk over your concerns with your physician.

If you have stopped infertility treatment and have never been pregnant, make sure you have a complete gynecological examination annually. Some physicians suggest a vaginal ultrasound at that time to monitor ovarian size and contours.

## WHEN THE PROBLEM IS HORMONAL

Using decision tree worksheets can help you evaluate the options related to receiving hormonal treatments for infertility. We have created the following decision tree based on a fictional couple, Jodi and Richard. Study the decision-making process in this example.

Jodi is 26 years old and her partner, Richard, is 29. Jodi has always had a weight problem and irregular menstrual cycles. Last year she was diagnosed

## PCOS—What's Next?

### Take a break from treatment while Jodi continues weight-loss program

Pros:
1. May improve fertility
2. Other health bonuses
3. No cost
4. Lower stress
5. Jodi is still young; we can afford to wait awhile

Cons:
1. Postpones plan to start a family
2. Puts pressure on Jodi

### Injectable medications with sexual intercourse or IUI

Pros:
1. May cause ovulation
2. We feel more aggressive with our treatment plan
3. Some insurance coverage

Cons:
1. May lead to hyperstimulation of Jodi's ovaries (her age and PCOS diagnosis are factors)
2. Risk of multiple gestation pregnancy
3. Opposed to pregnancy reduction
4. Cost

### ART

Pros:
1. May cause ovulation
2. We feel more aggressive with our treatment plan
3. Some insurance coverage
4. Can control number of embryos transferred to Jodi's uterus
5. May have extra embryos to freeze for later attempt

Cons:
1. Hyperstimulation still a concern
2. Some coverage but higher cost

with polycystic ovarian syndrome (PCOS). (Note: Not all PCOS patients are overweight. A recent study, however, has shown that those who are can improve their fertility by losing weight.) Richard has no diagnosed fertility problems.

Jodi's health insurance covered her diagnosis and will cover treatment with clomiphene citrate. It will also cover the monitoring for three cycles of injectable ovulatory medication and intrauterine insemination (IUI), but it will not cover the cost of the drugs or assisted reproductive technology (ART).

The treatment plan the couple has devised with their physician is to try up to six cycles of clomiphene citrate and then to consider injectable medications, if necessary. They have tried three cycles of clomiphene, but Jodi has not ovulated, even after the dosage was increased. Jodi is on a weight-loss program, but finds it very difficult because the infertility experience is so stressful. Jodi's younger sister just had a baby, and several of her friends are pregnant.

**Decision:** The couple has decided to take a break from treatment while Jodi continues her fitness and weight-loss program. She has enlisted the help of empathetic RESOLVE friends to help shield her from baby showers and other emotionally painful events. She and Richard will save toward IVF treatment in the event they are not able to conceive within 2 years.

What decisions are *you* facing? Create your own decision tree to evaluate all the options available to you and your partner.

## POSITIVE STEPS YOU CAN TAKE FROM CHAPTER 6

**Feel comfortable.** Your hormonal status will be thoroughly evaluated by your healthcare team.

**Know the effects of medications you take.** If medications are ordered, make sure you understand why and how the medications will act in your body. Know the warning signs of ovarian hyperstimulation syndrome, and report symptoms immediately to your physician.

**Be informed about the risks for multiple gestation pregnancy.** Become familiar with the possible risks and factors involved with multiple gestation pregnancy. For more about multiple gestation pregnancy, see chapter 16, "Surviving Infertility and Moving Forward."

# 7 The Female: Structural Problems, Age-Related Factors, and Treatment

This chapter covers structural problems that may lead to female fertility problems, as well as age-related factors, and available treatments. The physiology of the female reproductive tract is intricate: For conception and a normal birth to take place, a complicated series of events must occur. If something goes wrong, anywhere along the way, infertility may result.

## ENDOMETRIOSIS

Endometriosis is a disease in which the endometrial cells that normally line the uterine cavity implant outside the uterus. Implants can appear on the ovaries, fallopian tubes, bladder, intestine, and pelvic side walls. In most cases, endometriosis is confined to the pelvic cavity, but on very rare occasions, it may be found in the lungs, within the muscle of the abdominal wall, and even in the brain. No matter where endometrial tissue is, it may respond to the hormones, estrogen and progesterone. Active endometrial cells bleed during menstruation, causing inflammation and scarring to surrounding tissue. As the disease progresses, deposits of endometriosis on the ovaries may bleed extensively and fail to be absorbed completely after menstruation, resulting in an accumulation of blood-filled cysts, sometimes called "chocolate cysts."

Millions of American women of reproductive age have endometriosis. This disease is prevalent in women 30 to 40 years of age, though it can begin as early as the teen years. About 40 percent of women with endometriosis may experience

## ENDOMETRIOSIS

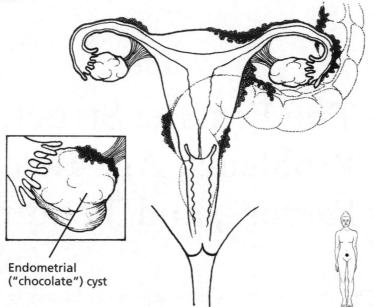

Endometrial
("chocolate") cyst

*Common sites of endometrial implants and adhesions.*

some degree of infertility. Endometriosis that causes severe pain may deplete a woman's energy, result in depression and anxiety, and interfere with many aspects of life. Adding infertility to the mix only increases the severity of these emotional symptoms and side effects.

Lack of agreement exists on what causes endometriosis, but there are a number of different theories:

- *Retrograde menstruation.* Endometriosis may occur because endometrial cells in menstrual fluid flow out the fallopian tubes and attach and grow outside of the uterus in the pelvic cavity, or rarely in the abdominal cavity, lung, or brain.
- *Endometrial conversion.* Endometriosis may begin because other embryonic tissues convert or give rise to endometrial cells that develop into implants that grow on fallopian tubes, ovaries, in the pelvic cavity, and sometimes on the bowel or bladder. This is known as metaplasia.
- *Vascular and lymphatic transmission.* Endometrial cells may reach sites outside the uterus by passing through the blood or lymph systems.

- *Combination theory.* It seems most likely that a combination of these theories and perhaps others is involved in the development of endometriosis.

## Endometriosis and Fertility

Substantial numbers of women with advanced endometriosis experience infertility. Even women with minimal to mild endometriosis, however, may have problems with fertility. Up to 27 percent of women with mild endometriosis have ovulatory dysfunction or luteal phase defect (LPD). There are several theories about the relationship between endometriosis and infertility, including the following:

- *Disruption of normal hormonal patterns and regular ovulation.* The last half of the menstrual cycle may be shorter in women with endometriosis. A few women with associated severe pelvic adhesions that encase the ovary may have a condition called luteinized unruptured follicle syndrome (LUF), in which the egg is not released from the follicle.
- *Scarring and adhesions.* An adhesion is scar tissue that may bind two or more organs together, such as a fallopian tube, ovary, and bowel. Adhesions can be filmy bands of tissue, or they can be dense and thick. A mild case of endometriosis may consist of scattered implants or minimal adhesions, with no involvement of fallopian tubes or ovaries. In severe endometriosis, the fallopian tubes and the ovaries may be affected, making it almost impossible for fertilization to occur. Adhesions and endometriosis are also associated with ectopic pregnancy. An ectopic pregnancy involves the implantation of the embryo outside the uterine cavity, usually in the fallopian tubes (see chapter 10, "Pregnancy Loss").
- *Secretion of prostaglandins.* Endometrial implants may act as miniature endocrine glands that secrete hormones called prostaglandins. These hormones may cause pelvic cramping and muscle spasms in reproductive organs and may play a role in preventing fertilization and implantation.
- *Autoimmune response.* Macrophages, a type of white blood cell, may be more prevalent in the pelvic fluid of women with endometriosis. These activated macrophages may explain increased prostaglandin production and adhesion formation and may contribute to poor implantation. Some women with endometriosis may produce antibodies known as antiphospholipid antibodies (APA), which are associated with miscarriages (see chapter 10, "Pregnancy Loss").
- *Inflammatory response.* It is possible that the lining of the pelvic cavity and

the lining of fallopian tubes in women who have endometriosis may have a generalized inflammatory response that damages or destroys sperm, eggs, and embryos. Such a phenomenon might explain the occurrence of infertility in women with mild endometriosis who have no ovarian or tubal involvement.

## Symptoms

In some women, endometriosis causes no symptoms. In about 40 percent of cases, the only problem is infertility. Other women experience severe menstrual cramps, heavy bleeding with or between menstrual periods, pain with sexual intercourse, pain at the time of ovulation (mittelschmerz), or low backache. Bowel and bladder pain can be present also. The amount or severity of pain does not always relate to the stage of disease. That is, some women with mild endometriosis may report a great deal of pain whereas others with severe disease may report no symptoms.

A physician may detect clues that endometriosis is present from a history of symptoms, family history of endometriosis, or during pelvic examination. An enlarged ovary can indicate disease, especially if the ovary is fixed by adhesions. Occasionally, endometrial implants may be visible in the vagina or the cervix.

## Diagnosis

In some cases, an endometrioma (chocolate cysts of the ovary) can be detected by vaginal ultrasound. However, the physician may want to confirm a suspected diagnosis of endometriosis with a laparoscopy. (For more information on laparoscopy, see chapter 5, "The Basic Infertility Work-up for Women and Men.") During laparoscopy, a tiny telescope is inserted into the abdominal cavity through a small incision near the navel. The surgeon can examine the outside of the uterus, fallopian tubes, ovaries, and other pelvic structures. A microscopic examination, or biopsy, of implants may be done.

Severity of endometriosis is assessed by stage. Points are assigned by criteria set by the American Society for Reproductive Medicine (ASRM)—considering implant size and extent, pelvic organ involvement, and scarring. Stage I indicates minimal or mild endometriosis, whereas more severe involvement ranges from stage II to IV. Some physicians simply describe what they see. Typical descriptions are as follows:

- Scattered implants in the pelvic cavity, but no adhesions or scarring.
- Endometriosis found on the ovaries and in the pelvic cavity.

LAPAROSCOPIC
VIEW OF PELVIC
ADHESIONS

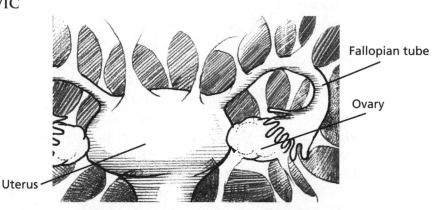

Fallopian tube

Ovary

Uterus

- Implants of endometriosis present on the ovaries with associated adhesions.
- Scarring involving the bladder and large intestine.
- Disease that resulted in implants and scarring affecting bowel, bladder, ovaries, and fallopian tubes.

Ultrasound, computerized tomography (CT) scans, or magnetic resonance imaging (MRI) can be used to obtain more information about the extent of endometriosis. A blood test for cancer cell surface antigen 125 (CA-125), used to diagnose and monitor ovarian cancer, can be used to monitor a woman for recurrence of endometriosis. There is no association between ovarian cancer and endometriosis, however.

## Treatment for Endometriosis

Treatment for endometriosis consists of surgery or hormonal medications, or a combination of the two approaches, and is determined by the severity of the disease and pain experienced, the woman's age, and whether reproduction is a goal.

### SURGICAL TREATMENT

If the physician finds endometriosis during a diagnostic laparoscopy, he or she will use a combination of laser, electrocautery, or surgical excision to remove the endometriosis implants and scar tissue.

For severe disease (stage III or IV), extensive surgery may be needed through either laparoscopy or a major surgical procedure called laparotomy. Some surgeons suggest that the woman take birth control pills or a gonadotropin-releasing hormone (GnRH) agonist before any surgery to treat endometriosis in the hope that these hormones will reduce the size of the endometrial implants and make surgical excision more complete.

### Preparing for Laparotomy

Laparotomy is major surgery that requires hospitalization for several days and a 4- to 6-week recovery period. Having any type of surgery that involves general anesthesia or hospitalization may be anxiety provoking. Being "put to sleep" may feel like the ultimate loss of control. In most cases, you will meet and talk with the anesthesiologist beforehand to discuss your concerns about the procedure and your medical history, including any prior surgeries. Right before surgery, an intravenous (IV) catheter is put in your arm, into which the anesthesiologist will put a sedative. You will fall asleep before general anesthesia is started. Special medications can be given to help prevent nausea and vomiting.

During laparotomy, the surgeon makes an incision to gain access to all the pelvic organs. In addition to removing endometrial implants, the surgeon may also suspend the uterus, returning it to its normal position within the pelvic cavity, if scarring or adhesions have displaced it. Special solutions or gauze to prevent future adhesions may be used during surgery. The gauzelike material is absorbed by the body and greatly reduces the risk of scar tissue developing. Microsurgical and laser techniques may decrease formation of scar tissue from surgery and shorten recovery after surgery. Selecting a physician who is an expert surgeon is important as effective use of these surgical techniques requires experience and expertise. Consult RESOLVE for names of physicians who have training and experience with microsurgical and laser procedures.

A presacral neurectomy also can be performed at the time of laparotomy or laparoscopy. By cutting a few nerves that transmit pain sensation, this procedure can offer relief to some women who have pain from their endometriosis.

Removal of endometriosis and scar tissue may improve pregnancy rates. Some physicians find that most women will conceive within the first 6 months after surgery for endometriosis, although many conceive after this. Pregnancy rates are best if the male partner's sperm count is normal, the couple has tried to conceive for less than 3 years, and the woman is younger than 35 years old. A birth rate of about 60 percent is expected after expert surgery in these women.

Controlled ovarian hyperstimulation (COH) and intrauterine insemination

(IUI) or assisted reproductive technology (ART) are other options used to enhance pregnancy rates in women with endometriosis.

Endometriosis can be a debilitating, devastating disease that may rob a woman of her vitality and potential fertility. Support through RESOLVE and the Endometriosis Association (see the Resources at the back of this book) can be a lifeline to education and better understanding of the disease. In some cases, if a woman or couple has completed family building or decided to end fertility treatment—and the disease is so severe that painful menstrual periods, painful sexual intercourse, or bowel or bladder symptoms are increasing—a hysterectomy with removal of both ovaries and as much endometriosis as is possible may be necessary to restore health.

### Voices

*Maureen is a 40-year-old single woman using donor sperm to have a child. After 4 months of trying through insemination, the physician discovered that Maureen's fallopian tubes and ovaries were completely encased with endometriosis. "It's been a frustrating and devastating process," Maureen remarks. "Having endometriosis makes the whole thing even more difficult. I never thought there would be so many hurdles. But I'm not giving up yet."*

### HORMONAL TREATMENTS FOR ENDOMETRIOSIS

Hormones are used to treat endometriosis by simulating a pseudopregnancy or pseudomenopause.

• *Oral contraceptives.* Oral contraceptives (OCs) can be given to simulate pseudopregnancy. A frequently used regimen is to take the pill continuously for 9 months to a year. This prevents ovulation and menstruation, which means that the endometrial implants do not have a chance to slough and bleed. Side effects may include nausea, water retention, weight gain, and irregular vaginal bleeding. More serious complications, such as stroke and cardiovascular problems, are rare. Women who smoke or have a history of blood clots should let their physician know before being considered for treatment with OCs. It may take several months for normal ovulatory patterns to resume after a woman stops taking birth-control therapy.

• *Danazol (Danocrine).* A synthetic derivative of the male hormone testosterone, danazol halts ovulation and puts the body into a pseudomenopausal state in which menstruation ceases. Danazol works to do this in several ways. First, it stops the production of estrogen and progesterone in the ovaries. Second, it blocks estrogen receptors from being stimulated by any remaining estrogen in the blood. Third, it prevents the pituitary from trying to compensate for estrogen by decreasing its production of follicle-stimulating hormone (FSH) and luteinizing hormone (LH). This three-pronged effect of danazol makes it an effective treatment for endometriosis, which requires estrogen stimulation to exist and grow. As with all hormonal treatments, however, symptoms often recur after stopping the medication.

- *Dosage:* For moderate to severe endometriosis, the usual dose of danazol, an oral medication, is 200 mg (milligrams) two to four times a day for 3 to 9 months. The medication is usually started on the first few days of a woman's menstrual bleed.
- *Monitoring:* A physical examination is often performed every 3 months to review symptoms of endometriosis.
- *Potential side effects:* The side effects of danazol may include hot flashes, sweating, vaginal dryness, and weight gain. Because it is a derivative of testosterone, it can also produce masculinizing effects, such as the growth of facial hair, deepening of the voice, decrease in breast size, and a rise in blood cholesterol levels. Side effects are dose-related and most decrease when the medication is stopped.
- *Contraindications:* Women who are pregnant should not use danazol as it may cause birth defects. Because the kidney and liver metabolize the drug, women with impaired kidney function should avoid using it.
- *Drugs used in combination:* None.

• *GnRH agonists (Lupron, Synarel).* Another class of drugs that cause pseudomenopause is GnRH agonists. See chapter 6, "The Female: Hormonal Disorders and Treatment," for a complete discussion of GnRH agonists and their use in treating endometriosis and fibroids, and as a component of ART. The longer-acting form of the drug, depot Lupron, can be given monthly by injection. A woman generally has a menstrual period 2 weeks after starting the medication. For treating endometriosis, the GnRH agonists are usually used for 4 to 6 months, and it may take up to 3 months for periods to resume after the medication is discontinued.

Hormone treatment for endometriosis can be given in combination with surgery, either preoperatively or postoperatively.

Symptoms of endometriosis often will stop during and shortly after a pregnancy. There is no known cure for endometriosis, however, and in some women the disease persists until menopause. Women need to monitor their symptoms and be followed by a physician who will evaluate their situation, recommending laparoscopy or other treatments when necessary.

# PELVIC INFLAMMATORY DISEASE (PID)

Each year in the United States, more than 1 million women are diagnosed with acute pelvic inflammatory disease (PID). PID is a name for any bacterial infection of the pelvic organs. Bacteria usually enter through the vagina and cervix. Infection may spread to the uterus, fallopian tubes, and ovaries. PID is a common and serious complication of sexually transmitted diseases (STDs). The most common STDs associated with PID are chlamydia and gonorrhea. Chlamydia is a particularly insidious disease because it is often a completely silent invader, causing no symptoms. Scarring from infection, however, can cause blocked fallopian tubes. Another way for infection to enter the pelvic cavity is through the use of an intrauterine device (IUD), a method of birth control widely used in the 1970s. PID can also occur as a complication of pregnancy loss, in which the cervix was dilated or the amniotic sac was broken for a prolonged time, or rarely from an infection introduced during childbirth, a D&C (dilation and curettage), or elective abortion performed under unsterile circumstances.

## Symptoms of PID

In many cases, no symptoms of PID are present, and a woman may not be aware that she has an infection. When symptoms are present, they may include lower abdominal pain, vaginal discharge, fever, painful sexual intercourse, and irregular bleeding. If PID is diagnosed, antibiotics will be prescribed, often for both the woman and her partner. If you know you have had PID in the past, your physician may perform a hysterosalpingogram (HSG) to document any tubal damage (more about tubal damage and HSG later in this chapter). Laparoscopy or laparotomy may be used to remove pelvic adhesions or to correct tubal damage in some cases. If the condition is too severe, surgery may not be warranted.

### Questions to Ask About PID

If you are concerned about whether you have PID, ask the following questions:

- Do I have pelvic pain or vaginal discharge that is discolored and has a foul odor?
- Has sexual intercourse ever been painful or caused spotting?
- If you are diagnosed with a pelvic infection, ask your physician whether your partner should be treated so that you do not reinfect each other.

### Other Infections

Bacterial infections of the vaginal canal can affect fertility: Vaginitis can change the quality of cervical mucus and interfere with sperm survival. Bacterial infection of the uterine lining, called endometritis, can cause inflammation and possible scarring, affecting normal implantation of an embryo.

### Diagnosis and Treatment

If your physician suspects bacterial infection, a culture of your vagina, cervical canal, or uterine lining can be taken or blood tests performed. If infection is found, your physician will prescribe one or more antibiotics (again, as for PID, often for both the woman and her partner). The medication may be taken systemically (orally) or vaginally.

## TUBAL FACTOR

The fallopian tubes are muscular tubes that receive the egg(s) from the ovaries and, if fertilization occurs, move the embryo to the uterus. Conditions that interfere with the proper functioning of the fallopian tubes may adversely affect fertility. This is the *tubal factor*.

**ANATOMY OF THE FALLOPIAN TUBE**

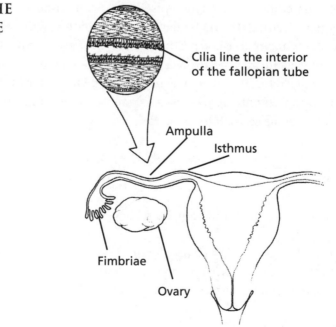

Cilia line the interior of the fallopian tube

Ampulla

Isthmus

Fimbriae

Ovary

### The Fallopian Tube

Two types of cells line the fallopian tube:

- Secretory cells, which produce mucus, glucose, and other substances necessary for nourishing the egg and the embryo.
- Tiny hairlike structures called cilia.

Each part of the fallopian tube has a different job to perform during the reproductive process:

- The fimbriae capture the egg during ovulation.
- The ampulla transports the egg, is believed to be a common site of fertilization, and allows the fertilized egg to mature.
- The isthmus serves as a conduit for sperm and transports the fertilized egg to the uterus.

Tubal factor problems include the following:

- *Congenital problems.* In very rare cases, a woman is born with an abnormality in the structure or functioning of her fallopian tubes.
- *Inflammation and infection (salpingitis).* Salpingitis means inflammation of the inside of the fallopian tube. Salpingitis infections cause no symptoms, and the damage is discovered only when a woman tries to become pregnant. Infection in the pelvic cavity surrounding the tubes may result in adhesions on the outside of the tubes, which can distort by pulling, causing kinks or narrowing of the tubes.

Another condition called salpingitis isthmica nodosa (SIN) is an abnormality of the muscular lining of the fallopian tube at the isthmic portion. Experts cannot agree whether this condition arises from infection or whether it is congenital. SIN may block the passage of sperm and may prevent the fertilized egg from entering the uterus. The affected portion of the tube may be surgically removed and the normal tubal segments reconnected to restore normal anatomy. Some women with tubal problems develop a hydrosalpinx, or fluid-filled bulge of the fallopian tube. If the hydrosalpinx is very large, both the lining and the musculature of the tube can be destroyed. In addition, researchers suspect that the fluid from the hydrosalpinx may seep out of the tube and have an adverse effect on implantation inside the uterus. Some studies suggest that pregnancy rates for women who undergo in vitro fertilization (IVF) are improved if such a tube is removed or tied off at the junction of the uterus.

- *Sterilization.* Approximately 1 million women in the United States each year undergo tubal ligation surgery as a form of birth control. Approximately 1 to 3 percent of these women eventually wish to reverse the surgery to attempt to restore fertility. Properly trained surgeons can reconstruct the tubes with excellent results.

## Diagnosis of Tubal Problems

The HSG is a procedure that involves injecting either an oil- or water-based dye into the uterine cavity and taking x-rays of the uterus and fallopian tubes. If the tubes are not blocked, the dye should pour through the tubes into the abdominal cavity. HSG can usually detect a hydrosalpinx. The test also can diagnose a common tubal problem, proximal tubal obstruction. In this condition, the tubes appear blocked where they join the uterus (near the isthmus). Problems resulting from proximal tubal obstruction may be minor (debris that plugs up the opening) but could indicate serious damage to the portion of the fallopian tube that joins the uterine wall. In addition, if a tube is blocked at the isthmus (proximal, or at the uterine-tubal junction), the dye will not flow through and the HSG cannot be used to diagnose problems further along the tube toward the fimbriated end (distal, or far, end of the fallopian tube). For that analysis, laparoscopy may be needed.

Laparoscopy can provide information about the fimbriated end of the tube, the exterior of the tubes, and the extent of any pelvic adhesions. During a laparoscopy, the physician may inject dye through the cervix and observe through the laparoscope to see whether it flows out the fallopian tubes.

Hysteroscopy allows for visualization of the inside of the uterine cavity, which is especially useful in diagnosing uterine problems discussed later in this chapter, but also in identifying any obstructions of the fallopian tubes at the utero-tubal junction. Hysteroscopy is often combined with laparoscopy, or it can be performed under local anesthesia at the physician's office.

Other techniques are now available to diagnose tubal problems. Selective salpingography involves the placement of a small catheter through the cervix into the fallopian tube. Dye is then injected and x-rays taken. The salpingoscope, or falloposcope, is a small optical device that the physician passes into the fimbriated end of the fallopian tube during laparoscopy, or it can be passed into the tube from the uterus. This procedure can be performed in the office or operating room.

For more information about diagnostic tests, see chapter 5, "The Basic Infertility Work-up for Women and Men."

## Treatment of Tubal Problems

If a tubal problem is diagnosed, choices must be made between attempting

**COMMON
TUBAL
BLOCKAGES**

Proximal tubal
obstruction

Hydrosalpinx

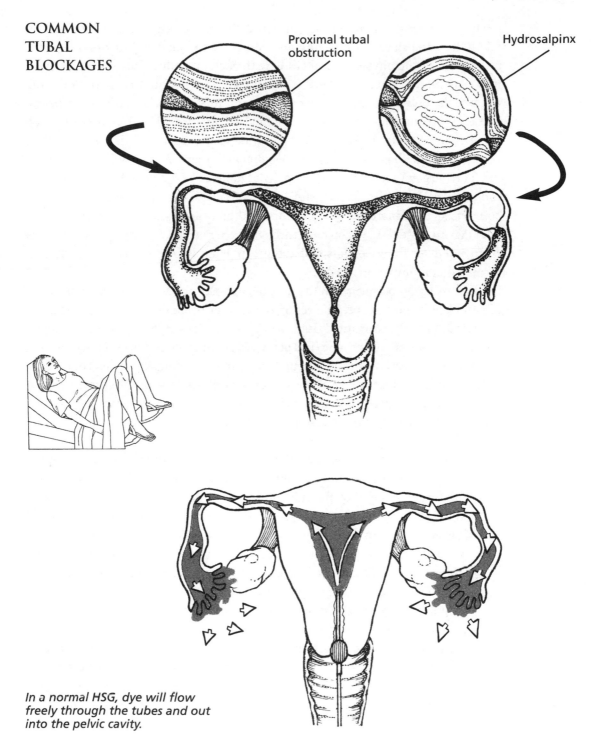

*In a normal HSG, dye will flow
freely through the tubes and out
into the pelvic cavity.*

to correct the problem surgically, or going directly to ART procedures, such as IVF. Often the decision depends on the extent of the tubal disorder and the experience of the physician and clinic with each procedure. Insurance coverage may play a role, as well. If there is a proximal obstruction where the tube connects to the uterus (isthmus), there are several surgical options, discussed below. If there is distal tubal blockage involving the fimbriated end of the tube, IVF may be your best option if the interior of the tube is seriously damaged. Talk to your physician about the risks and benefits of surgery versus IVF.

The surgical techniques for repairing damaged or blocked tubes are quite sophisticated and often successful. Microsurgical or laser techniques are now being used with increased success for tubal blockages and reversal of sterilization. Microsurgery is performed through either a laparotomy (major surgery requiring 1 to 2 days of hospitalization) or laparoscopy (surgery usually performed on an outpatient basis).

Laser surgery performed at the time of laparoscopy uses amplified light waves, mirrors, and a microscope. The action of the laser beam on cells causes the intracellular fluid in the unwanted tissue to vaporize. The surgeon controls the depth and amount of tissue destroyed. The perceived advantages of the laser are decreased bleeding and a decrease in swelling and adjacent tissue damage, which could result in less scar tissue formation. The experience and expertise of the surgeon in performing microsurgical and laser techniques are an important factor; choose a surgeon who performs these procedures on a regular basis.

- *Salpingolysis/Fimbriolysis.* Salpingolysis is a technique for cutting away adhesions from the tubes. Fimbriolysis is used to remove adhesions from the fimbriated end of the tube. Research shows pregnancy rates of about 40 to 60 percent after these procedures are performed (fimbriolysis has a higher success rate than salpingolysis). The risk of ectopic pregnancy is 5 to 10 percent after these procedures (see chapter 10, "Pregnancy Loss").
- *Fimbrioplasty.* This procedure is designed to repair damaged fimbria and a partially blocked tube by separating the fimbria surgically. Research shows pregnancy rates of about 40 to 60 percent after fimbrioplasty. The risk of ectopic pregnancy is about 10 percent.
- *Salpingostomy.* Salpingostomy is a surgical procedure performed to open a tube that is blocked at the distal (far) fimbriated end, toward the ovary. Depending on the extent of the damage, the pregnancy rate after salpingostomy is about 25 to 40 percent. The risk of ectopic pregnancy is approximately 10 percent.

- *Tubal anastomosis.* Removing a blocked portion of the fallopian tube and then rejoining the opened ends is called tubal anastomosis. This procedure is effective for women who have had tubal ligation. Pregnancy rates are 60 to 80 percent after surgery. Restoration of a woman's fertility by reversal of tubal ligation will depend on many factors, including the surgical procedure used at time of sterilization, the skill of the surgeon performing the reversal, the age of the woman at the time of attempted reversal, other coexisting problems such as pelvic scar tissue, and the status of the partner's sperm. The risk of ectopic pregnancy is about 5 percent.

- *Tubal catheterization.* Also known as tubal cannulation, this procedure is helpful for removing blockage from the proximal end of the tube, the isthmus. A surgeon usually performs this procedure during a standard HSG or hysteroscopy by flushing fluid through a catheter inserted into the fallopian tube. Another technique involves using a tiny balloon that is inflated within the tube itself, thereby stretching the tube open at the site of its blockage. If these methods fail, or repeat HSG indicates that a blockage still exists, further diagnostic testing and treatment may be necessary.

### Questions to Ask to Decide Between Tubal Procedures or IVF

If you are trying to decide between microsurgery or IVF, ask your physician the following questions. It is your right to seek a second medical opinion to confirm your diagnosis and treatment options.

- Is there a hydrosalpinx (thickness and ballooning out of the tubal wall)?
- Is there a problem at both ends of the tubes (bilateral blockage), which will lower significantly the success rate of microsurgery?
- What are my risks for an ectopic pregnancy?
- Should I have my male partner's semen analysis rechecked before surgery?
- Will there be any anti-adhesion techniques used during surgery that may help lessen scar tissue formation?
- When are my best chances to conceive after surgery?
- Are there any treatments (drugs, timing of ovulation, etc.) that will increase my chances of getting pregnant after surgery?
- Will I need a follow-up laparoscopy to remove adhesions after the microsurgical repair? If so, when?

TUBAL
CANNULATION
USING
HYSTEROSCOPY

Normal tube,
no blockage

Proximal tubal
obstruction

Proximal tubal
obstruction

Balloon inflates
to open tube
at the site of
blockage

## EXPOSURE TO DES

In 1938, physicians began prescribing diethylstilbestrol (DES), a synthetic estrogen, for pregnant women under the belief that the drug helped prevent miscarriage. Unfortunately, this drug caused birth defects in some offspring of mothers who took it while pregnant. About 1 in 1,000 women exposed to DES in utero develop precancerous lesions (dysplasia) or cancer of the cervix or vagina, and about 50 percent have structural abnormalities of the vagina, cervix, uterus, and fallopian tubes. These problems occur because the drug caused changes in the Müllerian ducts, the tubal structures that join together in the developing fetus to form the uterus. Abnormalities seem to be related to *when* and *how much*, not how long, the pregnant woman took DES. If she took DES in the first and second trimester of pregnancy, it is more likely that her daughter might develop structural abnormalities of the reproductive system—or that her son will have low sperm counts related to this DES exposure in utero (see chapter 8, "The Male: Diagnosis and Treatment," for more about male factor infertility).

## DES and Infertility

Women exposed to DES in utero are at higher risk for a number of fertility problems. They include the following:

- *Cervical problems.* Adenosis is a condition in which glandular tissue forms on the outside of the cervix. Cervical problems may include poor cervical muscle tone, reduced cervical mucus, or cervical stenosis (narrowing) often resulting from surgery to correct cervical dysplasia (abnormal change in tissue structure). About 75 percent of women exposed to DES who have cervical abnormalities also have other structural problems, often of the uterus and sometimes fallopian tubes.
- *Uterine problems.* The most common uterine abnormalities associated with DES exposure are small, internally T-shaped uterus; unusual bands of tissue within the uterine cavity; and a rough, irregular uterine lining. Some women exposed to DES have a hypoplastic (underdeveloped) uterus.

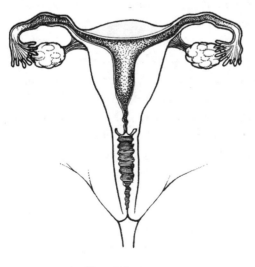

*Normal uterus*

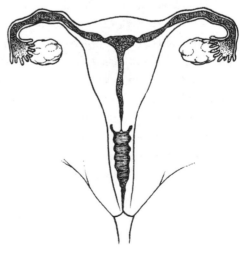

*DES: T-shaped uterus*

- *Tubal problems.* Some women exposed to DES have tubes with strictures at the junction of the uterus and tubes, and others have tubes that are smaller than normal. Some have a condition called "withered tubes" in which the tubes are convoluted, slightly twisted, and have few, if any, fimbria (the hairlike projections that capture the egg as it leaves the ovary).
- *Irregular menstrual cycles.* Several studies have documented higher than average irregular menstrual cycles in women exposed to DES.
- *Increased risk of endometriosis.* Women exposed to DES may have a higher incidence of endometriosis, which may be related to retrograde menstruation because of a narrowed cervical opening or small uterus.
- *Higher risk of pregnancy loss.* Pregnancy loss is common in women exposed to DES. This may be caused by the irregular uterine lining or abnormalities in the shape and size of the uterus, resulting in early miscarriage or premature labor before 37 weeks of pregnancy. Ectopic pregnancy rates are four to five times higher in women exposed to DES.
- *Increased risk of premature delivery.* The small uterine cavity and the lack of muscle tone in the cervical and uterine muscles often found in women exposed to DES contribute to higher than normal rates of premature labor and delivery.

### Voices

*Katherine's mother took DES while pregnant with her in the early 1960s. At the age of 24, Katherine's gynecologist diagnosed her with dysplasia. She had the abnormal cells removed with laser surgery, but—as is common with DES daughters—the dysplasia recurred and surgery was once again necessary. At the age of 28, after she and her husband had tried for a year to have a baby, Katherine saw a specialist, who diagnosed her with cervical stenosis—an abnormal narrowing of the cervical opening probably caused by the surgery to remove the dysplasia. "At this point, I've already been through 5 years of medical treatment, and, apparently, we're just getting started," Katherine recounts. "Now, tests show that I'm not ovulating regularly either, which may or may not be due to the DES. It amazes and humbles me that a drug that physicians thought would help women have babies may end up preventing me from doing so. It's sad and it's frustrating."*

*As Katherine continues to struggle through her infertility journey, she wonders how her mother is dealing with the situation. "I know my mother feels responsible for my infertility. I know she would do anything to turn back the clock. Mostly, she blames her physician who, by the time she took the drug in 1963, should have known better than to give her DES. Now I am paying the price."*

### Treatment for DES-Related Problems

If you are a woman who was exposed to DES and are trying to get pregnant, find a physician who is familiar with the problems associated with DES exposure. An HSG may be performed to evaluate your uterus and fallopian tubes, and a laparoscopy, to evaluate the pelvic cavity and uterus. If scanty cervical mucus is present, the physician may suggest IUI. Surgery to correct certain abnormalities or hormone treatment to correct cycle irregularities may be prescribed.

Women exposed to DES may also benefit from ART procedures, such as IVF, gamete intrafallopian transfer (GIFT), and zygote intrafallopian transfer (ZIFT), when appropriate (see chapter 9, "Assisted Reproductive Technology [ART]"). Although rates of egg retrieval and fertilization are similar to those of unaffected women in the same age group, viable pregnancy rates are lower, probably because of the higher incidence of early miscarriage in women exposed to DES. Also, premature labor from multiple gestation pregnancy is a serious potential problem in a woman with a small uterine cavity, so the number of embryos transferred back to the uterus of a woman exposed to DES during IVF should be few.

Women exposed to DES who do get pregnant require careful monitoring. After 10 to 12 weeks, the physician should evaluate the cervix for signs of premature dilation. If this occurs, a surgical procedure called a cerclage (stitches placed in the cervical muscle) may be considered to keep the cervix closed.

In addition to using RESOLVE's resources, an excellent resource is the local chapter of DES Action. This organization offers support groups that can help provide education and emotional support (see the Resources at the back of this book).

## UTERINE PROBLEMS

Fertility problems of the uterus include uterine fibroids, congenital abnormalities, Asherman syndrome, and adenomyosis.

### Uterine Fibroids

Fibroid tumors are noncancerous growths in the walls of the uterus and are frequently found in women between the ages of 30 to 45 years. Fibroids can occur anywhere in the pelvic cavity. Fibroids may be in the uterine walls (intramural), grow into the uterine cavity (submucosal), or be on the surface or attached to the uterine wall in the pelvic cavity (subserosal). Some women have only one small fibroid whereas others have many, ranging in size from small to large.

## UTERINE FIBROIDS

Subserosal fibroids

Intramural fibroids

Submucosal fibroids

The position of fibroids may cause problems with implantation of an embryo. If the fibroid bulges into the uterine cavity, then it may obstruct one of the utero-tubal openings or it may present a barrier to implantation. If the fibroid has invaded the wall of the uterus, it might interfere with blood supply to the uterine lining and affect implantation. If the fibroid is predominantly on the outside of the uterus with projection into the pelvis and abdomen, then it may outgrow its own blood supply and degenerate or become infected. Fibroids may grow with the stimulation of pregnancy hormones, causing pressure on the uterus, discomfort, and even premature labor.

Symptoms vary in relation to the size, number, and location of the fibroids. A fibroid within the uterine cavity may irritate the endometrium and cause it to bleed heavily. A small fibroid buried deep in the uterine wall may not produce any symptoms, whereas a grapefruit-sized fibroid on the exterior back wall of the uterus might cause severe constipation, urinary tract problems, or heavy menstrual periods. In general, larger fibroids are associated with heavy, painful menstrual periods, irregular bleeding, pain with sexual intercourse, and pelvic pressure.

## Diagnosis of Uterine Fibroids

Fibroids are fairly easy to diagnose. In some cases, a pelvic examination will allow the physician to gauge the size of the uterus. A normal uterus is about the size of a pear or an apple (see the illustration of the female reproductive tract in chapter 2, "Normal Fertility"). A uterus with a fibroid, however, may feel much larger on examination. Ultrasound, sonohysterography (a vaginal ultrasound using sterile salt water inside the uterus), hysteroscopy, and MRI are all tools used to diagnose and evaluate fibroids.

Hysteroscopy is useful for visualizing fibroids in the uterine cavity. A hysteroscope, a thin surgical instrument approximately ⅙ of an inch in diameter, is passed through the vagina and cervix into the uterine cavity; looking through the hysteroscope lens, the physician can view the interior of the uterus. Surgical procedures to correct certain uterine problems can be performed through hysteroscopy.

Because the uterus is flat and its inner walls in direct contact with one another, it is necessary to distend the uterus by carbon dioxide gas or saline solution during an operative hysteroscopy. The recovery time for operative hysteroscopy is about the same as for diagnostic laparoscopy. A woman may have some vaginal bleeding and some cramping for a few days after an operative hysteroscopy.

## Treatment of Uterine Fibroids

Many fibroids do not seem to interfere with fertility, and should not be removed unless a reproductive problem is identified and all other causes of infertility have been treated. When fibroids are large, the physician may first prescribe drug therapy, consisting of leuprolide acetate depot (Lupron), a GnRH agonist that puts a woman's body into a pseudomenopause and shrinks the uterine fibroids. Shrinking the fibroids may allow a surgeon to remove them more easily. Surgeons can remove fibroids using hysteroscopy, laparoscopy, or laparotomy. Surgical removal of fibroid(s) through laparoscopy or laparotomy is called a myomectomy.

- *Myomectomy.* During myomectomy by laparotomy, the surgeon will make an incision through the abdominal wall or vagina to gain access to the uterus and then remove the fibroids. Because this is major surgery and blood loss is a possibility, many physicians ask the woman to bank some of her own blood a few weeks before the operation. After myomectomy, many physicians recommend a 3- to 6-month healing period before trying to conceive. Similarly, cesarean section is usually recommended after a myomectomy because of concern about uterine rupture during labor.
- *Myolysis, cryomyolysis, and arterial embolization.* Myolysis and cryomyolysis are techniques performed during a laparoscopy and involve inserting a

probe into the fibroids to destroy them by heating or freezing the tissue. Arterial embolization of uterine fibroids is performed by a radiologist. This technique blocks the flow of blood to the vessels feeding the fibroid, and is reserved for women who have decided not to try to become pregnant because it may disrupt blood flow to the uterine lining as well.

- *Hysterectomy.* Hysterectomy is the surgical removal of the uterus. Benign conditions including uterine fibroids, abnormal uterine bleeding, and chronic pelvic pain account for about two of every three of the approximately 600,000 hysterectomies performed in the United States each year.

## Congenital Abnormalities of the Uterus

Between weeks 9 and 16 of pregnancy, the tubular systems forming in the fetus called the Müllerian ducts fuse together to form the uterus. If the fetus's Müllerian ducts do not develop normally, congenital abnormalities of the uterus can occur. Depending on how severe the uterine abnormality is, it may be possible for a woman to get pregnant and give birth.

- *Mayer-Rokitansky-Küster-Hauser syndrome.* This severe congenital problem occurs when the Müllerian cells fail to develop the tubes that must fuse to create a uterus. A woman born with this condition has no uterus and will never be able to carry a child.
- *Uterine didelphys.* Women with this rare congenital condition have a uterus with two distinct parts with a wall between them, as well as a double cervix and, often, a septum made of fibrous tissue that divides the vaginal canal down the middle. Pregnancy is difficult because the uterine cavities often are very small and do not expand normally.
- *Bicornate uterus and septate uterus.* A failure of the Müllerian ducts to fuse causes a division of the uterus, although other parts of the reproductive system develop normally. Often, one uterine cavity is larger than the other. If only a simple septum divides the cavity, it may be surgically removed. The septate uterus is associated with pregnancy loss. About 80 percent of these women carry their pregnancies successfully after surgical removal of the septum.

## Asherman Syndrome and Adenomyosis

When the uterine cavity has scar tissue within it (intrauterine adhesions), it is called Asherman syndrome. It can be severe, in which case the whole uter-

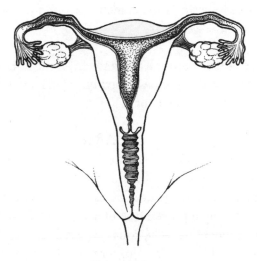

*Normal uterus*

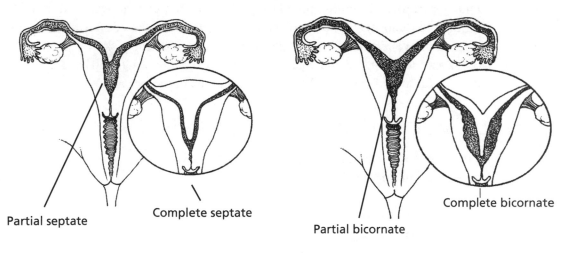

Partial septate

Complete septate

*Septate uterus*

Partial bicornate

Complete bicornate

*Bicornate uterus*

ine cavity is scarred and the woman does not menstruate, or mild, with only a few bands of scar tissue present. These women may have light periods. Some causes of Asherman syndrome include the following:

- Scar tissue resulting from a vigorous D&C after a miscarriage.

• Scar tissue resulting from infection from a therapeutic abortion, or from PID.

Adenomyosis is the growth of glands from the endometrium into the muscle wall of the uterus (called the myometrium). This condition can lead to excessive menstrual bleeding and pelvic pain.

### Treatment of Asherman Syndrome and Adenomyosis

Removal of adhesions within the uterus is performed by hysteroscopy. A semirigid scissors is inserted through the hysteroscope to cut through the scar tissue. Postoperatively, a high dose of estrogen may be prescribed and/or an IUD may be inserted to help prevent the uterine walls from healing together.

For mild to moderate adhesions, expect a 60 to 80 percent chance of successful pregnancy after repair. For more extensive adhesions, the chance of successful pregnancy is lower. If a pregnancy does occur after repair of Asherman syndrome, there is a greater chance of preterm labor and delivery, placenta accreta (a condition in which the placenta invades the uterine wall and becomes difficult to remove) and postpartum hemorrhage (heavy bleeding after the delivery of a baby). The pregnancies should be considered high risk.

Treatment for adenomyosis is similar to that for endometriosis and may involve the use of drugs such as GnRH agonists, danazol, or OCs.

## CERVICAL MUCUS AND SPERM TRANSPORT PROBLEMS

There are several conditions and procedures that can cause poor cervical mucus quality, including the following conditions:

• Cervical infection or the presence of cervical sperm antibodies.
• Exposure in utero to DES.
• Surgical procedures performed on the cervix, such as treatment for dysplasia.
• In some cases, treatment with the fertility drug clomiphene citrate, which can cause the cervical mucus to become scanty and thick.

Cervical mucus transports sperm from the vaginal canal through the cervix up into the uterus. Poor mucus quality can adversely affect the sperm's ability to reach the egg.

## Problems Caused by Infections

The postcoital test (PCT) is used to evaluate sperm-mucus interaction (see chapter 5, "The Basic Infertility Work-up for Women and Men," for more information about the PCT). If the physician finds dead sperm and white blood cells, a culture of the mucus may be taken to identify specific microorganisms. If infection is found, both partners must be treated with antibiotics. After antibiotic treatment (usually for 7 to 10 days, depending on the type of infection and medication used to treat it), the physician will repeat the PCT to see whether this treatment solved the sperm-mucus interaction problem.

## Antisperm Antibodies

Antibodies are cells that act as a line of defense against foreign organisms, such as viruses and bacteria. About 30 percent of women with unexplained infertility may produce antibodies against their partner's sperm. These antibodies can cause the sperm to clump and immobilize. Diagnosis of antisperm antibodies may require testing of the man's sperm and the woman's cervical mucus, as well as blood tests for both partners.

In cases in which antisperm antibodies are confirmed in the woman's cervical mucus, a physician may recommend IUI. This treatment allows the sperm to enter the uterus directly, thereby bypassing the vaginal canal and cervix altogether (as opposed to cervical insemination, in which sperm are deposited at the woman's cervix and must still travel through the cervical mucus to the uterus). IVF can also be used successfully in couples with antisperm antibody problems.

# INTRAUTERINE INSEMINATION (IUI) AS A TREATMENT OPTION

IUI is a procedure used for couples with unexplained infertility, minimal male factor infertility (see chapter 8, "The Male: Diagnosis and Treatment"), women with cervical mucus problems, and in conjunction with ovulation-stimulating drugs (see chapter 6, "The Female: Hormonal Disorders and Treatment"). Before IUI, the woman should be treated for any hormonal imbalance and for infection. She should also have an HSG to confirm a normal reproductive system. If there is a structural problem, corrective surgery also should be done before the IUI procedure.

Sperm from the male partner or third-party donor are prepared for IUI by being "washed" or centrifuged. (For more information on donor insemination

[DI] using a third-party sperm donor, see chapter 15, "Exploring Other Family-Building Options.") The sperm washing process removes prostaglandins and other debris from the specimen. Various techniques and special solutions are used to concentrate the highest quality, motile sperm. The washed specimen is then placed by the physician into a soft catheter that is passed through a speculum directly into the woman's uterus at the time of ovulation. Ovulation will be predicted either by a urine test kit or by blood testing and ultrasound. Insemination is usually performed within 24 to 36 hours after the LH surge is detected, or after the "trigger" injection of human chorionic gonadotropin (hCG) is administered. It is important to ask whether the clinic or physician's office is open over weekends and holidays, in the event you need an IUI treatment then.

The physician may recommend one or two inseminations per menstrual cycle. Studies evaluating success rates for one versus two inseminations per cycle vary, and each clinic has its own protocol (guidelines) about the number of inseminations per cycle that is recommended.

IUI may be used in conjunction with ovulatory medications, such as clomiphene citrate, gonadotropins, or urofollitropins. If injectable ovulation-stimulating drugs (gonadotropins or urofollitropins) are used in an IUI cycle, careful monitoring is essential. Monitoring includes periodic ultrasound evaluation and blood tests, started on or about day 6 of the woman's cycle. Blood will be drawn to determine the estradiol level (a form of estrogen produced by the follicles). This level is used to individualize medication treatment. Results of the ultrasound and blood test monitoring will indicate when eggs are mature. At that time, an hCG shot will be given to cause the release of the eggs(s).

If follicular development has been too vigorous and estradiol levels indicate that multiple eggs may be released, the physician may advise the woman *not* to take hCG and to cancel the cycle to prevent the possibility of multiple gestation pregnancy. In some cases, the cycle may become an IVF cycle in which the eggs are removed and fertilized in the laboratory and a limited number of embryos (usually no more than three or four) are returned to the woman's uterus (see chapter 9, "Assisted Reproductive Technology [ART]").

IUI should not be painful, although some women report discomfort and mild cramping after the procedure. Some clinics ask the woman to remain lying down for 20 minutes after an IUI. A tampon device may be used to prevent fluid from seeping out vaginally. If a woman develops abdominal tenderness, fever, or foul-smelling vaginal discharge after an IUI, she should contact her physician at once. Infection is rare after IUI, but possible.

## INTRAUTERINE
## INSEMINATION (IUI)

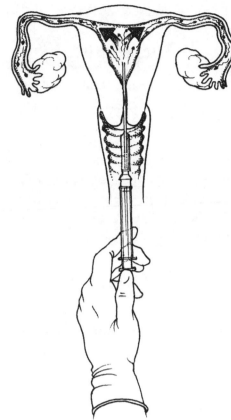

Individuals and couples who fail to conceive within three medicated IUI cycles should review their treatment plans with their physicians, and may want to consider ART procedures, such as IVF.

### Success Rates for IUI

A study of pregnancy rates among 9,963 consecutive IUI cycles performed between January 1991 and December 1996, conducted by the Institute for Fertility Research, reveals that IUI success rates have increased from 5.8 percent per cycle in 1991 to 13.4 percent per cycle in 1996—even considering an increase in the average age of the woman receiving the procedure, which rose from 36 to 39 years of age during the period of study. Researchers noted, however, that the age of the woman at the time of the IUI cycle remains the most important factor affecting fertility, and women studied who were older than 32 years showed a lower pregnancy rate. IUI success also is affected by the number of follicles at the time of insemination, the quality of the eggs, and the male partner's sperm count.

## A WOMAN'S AGE AND INFERTILITY

If you are older than 35 years and attempting to start a family, you are not alone. In fact, about 20 percent of first children are now being born to women older than 35 years of age. Although some women in their late 30s and early 40s give birth to healthy babies without requiring medical intervention, many face difficulties. Not only is it often difficult to get pregnant at an older age, but also the risk of miscarriage increases.

### Voices

*"It seemed like it should be so easy—movie stars had done it," asserts Alison. "Just look at them all: Bette Midler had married late and had her first child at 40, Sigourney Weaver had her first at 40, too, and Glenn Close. My own mother had been in her 30s when she had me, and her mother had had her at 42. My husband's mom had him when she was 41. Yes, we'd waited until we were both emotionally and economically ready for a planned pregnancy and parenthood. Now, I was ready to join the ranks of first-time mothers at 40. I didn't know it would prove to be so hard. I thought it was inevitable, natural, easy."*

The decline in fertility with age results from one or more of the following conditions:

- *Ovulatory dysfunction or failure.* At about age 35, a woman's ovarian function changes. The number of healthy eggs remaining in her ovaries has decreased, and thus, her ovarian reserve has declined. Ovarian reserve is measured by a menstrual cycle day 3 blood test to measure FSH and estradiol (estrogen) levels. As a woman ages, her day 3 FSH or estradiol levels may begin to rise. When this occurs, her ovaries may become resistant to stimulation and thus produce fewer follicles (an indicator to physicians of how well the woman will respond to ovulation induction) and produce poorer quality eggs and embryos. There is no effective treatment for rising FSH and estradiol levels because of aging.
- *Luteal phase defect (LPD).* Older women tend to have a higher incidence of LPD, which means that the endometrium is inadequately prepared for the implantation of a fertilized egg either because the secretion of the hormone progesterone is low or the response of the endometrium is inadequate. Treatment with progesterone and ovulation-stimulating drugs can help to compensate for this defect.
- *Chromosomal abnormalities.* Older women's embryos tend to have higher incidences of chromosomal abnormalities. Chromosomal abnormalities are a leading cause of miscarriages in older women. In addition, women in their late 30s and early 40s have an increased risk of having genetically abnormal babies, for example, infants with Down syndrome. The incidence of Down syndrome is approximately 1 in 100 children at maternal age 40.

If you are an older woman attempting to become pregnant, talk about the potential impact of your age on your fertility with your physician and know what to expect. Many women assume that because they have had no gynecologic problems in the past and because their menstrual cycles have always been regular, they can become pregnant easily in their late 30s. It is with shock and sadness that many women hear the news from their physicians that their "biological clocks" are running out. Suddenly, a woman or couple is confronted with social pressure to pursue more aggressive treatment. Priorities suddenly shift as the couple may face the expense and stress of so-called high-tech treatment. Take the time to review your options carefully. Think about a second medical opinion if you are faced with such stark news about your fertility. You may want to speak with other RESOLVE members who have faced similar choices and talk with them about their resolutions, including treatment with ART procedures using the woman's own eggs, adoption, treatment with ART procedures using donor eggs (DE), and childfree living. Help from a therapist experienced with infertility issues is often beneficial; limited counseling is available through some insurance plans.

## UNEXPLAINED INFERTILITY

Most cases of infertility can be diagnosed after thorough evaluation. However, 10 percent of those experiencing infertility will never have a definitive diagnosis. Approximately 40 to 60 percent of couples with unexplained infertility eventually achieve pregnancy either with or without medical treatment within 4 years.

---

### *Voices*

*"It's the not knowing that's the worst," admits Naomi, a 28-year-old woman with unexplained infertility. Her physician removed some endometriosis and scar tissue, then gave Naomi and her husband the "all clear." They have tried four cycles of IUI and tried on their own for several months, but so far, they are not pregnant. "If the doctor told me there wasn't a chance, I could move on. But knowing I can get pregnant makes it very difficult; I don't want to stop, I just want to keep trying. Every month, I have hope. Some months, my period comes and I just shrug and say well, maybe next month. Other times, I fall apart."*

---

If you are experiencing unexplained infertility, consider taking your medical records, operative notes, laboratory data, and x-ray films to another physician to seek a second medical opinion.

---

### *Questions to Ask About Unexplained Infertility*

If, after completing your infertility work-up, you and your partner are facing unexplained infertility, you may find the following questions helpful. Not all tests or procedures are appropriate for all couples. Consult your physician about pursuing the best options for your unique set of circumstances.

- Has your partner had a recent semen analysis?
- Has a sperm antibody test been performed on both you and your partner?
- Have mycoplasma cultures been taken from both partners to rule out infection?
- Are ovulatory cycles normal? Is the luteal phase normal and, if not, has this been treated and then reassessed with an endometrial biopsy or progesterone blood serum levels?
- Has a cycle day 3 FSH level been taken? Even if the level is normal, it should be retested in a future cycle.

- Has the physician performed a series of ultrasounds to document that the follicle does rupture and release an egg?
- Have you discussed with your physician the possibility that you may be having very early miscarriages before you get your menstrual period?

In many cases of unexplained infertility, medicated IUI or ART procedures, such as IVF, ZIFT, or GIFT, may be options for some couples (see chapter 9, "Assisted Reproductive Technology [ART]"). Before beginning ovulation-stimulating treatment with gonadotropins or undergoing ART procedures, a diagnostic laparoscopy may be performed on the woman.

IVF can document that fertilization is possible and allows the physician to evaluate the quality of the woman's eggs. ZIFT, in which an embryo develops to an early stage before transfer to the woman's fallopian tube, also provides the healthcare team with information about fertilization. If you and your partner are considering GIFT or ZIFT, an HSG or other tubal evaluation should first be done to document that the lining of the fallopian tube is normal.

When facing unexplained infertility, couples—and their physicians—may find it hard to answer the question, *when is enough, enough?* Unexplained infertility can be wrenching because it is so difficult to know when to stop infertility treatments or to consider other family-building options. If you find the decision-making process has become anguishing for you and your partner, consider talking to a therapist or counselor. A professional therapist may be able to help you work through the emotions of your situation, assess all the options available, and arrive at a plan to resolve infertility that works for you (see chapters 11 and 15, "Staying Centered" and "Exploring Other Family-Building Options," respectively).

## WHEN THE PROBLEM MAY BE STRUCTURAL

To help you through the decision-making process when structural and age-related factors may be contributing to infertility, we have created the following decision tree based on the fictional single woman Valerie, 36 years old.

Valerie has known since she was a teenager that her mother took DES when she was pregnant with Valerie, and she has been vigilant about monitoring her reproductive health, with annual pelvic examinations and Pap smears. She has a moderately T-shaped uterus and has had two miscarriages since beginning treatment with DI about 2 years ago. Valerie conceived easily the first time, but miscarried at 6 weeks. It took eight cycles of DI to become pregnant the second time; unfortunately she miscarried after 8 weeks. Her specialist believes she still could carry a pregnancy and that her losses were unfortunate but random and unrelated to her uterine problem.

Here is Valerie's decision tree.

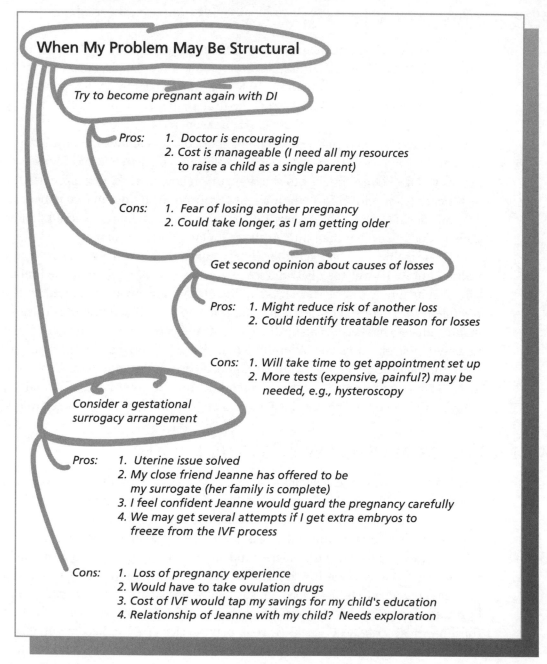

**When My Problem May Be Structural**

*Try to become pregnant again with DI*

*Pros:*    1.  Doctor is encouraging
2. Cost is manageable (I need all my resources to raise a child as a single parent)

*Cons:*    1.  Fear of losing another pregnancy
2. Could take longer, as I am getting older

*Get second opinion about causes of losses*

*Pros:*    1. Might reduce risk of another loss
2. Could identify treatable reason for losses

*Cons:*    1. Will take time to get appointment set up
2. More tests (expensive, painful?) may be needed, e.g., hysteroscopy

*Consider a gestational surrogacy arrangement*

*Pros:*    1.  Uterine issue solved
2. My close friend Jeanne has offered to be my surrogate (her family is complete)
3. I feel confident Jeanne would guard the pregnancy carefully
4. We may get several attempts if I get extra embryos to freeze from the IVF process

*Cons:*    1.  Loss of pregnancy experience
2. Would have to take ovulation drugs
3. Cost of IVF would tap my savings for my child's education
4. Relationship of Jeanne with my child? Needs exploration

**Decision:** Valerie has decided to take her medical records to another specialist for a second opinion. She has also made an appointment with an attorney who specializes in surrogacy contracts to discuss her friend's generous offer.

## POSITIVE STEPS YOU CAN TAKE FROM CHAPTER 7

**Explore your treatment options.** Effective surgical and hormonal treatments exist today for a wide range of problems affecting women's fertility. Selection of a competent and experienced medical team will improve your chances of overcoming obstacles to fertility.

**Consider IUI and ART.** Techniques such as IUI and ART are available to circumvent structural and immunologic problems, and can be used effectively in cases of unexplained infertility. Knowing when these techniques are appropriate can help you participate with your physician in devising a medically sound and cost-effective treatment plan.

**Learn more about your options when the woman's age is a factor.** Age-related infertility—from ovulatory dysfunction or failure—can be devastating. Learning as much as you can about the biology of human fertility may help you make decisions about continued pregnancy attempts using your own eggs and about when to consider alternative family-building options (see chapter 15, "Exploring Other Family-Building Options").

# 8 The Male: Diagnosis and Treatment

In this chapter, we will examine what could be causing a male factor infertility problem and explore available treatments. Throughout the text of this chapter, we will address the male partner of the couple.

Many of you reading this will work with physicians to find and solve your medical problem. The solution could be a surgical procedure. Another option may be one of the more sophisticated assisted reproductive technologies (ART) available to overcome the problem and fertilize your partner's eggs, or treatment could involve complex and intricate micromanipulation techniques to enhance fertilization. Some may opt to use donor sperm to create a family. Each couple will find the solution that best fits their own needs.

The options for biological family building, even in cases of severe male factor infertility, have never been better. Yet some techniques are expensive and may not be well covered by most insurance plans (see chapter 14, "Creating a Financial Game Plan and Getting Through the Insurance Maze"), and none is guaranteed successful. You and your partner may decide to explore both medical treatment and other paths to resolution, such as donor sperm insemination (DI), adoption, and childfree living, while you are on this journey. You will want to take a close look at the infertility decision tree at the end of this chapter, and create your own decision tree to help guide you through your very personal set of circumstances.

Do not be surprised if the male's experience is an emotional one. Just as a woman's feelings of self-worth and femininity may be wrapped up in issues of fertility and motherhood, so, too, may a man's sense of masculinity be associated with his ability to conceive a child. Some men may feel that a finding of low sperm count or poor sperm quality makes them somehow "less of a man" or not as virile. Feelings of guilt, anger, and low self-esteem may be quite profound, affecting every aspect of your life. Throughout this chapter, you will hear the voices of couples who have experienced male factor problems and learn from their experiences. In part 3, "Coping with Infertility," we offer more suggestions that can help you and your partner work through these emotions so that you can stay focused during this difficult time. As always, communication, being able to talk about your situation and the feelings you have about it, with the people you love most—and with your healthcare team, too—is an important element of going through infertility treatment. Discussing infertility issues in the supportive context of a RESOLVE group can also be beneficial.

---

### *Voices*

*Henry, a 34-year-old man, who with his wife, Pauline, went through years of treatment for male factor infertility and recently resolved to be childfree, says, "I found that if you don't say anything, you also don't learn anything. By talking about what was happening to us in a support group, I learned a lot from people who were also going through infertility treatments, or who knew someone who was. The more you talk, the more you learn."*

---

## THE DIAGNOSTIC WORK-UP FOR MEN

Your basic infertility work-up (see chapter 5, "The Basic Infertility Work-up for Women and Men"), includes a physical examination, semen analyses, and hormone-level blood testing. Other diagnostic tests will also need to be performed. You can review the normal values for male factor infertility tests by consulting the worksheet for men at the back of this book. You will want to use the worksheet to record the tests you have received and their results.

Sperm testing will determine whether you are producing sperm and, if so, how healthy that sperm is and how capable it is of penetrating and fertilizing an egg. The following terms are used to describe problems with sperm production or quality.

- **Aspermia** usually indicates a malfunction or obstruction of the glands that provide seminal fluid: the prostate and the seminal vesicles. No ejaculate is produced.

- **Azoospermia** means that there is a complete absence of sperm in your semen. This lack of sperm in the ejaculate could be caused by an obstruction of the vas deferens or epididymis that prevents the passage of sperm, or by failure of sperm to form or mature in the testes.
- **Oligospermia** is a term to describe a reduced number of normal sperm cells in your ejaculate.
- **Asthenospermia** describes poor motility and sperm that do not swim forward.

### Voices

*The pressure to attribute a source to an infertility problem can be tough for couples to deal with. After several miscarriages, Tina and Mark's physician suggested that Mark be tested. Tina recalls: "The tests came back with mixed results. The count was good, but the sperm didn't look good or swim well. So there was a male factor as well. I felt, thank goodness—it took the pressure off me a little bit. I'm sure Mark was frustrated with me, blamed me a little, but he was always supportive. Then, when he got his test results back, he felt the guilt the same way that I did. He just didn't take the weight of it the same way I did." Much of the time, there is not one clear-cut source of infertility, and couples learn that they must work together toward their goal of having a child, without placing blame or shouldering the burden of unreasonable guilt.*

If you receive a diagnosis of aspermia, azoospermia, oligospermia, or asthenospermia, your physician will perform additional tests. If you have no sperm in your semen analysis, the laboratory will check to see whether fructose is present in the semen. If none is present, absent vas deferens or blocked ejaculatory ducts are likely. Other laboratory tests to assist in the search for your diagnosis may include blood levels for the hormones follicle-stimulating hormone (FSH), luteinizing hormone (LH), testosterone, and prolactin.

If your sperm analysis is very poor but your hormone levels are normal, your physician may recommend other, more invasive, diagnostic tests described below.

## Testicular Biopsy

In most cases, the testicular biopsy is performed in a hospital as an outpatient day surgery under general or local anesthesia. During the procedure, the physician removes a small sample of tissue from each testicle and sends it out to a pathologist for microscopic examination to see whether the cells are producing adequate numbers of healthy sperm. A biopsy will show whether cells in the testicles are producing immature sperm cells, whether all sperm cells are absent (in which case only Sertoli cells or "support cells" will be seen), and whether other cells called Leydig cells, which produce testosterone, are also present and normal appearing.

Preliminary test results are available almost immediately, but it can take about a week to get the final report from the laboratory. If many sperm are present in the testicles, but not in the ejaculate, then a blockage probably exists somewhere in the epididymis or vas deferens (the gland and tubes that connect the testicles to the penis). To find the site of blockage, your physician may inspect the vas deferens under a microscope and take a sample of fluid directly from the duct itself. If sperm are present there, but not in the semen, then the tube is blocked. Another technique involves injecting saline into the vas deferens and, if the liquid does not flow freely into the bladder, then a blockage exists near the prostate. A catheter or nylon thread can be threaded through the vas deferens to find the blockage. For example, the thread will stop at the site of a prior hernia operation in the groin if the vas deferens was obstructed inadvertently during the hernia repair.

## Vasography

If these tests are inconclusive, a vasogram may be suggested. This technique involves sophisticated, invasive x-ray and should be done only if a testicular biopsy reveals normal sperm production. Under local or general anesthesia, the physician will make a small incision in the scrotum to expose the vas deferens and, using a microscope to avoid injuring the tiny vas, will inject contrast dye into the vas deferens or the ejaculatory duct and take x-rays. Obstructions or blockage can be identified by the patterns of the dye flow. Vasography should be done at the time microsurgery is performed to fix a blockage. This is because a vasogram itself can block the tiny (½ mm [millimeter]) passage inside of the vas deferens.

## Microsurgical Reconstruction and Sperm Retrieval

Incredible advances in the use of microsurgical techniques have brought new hope to men once considered permanently infertile. If you have a condition that prevents sperm from entering the seminal fluid or from leaving the penis, microsurgical reconstruction or sperm aspiration using microsurgical techniques is available.

- An obstructed epididymis or vas deferens can often be reconstructed using the latest microsurgical instruments. This procedure is done on an outpatient basis with a very short recuperation.
- Microsurgical epididymal sperm aspiration (MESA) allows a skilled urologic microsurgeon to retrieve sperm from the epididymis (the duct leading out from the testes where sperm mature).
- Testicular sperm extraction (TESE) is an offshoot of a testicular biopsy in which sperm are obtained from the tissue retrieved for the biopsy. If your sperm analysis shows that you are producing no sperm at all, your physician may perform TESE, which involves searching for small areas of sperm production in the testes and extracting the sperm from testicular tissue.

If MESA or TESE are used, the retrieved sperm are either frozen for future use or used immediately for in vitro fertilization (IVF) with intracytoplasmic sperm injection (ICSI)(see chapter 9, "Assisted Reproductive Technology (ART)").

If you produce a sperm count but it is very low, your physician may suggest the use of the sperm you have for IVF with ICSI.

## MALE FACTOR PROBLEMS

Your physician will structure your work-up on the basis of the following general categories of male factor issues:

- *Structural abnormalities.* Abnormalities of the reproductive tract that consist mainly of obstructions that partially or totally block the flow of sperm and/or seminal fluid. Some of these abnormalities may be present at birth (congenital), others may have occurred after infection of the urogenital tract, whereas others may result from previous surgery.
- *Sperm production disorders.* The production of sperm is inhibited.
- *Ejaculatory disturbances.* These disturbances prevent sperm from reaching the female.
- *Immunologic disorders.* These disorders prevent sperm from meeting and successfully penetrating the egg in the female genital tract.

### Congenital Abnormalities

In some cases, problems that were present at birth can affect a man's fertility. Surgery performed during childhood to correct the abnormalities in the reproductive system can affect fertility, as well.

- *Congenital absence of the vas deferens (CAVD).* A rare condition in which the vas deferens, the tube that leads out from the testicle, is absent from birth. Although testicular function is normal, the vas deferens is not present to contribute sperm to the ejaculate, which means that no sperm can leave the body. In such cases, sperm can be collected directly from the epididymis and used for IVF with ICSI. Many men with absent vasa deferentia are carriers of a mutation of the cystic fibrosis gene. These men do not have cystic fibrosis themselves but may pass the gene to their offspring. After testing, genetic counseling may be recommended.

- *Undescended testes.* Undescended testes, a condition also called *cryptorchidism*, is the absence at birth of one or both of the testes. The testis may be malpositioned within the groin or abdomen or, less commonly, absent altogether. This condition is more common in premature infants because the testes do not fully descend until after the seventh month of gestation. Sometimes, hormones are given to a child to bring the undescended testis into place. If the testes have not descended by the child's first birthday, they will not do so spontaneously, and the condition is treated surgically (orchiopexy) at 12 to 15 months of age. If left untreated, the testis can shrivel and atrophy, which can lead to irreversible infertility in adulthood. Men with cryptorchidism, even after corrective surgery, have a higher incidence of testicular cancer.

- *Hypospadias.* In this congenital defect, which affects about 1 in 500 newborns, the urethral opening (meatus) is not in its normal position at the tip of the penis. In its mildest form, the opening is on the underside of the penis; in its most severe form, it may be as far away as the scrotum. Meatal misplacement is often associated with a condition that causes the penis to curve downward; the more severe the degree of hypospadias, the more curved the penis.

  Hypospadias can be treated surgically if the condition is severe and the penis is deformed. However, mild cases may go unnoticed and affect fertility later. Because the opening of the urethra is farther up on the shaft of the penis in a man with hypospadias, he is unable to deposit his sperm as deep in the vagina as he would if he had a normal urethral opening. If the hypospadias is mild to moderate, it can usually be corrected even in adulthood. If not, intrauterine insemination (IUI) may be the best option.

Other conditions present at birth that affect male fertility include the following:

- *Kallmann's syndrome*, which is a hypothalamic failure resulting in lack of the essential hormone gonadotropin-releasing hormone (GnRH) for sperm production. We will discuss this condition in greater detail later in this chapter in the context of hormonal problems.
- *Klinefelter's syndrome*, in which an extra X chromosome is present. This results in the individual having very small, poorly functioning testes, azoospermia, and, often, mild breast enlargement and testosterone deficiency. Men with Klinefelter's syndrome also tend to have long arms and legs, little body or facial hair, and wide hips.
- *Sertoli-cell only syndrome*, is the complete absence of germ cells (sperm-producing cells). In these rare cases, men are born without any germ cells at all (or very few) in their testes, which means that they cannot produce sperm.

In both Klinefelter's syndrome and Sertoli-cell only syndrome, no medical treatment is available, but in a few cases small pockets of sperm production can sometimes be identified and sperm extraction performed. The sperm can then be used for IVF with ICSI.

## Infections and Previous Surgery

Both infections and previous surgeries in the urogenital tract may lead to scarring that blocks the transport of sperm or seminal fluid. In more than half the cases, microsurgery can help clear the blockage, but often sperm must be retrieved directly from the vas deferens, epididymis, or testes for IVF with ICSI. To diagnose a blockage, testicular biopsy and a vasogram are useful.

### For Your Information

Sperm production is negatively affected by external influences, especially heat. Your sperm count may be lower immediately after an illness accompanied by a high fever. Therefore, you should have a repeat semen analysis in 3 months.

## Retrograde Ejaculation

Retrograde ejaculation is a fairly unusual phenomenon in which the semen, rather than being ejaculated from the penis, enters the bladder during orgasm. Various conditions can cause retrograde ejaculation, including diabetes, prostate surgery, bladder surgery as a child, and use of certain medications such as those used to treat high blood pressure and mood disorders. It occurs because these conditions sometimes weaken the nerves that would normally close down the bladder's sphincter muscle to keep urine from entering the ejaculate and the ejaculate from flowing back into the bladder. Men with spinal cord injuries may also have retrograde ejaculation.

Your physician will suspect retrograde ejaculation if after ejaculation you produce a small amount of semen with a low sperm count, or if your urine looks milky when you void shortly after orgasm and ejaculation. A diagnosis is confirmed if a large quantity of sperm cells is found in a detailed urinalysis.

Treatment with common cold medicines, such as Sudafed, can sometimes correct the problem, helping to close the bladder more effectively during ejaculation. In addition, your physician may put you on oral alkalinizing agents to decrease the acidic quality of your urine, and thus prevent the urine from killing sperm. After orgasm, the urine can be removed from the bladder either by having you void or through the use of a special catheter, and the sperm can then be separated from the urine. The sperm may then be used with an IUI or an IVF procedure.

## Impotence

Approximately 25 to 30 million American men suffer from impotence, yet according to the Impotence Resource Center, only 5 percent ever seek treatment. Impotence, also known as erectile dysfunction (ED), is the inability to achieve or maintain an adequate erection during sexual intercourse. It is important to realize that an occasional episode of impotence occurs for most men, is perfectly normal, and is no cause for alarm—and that is especially true as you continue along the infertility journey. As we will discuss further in chapter 13, "Enhancing Your Relationship: Sexuality, Intimacy, and Infertility," your sexual relationship with your partner may well change when getting pregnant, rather than sensual pleasure, becomes the primary motivation for sex.

When impotence proves to be a pattern or a persistent problem, it may indicate the presence of a medical disorder or a psychological problem. Contrary to popular belief, impotence is neither strictly a disease of aging nor is it primarily caused by psychological factors. Only 15 percent of impotence cases can be attributed entirely to depression, stress, or anxiety. Usually, it is a secondary problem brought on by physical conditions, and often it is a combination of physical and psychological factors. If you are having a problem getting or maintaining an erection, do not assume it is caused by stress—even if you are under a great deal of it. Instead, see a physician for an evaluation and advice.

If your fertility problem stems solely from ED, talk with your physician about counseling, breaking certain lifestyle habits, changing medications, or treatment with sildenafil (Viagra). Treatment with Viagra may be helpful for impotency that affects fertility. Your physician will decide whether Viagra is appropriate for you and will explain the possible (sometimes serious) complications and side effects. But remember that impotence is rarely the cause of primary infertility. However, during infertility treatments, such as inseminations or ART, when the male is under pressure to produce a semen specimen, impotency can be an issue.

# VASECTOMY AND VARICOCELE

Several conditions can impede or prevent the development of healthy sperm or the ejaculation of sperm. They include voluntary sterilization and problems of poor circulation in the testes.

## Vasectomy

One of the most common structural disruptions of the male ductal system is caused by voluntary vasectomy. Each year, more than 500,000 American men undergo this simple surgical procedure as a birth control method—and about 5 percent or more will later change their minds. The vasectomy procedure is actually quite simple: A surgeon removes about a ½- to 1-inch segment of the vas deferens and seals the end of the vas deferens with stitches, heat, or nonreactive clips (staples). Once severed, the vas deferens can no longer contribute sperm to the ejaculate, and thus no sperm can enter the female reproductive tract.

Today, thanks in large part to microsurgical techniques, many men who have had vasectomies can have the effects of those surgeries reversed through a procedure called *vasovasostomy*, or vasectomy reversal. During vasectomy reversal, the surgeon will use microsurgical techniques to check for the presence of sperm, then rejoin the severed vas deferens. If no sperm are found or they are of poor quality, the surgeon can check for blockage that may have occurred in the epididymis. Such blockages may be repaired microsurgically and, if sperm are found, the vas deferens can be sewn to an open epididymal tubule (vaso epididymovasostomy). This surgery is more difficult to perform because the epididymal tubules are very thin and delicate. Most microsurgeons recommend collecting motile sperm from the epididymis at the time of surgery and freezing it for use in case the surgery fails. This type of surgery is very difficult and should only be done by surgeons who do many of these operations.

## VASECTOMY
## VASOVASOSTOMY

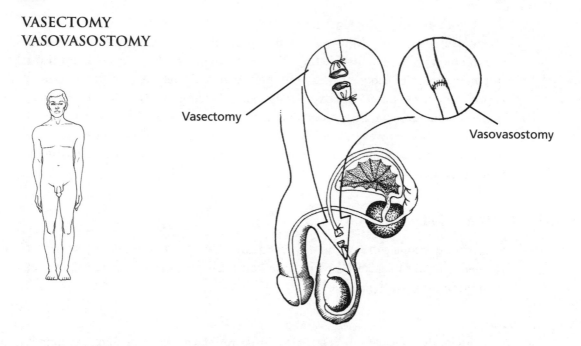

Vasectomy

Vasovasostomy

One factor that works against successful reversal is the length of time between the vasectomy and the surgery to reverse it. As this time interval increases, the likelihood of success from a vas to vas reconnection decreases. In addition, it appears that vasectomies may cause sperm antibodies to form, which can interfere with sperm motility or block the sperm from attaching to the egg. If this occurs, it means that even if a surgeon successfully reverses the vasectomy and you have sperm in your ejaculate, you may still have diminished fertility. However, the presence of antisperm antibodies does not necessarily mean that fertilization will not occur (see the discussion of antisperm antibodies later in this chapter).

### Questions to Ask

If you are thinking about having a vasovasostomy, ask your physician the following questions:

- How many vasovasostomies do you perform in 1 year? How many vaso epididymovasostomies in 1 year?
- Do you aspirate sperm for use during an IVF procedure?
- Can you freeze sperm extracted during an operation for future use?

## Varicocele

A varicocele is a bundle of enlarged (varicose) veins located around the testicle. Most varicoceles (up to about 60 percent) are found only on the left side, but many men have bilateral varicoceles.

Scientists still are not sure exactly what the connection is between varicoceles and infertility. Varicocele is caused by defects in the valves in the veins of the testicle. This produces an abnormal backflow of blood from the abdomen into the scrotum resulting in a rise in temperature in the testes that may interfere with testosterone levels and the production and maturation of sperm. Varicoceles are very common in both the fertile and infertile population: It is possible that up to 10 to 15 percent of the male population may have a varicocele. Small varicoceles can affect fertility in some men; in others with large varicoceles, there is no compromised fertility. Approximately 40 to 50 percent of men evaluated for infertility are found to have a varicocele.

Your physician may suspect that your varicocele is causing a problem if your sperm analysis reveals an increased number of abnormally shaped sperm or poor sperm motility. This typical pattern seen in men with varicocele and other cases of impaired sperm production is called the "stress pattern." It is often a challenge to the laboratory to differentiate between the immature cells frequently seen in the patient with a varicocele and white blood cells found when there is infection. Special tests are used to differentiate these very similar appearing cells.

## VARICOCELE

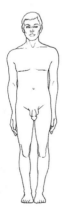
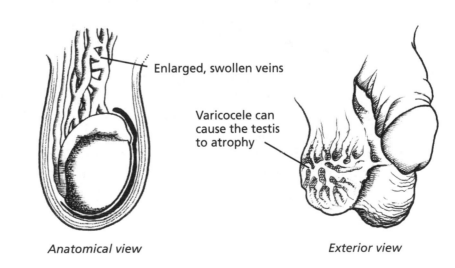

Enlarged, swollen veins

Varicocele can cause the testis to atrophy

*Anatomical view*

*Exterior view*

Some varicoceles are large enough for a physician to feel during the physical examination portion of the basic infertility work-up (see chapter 5, "The Basic Infertility Work-up for Women and Men"). Ultrasound or a Doppler stethoscope, which magnifies the sound of blood traveling through the testicular veins, may also be used for harder-to-find though suspected varicoceles. Other techniques include a thermogram, a device that identifies pockets of heat in the testicles such as those that occur with varicoceles, and venography, a procedure in which radiopaque dye is injected through veins in the groin and x-rays are taken to document the blood flow in the testicle.

Chances are you will not know that you have a varicocele until your physician examines you. In severe cases, the testicle may be atrophic (small) and feel tender, or heavy, especially after exercise or standing for a long time. The presence of a varicocele does not mean that surgical correction is required. However, if there is a low sperm count and atrophy (shrinkage) of the affected testicle, surgery is usually recommended. If, on the other hand, your sperm analysis was marginal and the varicocele is not evident on the physical examination (that is, your physician finds it only on ultrasound), surgical correction may not be recommended.

### Voices

*Greg just underwent surgery to repair a varicocele. "Guys aren't supposed to show their emotions. I have to be supportive of my wife and I have to stay calm and not feel my stuff until later," Greg asserts. "Society says it shouldn't be as hard for me as it is for her. But it is hard to fail. Every month was failing, every cycle a failure. Then it became like a challenge, like 'I'm going to beat this.' And then it became more of an issue of not failing than it was about a baby. These days, one day I feel great and the next.... Now with the surgery—it's something I can do. The waiting, though, to see if this will work for Jena and me is hard."*

## Treatment of Varicocele: Varicocelectomy

If your physician determines that a varicocele may be the cause of your poor sperm analysis, you may elect surgery to correct the condition. There are three approaches for the treatment of a varicocele: conventional surgery, microsurgery, or nonsurgical techniques to block the vein using a small balloon or special substances (occluding agents) injected into the vein to cause it to close. The method your physician and surgeon choose depends on the size and location of the varicocele, among other factors. The procedures include the following:

• *Conventional surgery.* If your surgeon decides to use the surgical approach, it can be either inguinal (in the middle of the groin) or subinguinal (just above the scrotal sac). The surgery takes place in a hospital, and you will be under either local or general anesthesia. The surgeon makes a 2- to 3-inch incision in your groin and lifts the spermatic cord out of the deeper tissue, identifies enlarged veins, and ties them off with sutures. This procedure corrects the abnormal blood flow in the swollen veins. The skin stitches may require removal about a week later or may be absorbable. It may take 1 to 2 weeks to recover completely. Some men, less than 10 percent, who have this surgery suffer recurrences and may have to have the vein occluded again at a later date. The surgery may infrequently cause complications such as the formation of a hydrocele, a collection of fluid around the testicle, or damage to the testicular artery that brings blood into the testicle. In the case of a hydrocele, which can form if too many of the tiny lymph ducts that run close to the veins are also tied, a later hydrocele repair may be elected. If damage to the testicular artery occurs, the organ will not necessarily suffer noticeable damage, as there are two other arteries supplying the testes. Loss of testicular size is a very infrequent problem.

• *Microsurgery.* Thanks to advances in microsurgical techniques, the treatment of varicocele has become much easier and less fraught with potential complications. The procedure can be performed under local anesthesia on an outpatient basis—which means you go home the same day. Using microsurgical equipment and an operating microscope, the surgeon can make an incision of less than an inch in the groin and then identify and tie off the veins that form the varicocele. No visible skin stitches are required. This method has a failure rate of only 1 percent.

• *Nonsurgical approaches (percutaneous occlusion).* Other techniques to repair a varicocele use small silicone balloons, coils, or occlusing agents to block off the veins. This type of repair, which does not require a general anesthetic, takes place in an outpatient setting. A specially trained radiologist makes a half-inch incision in the groin, threads a tiny catheter into a large vein in the thigh, up into a kidney vein, and down again into the testicular vein. Using a sophisticated x-ray, the radiologist passes an even tinier balloon or coil through the catheter until it reaches the varicocele, then inflates the balloon or releases the coil to obstruct the abnormal veins and allow blood to flow out of the testicle in a normal way. These devices remain in place permanently. It should be noted that there are risks with these types of repair: If the device (balloon or coil) becomes dislodged, damage to other tissues could occur. Although this complication is rare, it can be quite serious. This method has a higher failure rate than microsurgical varicocele repair (15 to 25 percent).

### Success Rates After Varicocele Repair

According to controlled studies reported in a 1995 issue of *Fertility and Sterility*, up to 70 percent of men will have improved sperm counts and better sperm motility after surgical varicocele repair, and thus can expect to improve their chances of fathering a child. Some studies site an average of 50 percent of the partners of men who have had varicocele will become pregnant within 2 years of surgery. Remember that it will take at least 3 months after surgery to see potential improvement in semen analysis, inasmuch as that is the time necessary for a man's reproductive system to produce entirely new sperm.

In rare cases, your physician may prescribe the drug clomiphene citrate (Clomid or Serophene) to help increase your sperm count after a varicocelectomy.

## HORMONAL IMBALANCES AND IMMUNE SYSTEM PROBLEMS

Other conditions that affect sperm production or maturation involve hormonal imbalances and immune system problems.

### Endocrine Disorders

A small percentage of infertile men—about 5 to 10 percent—have a disturbance of their hormonal systems. As discussed in chapter 2, "Normal Fertility," the male reproductive system is controlled by three main hormones. GnRH, released by the hypothalamus, stimulates the pituitary gland to secrete LH and FSH. In turn, LH and FSH stimulate the maturation of the testes and the production of sperm. Specifically, LH triggers the Leydig cells of the testes to manufacture testosterone, whereas FSH influences the Sertoli cells, which support and nurture sperm cells. Another hormone, prolactin, is also potentially involved in infertility. If present in excess, prolactin can interfere with LH stimulation of the Leydig cells, which in turns slows down the production of testosterone and interferes with sperm production.

Treatment of hormonal disorders in men involves the use of the same drugs that women take to correct their hormonal disorders, namely clomiphene citrate, human menopausal gonadotropin (hMG), human chorionic gonadotropin (hCG), FSH, or bromocriptine. Here is a description of some of the conditions involving hormonal disruption and how these conditions might be treated.

• *Kallmann's syndrome and other cases of hypogonadotropic hypogonadism.* Rarely, infertility can result from a failure of the hypothalamus to produce and release GnRH, which results in a complete lack of FSH, LH, and, hence, testosterone and sperm. In such cases, secondary sex characteristics, such as facial and body hair, may also be affected. Fortunately, fertility can often be restored with drug therapy. If you suffer from Kallmann's syndrome, your physician will most likely suggest that you start by taking hCG injections, probably 3 times a week for about 6 months. The hCG will help stimulate the production of testosterone. If your testosterone reaches normal levels, you will then start to add hMG, FSH, or FSH/LH to stimulate the production of sperm. Possible side effects, reported by men using these drugs, include soreness at the injection site and, rarely, breast enlargement.

• *Hypothyroidism or pituitary tumors.* The thyroid plays a role in regulating many glands in your body. Blood tests may be done to document normal thyroid-stimulating hormone (TSH) levels, even though abnormal levels of TSH produce only a rare case of male infertility. In some men, the hormone prolactin can be elevated, which may affect sperm count and/or quality.

• *Unexplained low levels of FSH, LH, or testosterone.* In many cases, physicians are unable to identify a cause for a hormonal imbalance in an infertile man. If you fall into this category and you have a low sperm count, your physician may prescribe hormone treatments to correct the problem. If your levels of FSH and LH are mildly reduced, for instance, taking a dose of clomiphene citrate once a day or once every other day for several months can sometimes boost the pituitary's release of these hormones. Rare side effects reported by men taking clomiphene include enlarged breasts and changes in their night vision. If your deficiency of FSH and LH is more severe, your physician might prescribe hMG for about 3 to 6 months. Finally, if you exhibit low levels of testosterone along with a low sperm count, your physician might suggest that you inject hCG 3 times a week. hCG may help stimulate the Leydig cells to produce testosterone, which may in turn increase sperm production from the testicles. However, it is important to note that only rarely does taking hormones significantly improve sperm production in men with unexplained infertility. Discuss the benefits of taking medication thoroughly with your physician before starting on a long course of drug therapy.

## Antisperm Antibodies

Some men produce antibodies (immunologic proteins that attack foreign cells) to their own sperm, resulting in poor sperm motility or agglutination (sperm are linked together by the head or tail and thus unable to fertilize an egg). Antibodies may also just coat the sperm, which means that sperm retain their motility but are unable to attach to the egg when they meet it. (Your partner can also produce antibodies against your sperm, which is a problem discussed in chapter 7, "The Female: Structural Problems, Age-Related Factors, and Treatment.")

In some cases, men begin to form antisperm antibodies if their vas deferens or epididymis is blocked on one side from surgery, such as following a hernia repair, or infection. When sperm are not ejaculated but are absorbed by the body, the immune system reacts to the sperm as a foreign invader, attacking the sperm as it would a bacteria or virus.

The most common cause for antisperm antibodies in men is vasectomy. In these men, the immune system produces not only cells that act to resolve the inflammation but also cells that mistakenly attach to the accumulating sperm. The production of sperm antibodies may persist, even if the vasectomy is reversed, which may, but not always, compromise sperm quality and function.

A specialized sperm analysis and other specific blood tests can detect antisperm antibodies. A test called the immunobead binding assay (IBD) is one of the most informative and specific of all tests currently available to detect antisperm antibodies bound to the surface of the sperm.

### Treatment of Antisperm Antibodies

Treatment of antisperm antibodies in men may include prescription of oral steroid drugs such as prednisone, which helps reduce the inflammation that can trigger antisperm antibody production and activity. However, if the condition is serious, most physicians recommend sperm washing followed by IUI, or IVF with ICSI.

## OTHER SPERM PRODUCTION PROBLEMS

Several other diseases or conditions, all fairly rare, may prevent or interfere with sperm production or maturation. They include the following:

• *Adult mumps infection.* Although all American children are now vaccinated against mumps, in the past, mumps was a common infection. If you had the mumps when you were a child, your symptoms may have been swollen salivary glands and a high fever. If infection occurred after puberty, however, the disease might have destroyed sperm-producing cells in the testes. In about 70 percent of these cases, only one testicle was affected, but some men were left permanently sterile from the disease if both testes became involved.

• *Trauma to the testicles.* In rare cases, a sports injury or accident can cause vessels that nourish the testicles to rupture, which reduces the oxygen supply to sperm-producing cells and may cause them to die. Such injuries require immediate surgery, or infertility could be the result. Another form of trauma is surgery to repair a hernia or to reposition an undescended testicle. If, during surgery, the blood supply is cut off for any reason, serious injury to the testes can result.

• *Prostate infection.* The prostate gland is vulnerable to infection, a condition called prostatitis, which can cause a decrease in sperm motility and sperm count while the infection is active. Unfortunately, even with antibiotics, the bacteria that cause the infection can remain in the lobes of the prostate and cause recurrent flare-ups. Usually, if the testicles are not involved in the infection, sperm production rebounds after a few months.

## INSEMINATION AS A TREATMENT OPTION

Artificial insemination with sperm from the male partner (sometimes called *husband insemination,* or AIH) is sometimes indicated in cases of otherwise untreated male factor infertility in the following situations:

- • when sperm are produced in abnormally low numbers,
- • when the number of healthy motile (swimming) sperm is reduced,
- • or when sperm do not survive in the cervical mucus.

### For Your Information

There are some products that fall under the category of nutritional supplements that may be of benefit to sperm count and quality. Ask your physician about these products.

Insemination involves the placement of specially prepared sperm into the woman's uterus in a procedure called IUI (For more on IUI, see chapter 7, "The Female: Structural Problems, Age-Related Factors, and Treatment"). The male partner or donor will produce a semen specimen, preferably at the clinic site or physician's office. The sperm are then prepared for IUI in a process called sperm washing or sperm separation. Separation selects out motile sperm from a man's ejaculate and concentrates them into a small volume. Sperm washing also cleanses the sperm of potentially toxic chemicals that may cause adverse reactions in the uterus. If the male partner is contributing sperm, the prepared sperm will be used immediately for IUI. Sperm collected from donors is prepared and frozen for future use.

***Voices***

*"I know this isn't true for all men," admits Dan, a 38-year-old man diagnosed with a very low sperm count. "But I never felt that having this problem made me less of a man—and neither did my wife. It was a medical problem, with a medical solution. I grieved over not being able to have my own biological child, but in the end, it was being a father that mattered. I'm a father to my two children, donor sperm or no donor sperm."*

Hundreds of thousands of couples choose to use sperm from a third-party donor to conceive their children. Although micromanipulation and IVF approaches help more and more couples with male factor infertility, for some, donor sperm remains the most affordable, successful, and readily available option. With donor sperm, you will choose a donor from among many offered at a sperm bank or fertility clinic. See chapter 15, "Exploring Other Family-Building Options," for information on third-party donor insemination (DI).

## ART, DI, or Adoption?

Today, there are more options for a couple with male factor infertility, a combination of male and female factor infertility, or unexplained infertility. If your situation falls into one of these categories, using decision tree worksheets can help you work through each available option. We offer the following sample decision tree, based on the fictional couple Amy and Sam, a couple with a combination of male and female factor infertility. Study the decision-making process in this example. Then, consider creating your own decision tree.

Amy and Sam are 28 and 35 years old and began trying to conceive right after their recent marriage. Amy has always had severe cramps with her menstrual cycle, but in recent years she has often been incapacitated with her period. The couple decided to consult an infertility specialist after 6 months of trying to become pregnant.

On the basis of Amy's symptoms and medical history, the physician quickly recommended laparoscopy, found severe endometriosis, and removed the disease and associated adhesions. Amy continued to experience pain, so the physician prescribed a birth control pill for several months, which has helped with the pain.

When Amy started treatment, Sam had a semen analysis. To the couple's shock, there were no sperm in Sam's semen. A testicular biopsy has confirmed the presence of healthy sperm, and the physician suspects blockage at the epididymis. The physician recommends IVF with TESE and ICSI as the most promising option for Amy and Sam to have a biological child.

The couple has thoroughly reviewed their health insurance policy, written a

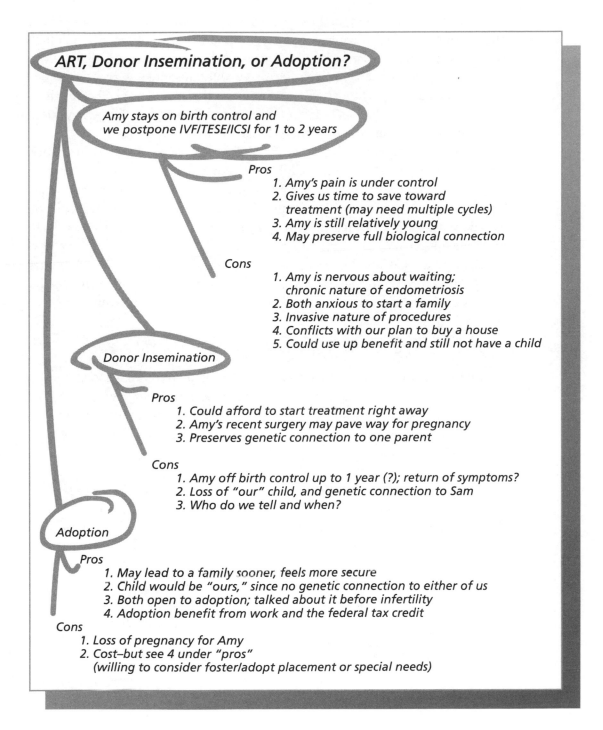

**ART, Donor Insemination, or Adoption?**

*Amy stays on birth control and
we postpone IVF/TESE/ICSI for 1 to 2 years*

Pros
1. Amy's pain is under control
2. Gives us time to save toward
   treatment (may need multiple cycles)
3. Amy is still relatively young
4. May preserve full biological connection

Cons
1. Amy is nervous about waiting;
   chronic nature of endometriosis
2. Both anxious to start a family
3. Invasive nature of procedures
4. Conflicts with our plan to buy a house
5. Could use up benefit and still not have a child

Donor Insemination

Pros
1. Could afford to start treatment right away
2. Amy's recent surgery may pave way for pregnancy
3. Preserves genetic connection to one parent

Cons
1. Amy off birth control up to 1 year (?); return of symptoms?
2. Loss of "our" child, and genetic connection to Sam
3. Who do we tell and when?

Adoption

Pros
1. May lead to a family sooner, feels more secure
2. Child would be "ours," since no genetic connection to either of us
3. Both open to adoption; talked about it before infertility
4. Adoption benefit from work and the federal tax credit

Cons
1. Loss of pregnancy for Amy
2. Cost—but see 4 under "pros"
   (willing to consider foster/adopt placement or special needs)

letter of predetermination, and found they have coverage for two cycles of IVF, but not for the TESE procedure. Amy's employer offers a $5,000 "family-building" benefit, which may be used toward uncovered infertility treatment or adoption.

After sketching their decision tree, Amy and Sam spoke with several couples who had children through DI; some had told their families and had plans to tell the children or had told them, some planned never to tell. They were impressed with the smooth transition all had made to parenting.

**Decision:** The couple went back to their infertility therapist to work through their options. Amy realized that the return of endometriosis symptoms terrified her and that she was more interested in parenting than in pregnancy. The couple decided to adopt. The financial assistance and tax relief available for adoption means they can reach a satisfying and more certain goal sooner. They may revisit a genetic option after they adopt their first child.

Remember that the decision-making process is unique to each individual and couple. In creating your own decision tree, you will work through the options in your own way to arrive at the decision that is best for you.

## POSITIVE STEPS YOU CAN TAKE FROM CHAPTER 8

**Explore treatment options.** Today, there are more treatment options open to men with male factor infertility than ever before. The most promising treatments require a skilled urologic surgeon or fertility specialist. Seeing the most experienced professional available to diagnose and treat your problem is the best investment of time and money you can make.

**Keep the lines of communication open.** Infertility can be an isolating experience to both you and your partner, even as you strive together to build your family. For some, that is especially true if they feel that the problem is their "fault." Make every effort to discuss how you are feeling and what you are thinking at each stage in the process.

**Stay current.** Research new breakthroughs by asking questions of your physician, reading, and joining RESOLVE. We are dedicated to educating you with the most current information about medical treatments available.

# 9 Assisted Reproductive Technology (ART)

If you are reading this chapter, you have probably started to consider high-tech treatment to improve your chances of getting pregnant. In this chapter, procedures and techniques used in the assisted reproductive technologies (ART) are explained.

## WHAT IS ART?

ART is defined by the U.S. Centers for Disease Control and Prevention (CDC) as "all treatments or procedures that involve the handling of human eggs and sperm for the purpose of helping a woman become pregnant." Types of ART include in vitro fertilization (IVF), gamete intrafallopian transfer (GIFT), zygote intrafallopian transfer (ZIFT), embryo cryopreservation, egg or embryo donation, and gestational carriers. Note that ART does *not* include intrauterine insemination (IUI), with either partner or donor sperm. Issues surrounding third-party parenting options, such as donor egg and embryo, donor sperm, and surrogacy, will be addressed in chapter 15, "Exploring Other Family-Building Options."

In this chapter, we will:

- *describe* the steps involved in an IVF, GIFT, and ZIFT procedure;
- *describe* micromanipulation techniques and the developing technique of preimplantation genetic diagnosis; and
- *help you understand* reported success rates in ART cycles.

Before committing to intensive ART therapy, you should review with your physician your condition and prior therapy. The decision to move from conventional therapy (such as IUI for some) to ART should be considered carefully in view of the time, expense, emotional aspects, and risks involved. One of the most important risks to consider is hyperstimulation of the ovaries from taking ovulatory medication, which is more likely to occur in younger patients (see chapter 6, "The Female: Hormonal Disorders and Treatment"). Factors that may influence your likelihood of success, such as your age and ovarian reserve, also should be reviewed with the physician (see chapter 7, "The Female: Structural Problems, Age-Related Factors, and Treatment"). Create a decision tree and use your journal to work through the complicated emotional, financial, and treatment issues associated with your situation and options.

### Voices

*Brenna, mother of a 2-year-old son, remembers, "We started down the road of trying an insemination, then drugs and insemination; we didn't have to go to IVF yet. But, based on the results of Bill's further sperm testing—sperm motility and sperm morphology—we became IVF and intracytoplasmic sperm injection (ICSI) candidates. We were beginning to think we might not be able to have biological children, but we still felt we had a long way to go before we'd reach that conclusion. Fortunately, the financial end wasn't an issue for us; we had good insurance and enough savings to cover the out-of-pocket expenses—at least for a couple of cycles. We were thrilled when we succeeded with the first cycle."*

*Sandro and his wife, Diana, have just decided to try two cycles of IVF. Sandro says, "Di and I have been very close through every single step. I was a little ahead of her on the IVF, but I feel strongly that we owe it to ourselves to try."*

## IN VITRO FERTILIZATION (IVF)

IVF gets its name from the fact that fertilization occurs outside of the body, in a laboratory dish, instead of in the woman's fallopian tube. (In vitro means *in glass*, although today the laboratory dishes are plastic.) If fertilization takes place, the physician transfers the embryo(s) into the woman's uterus for possible implantation.

IVF was developed as a technique to assist women who had blocked or absent fallopian tubes to become pregnant. The first successful IVF procedure was done in the United Kingdom and resulted in the birth of Louise Brown in 1978. In the two decades since her birth, IVF and other ART procedures have

IVF

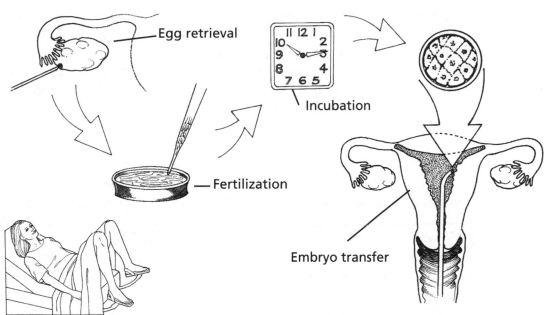

become a growing and important part of infertility treatment. Today, they are used to treat many infertility problems, including tubal factor, endometriosis, male factor, and unexplained infertility. In the United States in 1996 (the most current reported data available at the time this book went to press), 300 clinics reported doing 64,036 ART cycles (92 percent of which were IVF), resulting in the birth of 20,659 babies.

## Preparing for an IVF Cycle

An IVF cycle involves the following preliminary steps:

- Before the first cycle, the physician may do a trial or mock embryo transfer. This involves passing a catheter through the cervix into the uterus to determine its path through the cervix and to measure the distance to the top (fundus) of the uterine cavity.
- IVF normally is preceded by the use of ovulation-stimulating drugs to increase the number of mature eggs that can be retrieved. Far less common is natural cycle, or unstimulated, IVF, in which an egg is retrieved from a woman during her normal menstrual cycle, without the use of drugs.
- The physician will perform a semen analysis of the male partner.

## Drug Regimens

There are several drug regimens that may be used. Lupron (by injection) or Synarel (by nasal spray), both gonadotropin-releasing hormone (GnRH) agonists, or Antagon (by injection), a GnRH antagonist, are given to suppress hormone function and reduce the risk of a premature surge in luteinizing hormone (LH), which could result in eggs being released into the pelvic cavity before the egg retrieval procedure. In the so-called down-regulation protocol, the GnRH agonist is started on day 21 of the menstrual cycle before the IVF cycle begins. When the ovulation-stimulating drugs are started, typically on day 2 or 3 of the IVF cycle, the dose of GnRH agonist may be reduced, but it is continued until the human chorionic gonadotropin (hCG) shot is given just before egg retrieval. In the "flare-up" protocol, the GnRH agonist is started on day 2 or 3 of the IVF cycle, at the same time ovulation-stimulating drugs are started. Sometimes low-dose birth control pills are used before GnRH agonist suppression and ovarian stimulation as well.

Ovulatory-stimulating medications known as gonadotropins, such as Pergonal, Humegon, Repronex, Fertinex, Follistim, or Gonal F, are used to stimulate the ovaries to produce mature eggs. Frequent early morning transvaginal ultrasound examinations and blood tests (about every 2 to 3 days) will allow the clinic to assess your response to the drugs, monitor for hyperstimulation of the ovaries, and adjust the dose as needed. When the largest follicles reach maturity, between 18 and 22 mm in diameter, estradiol levels are usually about 150 to 400 pg/mL (picograms per milliliter) per mature follicle. At that time, a shot of hCG (Profasi, Pregnyl, or Novarel) will be ordered to trigger the release of the mature eggs. Egg retrieval will be scheduled for approximately 32 to 36 hours later. (See chapter 6, "The Female: Hormonal Disorders and Treatment," for a full discussion of these medications.)

Cancellation of a cycle of ART occurs in 10 to 20 percent of cases, either because a woman has not stimulated well or has overstimulated. Standard doses of ovulatory drugs are selected by the physician on the basis of clinical experience, and then individualized for particular patients. Occasionally, women overrespond to ovulatory medication, risking hyperstimulation of the ovaries. Sometimes this is managed by withdrawing drugs for a few days, known as "coasting." Other instances require cancellation of the cycle.

### Voices

*"I have become bloated from a mild hyperstimulation reaction, and I liken myself to the girl in* Willy Wonka and the Chocolate Factory *who blew up like a blueberry,"* says Jane. *"You get the point . . . it is hard to create funny moments here, but Aaron*

*and I try to maintain a sense of humor to get through it all. Humor and love are the keys to dealing with life and all crises, including this ongoing one, which hopefully is soon to be resolved."*

## Egg Retrieval

Egg retrieval is done in the physician's office or outpatient procedure room, often under intravenous sedation. Using transvaginal ultrasound to visualize the follicles in the ovaries, the physician inserts a needle through the vagina to aspirate the eggs out of the follicles. The procedure takes 15 to 60 minutes and, except for grogginess and some mild pelvic discomfort, there should be no after-effects. Although there is a very small risk of ovarian bleeding or infection, this complication is rare.

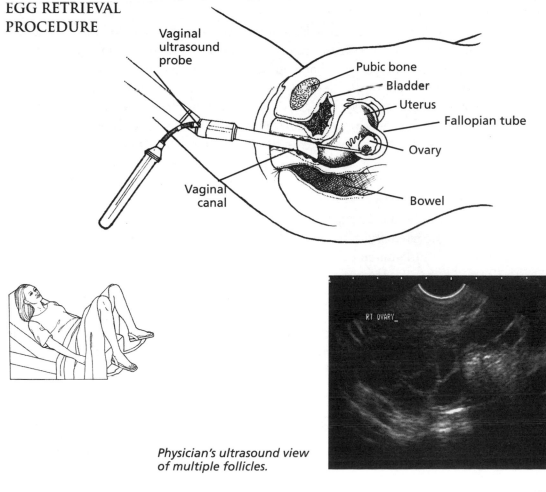

**EGG RETRIEVAL PROCEDURE**

Vaginal ultrasound probe

Pubic bone

Bladder

Uterus

Fallopian tube

Ovary

Bowel

Vaginal canal

RT OVARY

*Physician's ultrasound view of multiple follicles.*

As soon as the eggs are retrieved, they are graded 1 to 5 by the embryologist. Grade 1 indicates the best development. The eggs are incubated for several hours in the Petri dish before the sperm cells are added. The combined egg and sperm are incubated and reevaluated in 12 to 18 hours for signs of fertilization. (See the section later in this chapter describing micromanipulation techniques used to promote or improve egg fertilization.) Within 18 hours, many embryos will have two pronuclei (one nucleus of chromosomes from the man and one from the woman) and will continue to grow and divide until the day of transfer. Between 18 and 20 hours after fertilization, the embryos are moved to a different culture medium. Some clinics add coculture to the medium—cells from the patient's fallopian tubes or endometrium, or bovine uterine or fallopian cells. Coculture is believed by some to enhance embryo quality.

## Embryo Grading

Most ART laboratories use a numerical grading system to evaluate and classify embryo quality. These numerical values vary among laboratories, and it is important to determine what grading system the laboratory uses. Embryologists evaluate an embryo by the color and texture of the cytoplasm—the material that surrounds the embryo's nucleus. Normal cytoplasm is straw-colored and has a homogeneous appearance. Embryos with dark yellow or brownish cytoplasm usually degenerate. Embryos resulting from immature eggs often have cytoplasm that is grainy or speckled, and this results in developmental failure. Other cytoplasmic abnormalities include vacuoles (sacs of water), inclusion (dark spots), and fragmentation.

Cytoplasmic fragmentation is probably the most common abnormality observed in embryos. It occurs when portions of the embryo's cytoplasm bud off to form little round balls that have no nucleus. If ICSI is used to fertilize eggs, moderate fragmentation of resulting embryos is common. Not all embryos in the same cycle will exhibit the same degree of fragmentation. Highly fragmented embryos have a much lower developmental potential than embryos with little or no fragmentation. Cell division is the other important factor that determines embryo quality. Usually cellular division results in embryos with 2 to 4 cells on the second day, and 5 to 10 cells on the third day.

### Voices

*Rhea and Doron, both 33 years old, are about to undergo their second IVF cycle. Rhea says, "Our problems are not in the carrying of the fetus, but rather in making embryos which develop well enough to become fetuses. Not being able to have our own offspring would be a traumatic failure for us; a very deep and life-defining disappointment. Still, I think I would ultimately decide that raising a child—even someone else's genetic offspring—is more important to me than never mothering anyone at all."*

## Embryo Transfer

Many clinics transfer embryos on day 3 after the retrieval, at the 4 to 8-cell stage of development. (Not all embryos reach this level of division, however, and most clinics have reported pregnancies and live birth after transfer of less well-developed embryos.) Another option is to continue to culture the embryos until the blastocyst stage is reached, usually 5 to 6 days after retrieval. (See the section later in this chapter describing micromanipulation techniques, including assisted hatching, which is thought by some clinics to increase implantation rates in selected patients.)

### Breakthroughs

During the late 1990s, scientists developed advanced culture media that allow embryos to develop in vitro to the blastocyst stage, or day 5 of development after egg retrieval and fertilization. Early studies have shown improved implantation rates with blastocyst transfer, with fewer blastocysts needed to establish pregnancy than when day three embryos are transferred. Limiting the number of embryos transferred minimizes the likelihood of multiple gestation pregnancy.

## HUMAN EMBRYO: BLASTOCYST

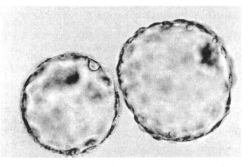

Embryo transfer is done without anesthesia. A speculum is placed in the vagina and the cervix is cleaned. The embryos are placed in a catheter attached to a syringe. The catheter is guided up through the cervix into the uterus. The embryos are pushed from the catheter into the uterus. Most physicians transfer two to five embryos, the number depending on embryo quality and the woman's age. If the embryos have been cultured to the blastocyst stage, fewer are transferred. Extra embryos may be cryopreserved (frozen) for use in future cycles.

Embryo transfer is an important topic to discuss with the physician at your initial consultation for IVF treatment. Discuss embryo transfer in the context of the clinic's rates for multiple births. Typically, 20 to 30 percent of ongoing pregnancies from IVF are multiple gestation, with about 5 percent of those triplets and 1 percent more than triplets. The medical risk of multiple gestation pregnancy and the individual's or couple's personal beliefs about multiple gestation pregnancy may influence the number of embryos transferred (see chapter 16, "Surviving Infertility and Moving Forward").

### Voices

*Christi asserts, "One of my friends who just had her first child after conceiving the very first month she attempted it has voiced the opinion that IVF skirts natural selection. I take major offense to that. I miscarried a presumably unhealthy embryo . . . if that isn't natural selection at work, I don't know what is. I feel strongly that everything wrong with me medically is biologically programmed that way, and that, if not today, then in the future, humankind will understand how to solve my problems."*

## After Embryo Transfer

Progesterone supplements are started the day after egg retrieval and continued until the pregnancy test is negative, or throughout the first trimester of pregnancy. Vaginal suppositories or gel, intramuscular injections, and oral capsules are the forms of progesterone used during IVF.

Instructions about activity after embryo transfer vary from clinic to clinic. Some suggest a few hours of bed rest and others suggest 2 to 3 days of minimal physical activity.

About 10 to 12 days after the embryo transfer, the physician will order a β-hCG test, which measures precisely the blood level of the β subunit of the placental hormone, hCG. A β subunit measurement greater than 5 mIU/mL (milli-International Units per milliliter) is considered positive for pregnancy, but borderline if it is less than about 50 mIU/mL. If the hCG level is borderline, another blood test will be taken in 2 to 3 days. The level should double every 2 to 3 days. Then, 5 weeks after the transfer, a sonogram is performed to document a heartbeat and confirm pregnancy.

Twenty percent of all pregnancies, regardless of how they are established, are lost. Very early pregnancies with no ultrasound confirmation of pregnancy tissue are called biochemical pregnancies, and losses at this stage are common. Unfortunately, a small number of ectopic, or tubal, pregnancies (less than 1 percent) occur after embryo transfer in an IVF cycle, resulting from embryos traveling out into the fallopian tube from the uterine cavity.

---

### Voices

*Laura is 31 and Will is 33; they have been trying for 5 years to have a baby. "We tried our second cycle of IVF and got ten embryos," says Laura. "We transferred five and froze the other half. Every one of them took. I carried them all for just under 20 weeks and then miscarried. We had a memorial service and a funeral and buried them in the local cemetery. It took me a long time to recover. We tried another cycle, and I'm pregnant again with twins. I'm 9 weeks." Will adds, "If this pregnancy doesn't work, I don't think we'll do this more than a few times more—we're both practical people and we'll think that if it hasn't happened by now it isn't meant to happen. Then, we'd go to adoption."*

---

## Embryo Cryopreservation

Extra embryos that are not transferred can be frozen (cryopreserved). Usually the clinic freezes only embryos that are good quality. They can be frozen and stored for years. The survival rate after thawing often depends on the quality of the embryos at the time of freezing. Pregnancy rates after transfer of cryopreserved embryos have been improving in recent years.

There are several ways to prepare the uterus for transfer of thawed embryos. Some clinics use a natural cycle, timing the transfer to match uterine development in a nonstimulated ovulatory cycle that has not been medicated. This often requires collecting daily urine and having frequent ultrasounds and blood tests performed. Other clinics may suppress the woman's natural cycle with GnRH agonist or birth control pills, and then give her estrogen and progesterone to prepare the endometrium for thawed embryo transfer. In all cases, supplemental progesterone will be used after the transfer.

---

### Voices

*Jerome, 32, and Hillary, 31, joke, "We have pictures of Jerome's sperm and my follicles on the refrigerator next to the pictures of all our friends' kids. If we're lucky enough to have enough good embryos to freeze, maybe we can expand the collection."*

---

### Questions to Ask If You Are Considering a
### Frozen Embryo Transfer Program

*Storage Issues*
- What criteria does the clinic use for embryos that can be frozen?
- Where are the embryos stored?

- What are the monthly/yearly fees?
- What is the clinic's policy for embryos that have been frozen longer than the clinic's stipulated guidelines?
- Can the couple request that embryos be transferred to another clinic? What are the fees?
- How does the clinic handle embryos from couples whom the clinic is unable to locate?
- What mechanism is in place for a couple who wants to donate their embryos to another couple or for research?

*The Transfer Cycle*
- What drugs will a woman take to prepare her uterus for transfer?
- Is a "mock" cycle done before a thawed embryo transfer to see how the uterus responds to the drugs used to prepare it?
- What is the minimum and maximum number of embryos transferred?
- Does the clinic do assisted hatching on thawed embryos?
- Will the clinic transfer thawed embryos that are very poor quality?

*The Written Contract*
- Will couples have to sign a consent form before each thawed transfer cycle?
- Does the written contract clarify issues about ownership of the embryos in case of divorce or death?

# GAMETE INTRAFALLOPIAN TRANSFER (GIFT)

In this ART procedure, conception takes place in the fallopian tube. GIFT should only be done when sperm quality is adequate and at least one fallopian tube is open and functional. The steps involved in GIFT are similar to IVF up to the egg retrieval. Egg retrieval is usually performed under general anesthesia, and eggs and sperm are transferred immediately to a catheter that is used to inject the eggs and sperm into the fallopian tube during laparoscopy. Unlike IVF, there is no ability to document fertilization or to evaluate embryo quality in a GIFT procedure. Progesterone supplements continue until the pregnancy test is negative or throughout the first trimester.

# ZYGOTE INTRAFALLOPIAN TRANSFER (ZIFT)

ZIFT is a combination of IVF and GIFT: A fertilized egg is transferred into the fallopian tubes. Fertilization takes place in a laboratory, and the zygotes (newly fertilized eggs) are transferred into the fallopian tubes at the time of laparoscopy. With ZIFT, fertilization is documented, but evaluation of the dividing embryo is not possible. Progesterone supplements are the same as for IVF and GIFT.

### Tips to Optimize Your Chances of Success with ART

*Women*

1. Avoid all pain medications other than Tylenol. If you are taking other prescription medications, check with your physician before beginning your treatment.
2. Do not smoke cigarettes or drink alcohol.
3. Avoid caffeine-containing beverages.
4. If you have active genital herpes report this to your physician at once.

*Men*

1. Report any fevers within 3 months before ART treatment, because such fevers may adversely affect sperm quality.
2. Avoid hot tubs or saunas for three months, because they can affect sperm function.
3. Avoid alcohol and drug use and cigarette smoking for 3 months before treatment and during the ART cycle.
4. Report all prescription drugs to your physician. If you have active genital herpes infection, report this to your physician.
5. Abstain from intercourse for 3 days, but not more than 7 days, before collection of semen for an ART cycle.

For more information for both women and men, see chapters 11 and 12, "Staying Centered" and "Staying Healthy."

## MICROMANIPULATION TECHNIQUES

If the clinic suspects that a woman's eggs will not fertilize well in vitro, or that implantation may not occur, micromanipulation techniques can be used to achieve or improve fertilization and implantation rates. These techniques also may be used to remove a cell from a developing embryo for assessment of the DNA before embryo transfer. Micromanipulators are tiny glass tools connected to motor-driven or hydraulically controlled robot arms, which are in turn linked to a microscope. Microtools are used to perform microsurgery on sperm, eggs, and embryonic cells. These cells and the tips of the tools are magnified 800 times and can be viewed on a television monitor.

### Intracytoplasmic Sperm Injection (ICSI)

Pioneered in Belgium to improve egg fertilization in couples with male factor infertility, ICSI has truly revolutionized treatment of male factor cases. Recently, it also has been used in cases of unexplained infertility and to enhance fertilization rates in older women and in women whose eggs produce thick zona pellucida (outer walls).

## INTRACYTOPLASMIC SPERM INJECTION (ICSI)

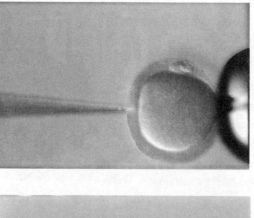

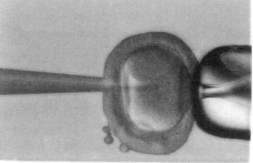

Once eggs are retrieved and sperm collected, the embryologist uses a tiny holding pipette to secure the egg and injects a single sperm into the egg's cytoplasm. Remarkably, when the injecting needle is withdrawn, the egg will reseal and assume its original shape. The resulting embryo is observed for normal cell division and, when appropriate, transferred to the woman's uterus. Several days of antibiotics and low-dose steroids may be given at the time of embryo transfer to reduce any chance of infection.

As long as a few living sperm are available, ICSI can be performed. Most men who produce no sperm in their ejaculate are candidates for invasive procedures to obtain sperm directly from the testicle (TESE) or from the epididymis (MESA).

## Testicular Sperm Extraction (TESE) and Microsurgical Epididymal Sperm Aspiration (MESA)

These procedures are used when the male has sperm in the testes or epididymis, but none in the ejaculate. (In these cases, where no obstruction is present, the physician may suggest genetic testing to detect genetically linked disease that could be passed on to offspring.) Sperm are collected, either through a testicular biopsy (TESE) or a needle inserted into the epididymis (MESA). These sperm are then used as part of an IVF/ICSI procedure (see chapter 8, "The Male: Diagnosis and Treatment").

## Assisted Hatching

Assisted hatching may be performed on the embryo in an effort to enhance implantation rates. A tiny opening is made in the outer layer of the embryo, the zona pellucida, just before transfer. This allows the embryo literally to hatch from the zona pellucida. Antibiotics and steroids are sometimes given to the woman at the time of embryo transfer and for several days after to enhance implantation and prevent infection. The effectiveness of assisted hatching is still being debated.

ASSISTED HATCHING

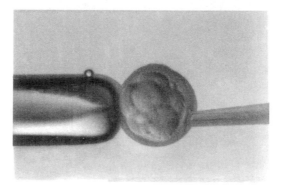

## Preimplantation Genetic Diagnosis

Preimplantation genetic diagnosis enables a physician to identify genetic diseases *before* embryo transfer to the uterus. This procedure could eliminate the need for possible pregnancy termination after prenatal tests indicating a genetically affected fetus. Sex-linked recessive diseases that are carried on the X chromosome, such as hemophilia and Duchenne muscular dystrophy, have been the major indication for preimplantation genetic diagnosis. In these cases, identification of the sex of the embryos allows transfer of only the unaffected XX, or female, embryos. Single gene defects and perhaps as many as 200 other X-linked diseases could also be diagnosed using these techniques.

Couples who are at exceptionally high risk of transmitting genetic disorders, such as Huntington disease and Tay-Sachs disease, would benefit from preimplantation genetic diagnosis, as well. These are autosomal dominant diseases in which 50 percent of offspring are affected.

The procedure involves removing one cell from a 4- to 8-cell embryo and analyzing the genetic material using a technique called polymerase chain reaction (PCR). All the embryos remain in culture and continue to divide, but only embryos with normal genes are transferred to the uterus.

Another technique, called polar body biopsy, can be performed on the egg before fertilization to diagnose a limited number of female-carried genetic diseases. In this technique, only the eggs with the normal gene are fertilized.

### *Mendelian Diagnoses*

Physicians can help identify the presence of the following conditions using current preimplantation diagnosis procedures:

- X-linked recessive disorder
- Hemophilia A
- Duchenne muscular dystrophy
- Huntington disease
- Tay-Sachs disease
- $\alpha_1$-Antitrypsin deficiency
- Cystic fibrosis
- Lesch-Nyhan syndrome
- Retinitis pigmentosa
- Alloimmune thrombocytopenia

## THE SUCCESS OF ART

The only fertility treatments for which pregnancy success rates are reported are those for ART cycles. In 1992, the U.S. Congress enacted the Fertility Clinic Success Rate and Certification Act, which requires each ART clinic in the United States to report annually its pregnancy success rates to the U.S. Centers for Disease Control and Prevention (CDC). The CDC uses data reported by clinics to the Society for Assisted Reproductive Technology (SART), an affiliate organization of the American Society for Reproductive Medicine (ASRM), to compile and publish these results. After consulting with RESOLVE and reviewing feedback on consumer issues, the CDC made the first such report available to the public in December 1997. (See the Resources Guide for information about obtaining the CDC report.)

The following statistics are compiled in the annual *ART Success Rates: National Summary and Fertility Clinic Reports* from data submitted by reporting clinics:

- ART cycles completed in the reporting year.
- Number of babies born as a result of ART cycles.
- The percentage of deliveries per egg retrieval and embryo transfer procedure for women using their own eggs.
- The delivery rate per embryo transfer procedure for women using donated eggs.

Statistics vary widely from clinic to clinic. Experts caution, however, that the success rates of any given clinic depend, in large part, on the number of patients treated, their ages, and their diagnoses. Statistics prove that older women have the lowest success rates. The best rates are for women younger than 35 years, and they drop significantly for women 39 and older. The report also provides data on the percentages of multiple births, information about the diagnoses of patients, and success rates categorized by age of the woman for each clinic.

These success rate reports provide a good overview of a clinic's record. However, it is always important to remember that—even at top-notch clinics and with the healthiest patients possible—ART procedures such as IVF have a limited chance of producing a viable pregnancy and baby from one treatment attempt. Your own chances of success are linked not only to the abilities of your physician and the clinic staff, but also to your specific infertility problem and, most importantly, the woman's age and ovarian reserve status.

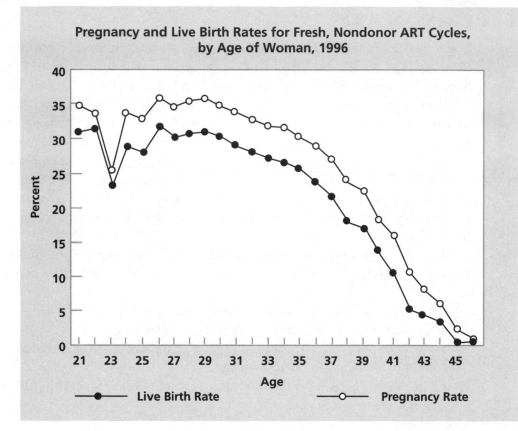

**Pregnancy and Live Birth Rates for Fresh, Nondonor ART Cycles, by Age of Woman, 1996**

*Percent* (y-axis) vs *Age* (x-axis)

● Live Birth Rate    ○ Pregnancy Rate

### Voices

*After trying IUI with drug therapy for several months with no success, Arlene and Bruce, both 30 years old, investigated adopting before deciding to try one cycle of IVF. Arlene recounts, "The IVF cycle was traumatic for us, and we are trying to stamp that feeling in our brains so we don't forget. You're sinking so much money, so much of your time, so much of your emotions into the effort—it changes your lifestyle. For my husband, it was giving me the shots—3 times a day at one point. I responded to the treatment really well. I had 20 eggs, 18 of which fertilized. They froze six immediately, and then two when they were a little more mature. They put three in, but none took. We're not sure we want to go ahead with another IVF cycle, but we have misgivings about leaving those embryos and not using them. We're not sure what our next step will be."*

Keep in mind that the statistics are not as straightforward as they may appear. Some clinics treat more young patients, who have a better chance of success. Others will take all patients, including older women or couples with long histories of infertility problems. Be sure to review a clinic's record for treating patients in your age group.

Finally, a clinic with a high pregnancy rate may be transferring multiple embryos in a single cycle. In many cases, the more embryos transferred, the greater chances that a successful pregnancy will occur. But that higher level of "success" must be balanced by the greater risk of multiple gestation pregnancy and birth that transferring a large number of embryos may entail. Because carrying more than one baby increases the risk of complications for both mother and infant, and because many potential parents would find it difficult to undergo multiple gestation reduction (MGR), the risks may outweigh the benefits for you (see chapter 16, "Surviving Infertility and Moving Forward").

## SHOULD WE TRY ART TREATMENT?

The decision to try ART treatment is a difficult one, involving complex medical, financial/insurance, and emotional issues and concerns. Putting everything down on a decision tree can help to clarify your decision-making process. We have created the following ART decision tree based on the fictional couple Virginia and Matt. Study the decision-making process in this example. Then, start your own ART decision tree.

### *Perspectives*

As you create your ART decision tree, also use your infertility journal to record the following:

- Your feelings, and those of your partner, about making an ART decision tree and exploring ART options.
- How you and your partner felt while working on the tree. Were you frustrated? Determined? Worried? Hopeful?
- How you and your partner feel about the decision you make regarding ART treatment. Have you reached a comfort zone?

Virginia, 36, and Matt, 39, have no children. They have been trying to have a baby for three years. Virginia has had open fallopian tubes, but a mild to moderate case of endometriosis. She had a recent laparoscopy to remove disease and adhesions. Matt's sperm count is on the low side of normal; motility and morphology are borderline. His semen analysis results improved after an operation for varicocele 2 years ago, but Virginia has not conceived. The couple's health insurance will cover four cycles of injectable ovulatory medication, for IUI or ART; the policy does not cover egg retrieval, laboratory costs, or transfers of egg/sperm or embryos. They have completed two cycles of medicated IUI. Matt's semen sample was adequate, although not optimum, each time. Virginia's response to medication was fair; she produced two mature follicles each cycle.

Virginia and Matt have worked closely with their physician and feel comfortable with the clinic staff. The clinic offers ART treatment. Virginia and Matt have created the following three decision trees to help them work through their complicated choices.

Virginia and Matt reviewed their finances, and they determined that they have enough savings, without borrowing or tapping into retirement funds, to try two cycles of IVF. They explored alternative decisions in their third decision tree that they could make if IVF using Virginia's eggs did not succeed.

**The final decision:** The couple has decided, with their physician, to try a cycle of IVF with Virginia's eggs and with ICSI. They understand their chance of having a baby after one cycle is about 25 to 30 percent. The treatment will help them to evaluate their fertility, even if they do not conceive and have a baby. Matt has agreed to go with Virginia to see a therapist who has expertise in counseling on infertility decision making and to discuss the adoption option. They will revisit their decision, if necessary, after the first cycle.

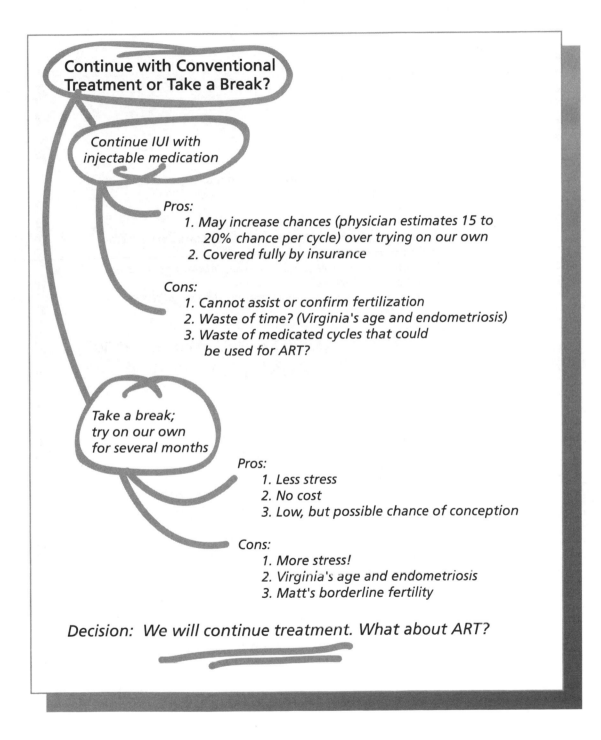

**Continue with Conventional Treatment or Take a Break?**

*Continue IUI with injectable medication*

*Pros:*
*1. May increase chances (physician estimates 15 to 20% chance per cycle) over trying on our own*
*2. Covered fully by insurance*

*Cons:*
*1. Cannot assist or confirm fertilization*
*2. Waste of time? (Virginia's age and endometriosis)*
*3. Waste of medicated cycles that could be used for ART?*

*Take a break; try on our own for several months*

*Pros:*
*1. Less stress*
*2. No cost*
*3. Low, but possible chance of conception*

*Cons:*
*1. More stress!*
*2. Virginia's age and endometriosis*
*3. Matt's borderline fertility*

*Decision: We will continue treatment. What about ART?*

**ART with Own Eggs**

**GIFT or ZIFT**

Pros:

1. Slightly higher average success rate: nationally and in
   Virginia's age group

Cons:

1. Cannot confirm fertilization with GIFT (Matt's male factor
   an issue)
2. No insurance coverage for retrievals, laboratory, transfers:
   ZIFT most expensive
3. Both require surgery and neither produces significant
   advantage over IVF

## Decision: We won't do GIFT or ZIFT. What about IVF?

**IVF**

Pros:

1. Partial insurance coverage
2. Can help fertilization (ICSI) and confirm it
3. Satisfy need to create our embryo or
4. Help with closure, if no fertilization occurs

Cons:

1. No coverage for egg retrieval, laboratory, embryo
   transfer
2. Time and emotional commitment
3. Virginia needs GnRH agonist and higher dose of
   ovulation medications (hyperstimulation of the ovaries
   is unlikely given Virginia's previous low response to
   medication) but
4. Virginia may not create many follicles or eggs even on
   higher dose (few or low quality potential embryos to
   transfer could lower prospects for success)

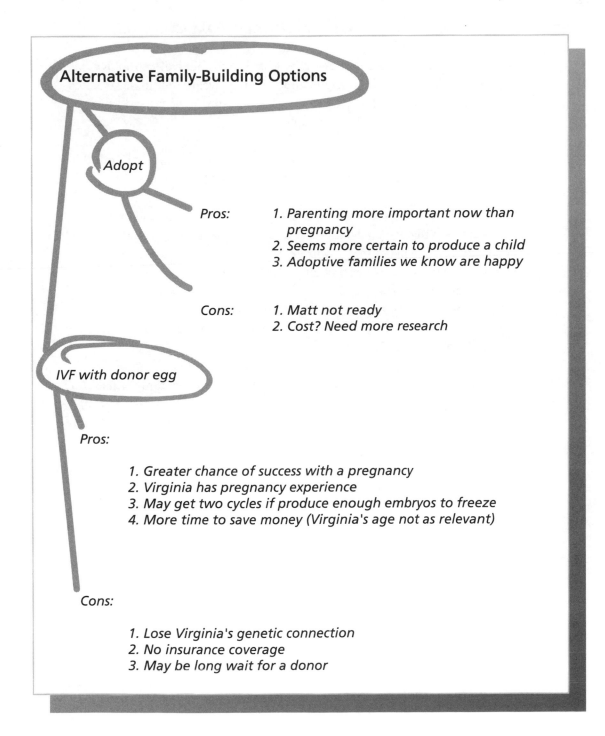

**Alternative Family-Building Options**

*Adopt*

*Pros:*
1. *Parenting more important now than pregnancy*
2. *Seems more certain to produce a child*
3. *Adoptive families we know are happy*

*Cons:*
1. *Matt not ready*
2. *Cost? Need more research*

*IVF with donor egg*

*Pros:*

1. *Greater chance of success with a pregnancy*
2. *Virginia has pregnancy experience*
3. *May get two cycles if produce enough embryos to freeze*
4. *More time to save money (Virginia's age not as relevant)*

*Cons:*

1. *Lose Virginia's genetic connection*
2. *No insurance coverage*
3. *May be long wait for a donor*

## POSITIVE STEPS YOU CAN TAKE FROM CHAPTER 9

**Consider all the pros and cons of ART.** Assisted reproductive technology has been helping people to build families for more than 20 years. Although it holds out hope for many, ART is intensive and involves substantial time and financial commitment for most individuals and couples.

**Understand ART procedures.** It is important to understand each step of ART treatment and to discuss with your physician such issues as:

- The likelihood of success with each cycle based on your age and diagnosis;
- The risks of ovulatory medications and multiple gestation pregnancy;
- The number of embryos to be transferred;
- The possible use of micromanipulation techniques;
- Embryo cryopreservation; and
- The number of cycles your physician would recommend you try.
- Any questions about consent forms that you will be required to sign (see chapter 4, "Choosing Your Medical Team").

**Do the research.** Assessing the "success" of ART treatment and clinics that offer it is an inexact science, at best. Review the national report and data offered in the CDC's *ART Success Rates Report and Important Factors to Consider When Using (Clinic Specific) Tables to Assess a Clinic* when you research this technology.

# 10 Pregnancy Loss

The grief and frustration experienced after a pregnancy loss is intense and nothing anyone can say will help to take those feelings of loss away. Miscarriage is a common occurrence. More than 15 percent of pregnant women experience a first trimester pregnancy loss. Experts believe that at least half of all fertilized eggs never progress to a viable pregnancy. Since a third of those losses occur between implantation and the sixth week of pregnancy, many women do not realize they have been pregnant or had a miscarriage.

In women under age 20, about 12 percent of first pregnancies end in miscarriage; after age 40, about 24 percent are lost. Recurrent or multiple miscarriages are also common. After two successive pregnancy losses, the miscarriage rate increases to approximately 25 percent.

As upsetting as those statistics may seem, especially if you have experienced your first or second miscarriage, remember that 60 percent of couples with four prior pregnancy losses go on to have a successful pregnancy and delivery.

Any discussion of miscarriage and infertility involves two issues. One is the medical aspect and the other is the emotional. But before we discuss pregnancy loss, and its potential causes and treatments, it is important to clarify a few terms.

The terms *spontaneous abortion, pregnancy loss,* and *miscarriage* are used interchangeably by medical professionals. Spontaneous abortion is the clinical term used by health care professionals in medical settings, while pregnancy loss and miscarriage are common lay terms. All three terms are defined medically as the loss of a pregnancy within the first 20 weeks. This is the most common type of pregnancy loss.

## Terms Associated with Pregnancy Loss

- **Blighted ovum (Embryonic pregnancy).** A pregnancy in which the embryo does not form.
- **Chemical pregnancy (Subclinical miscarriage).** An early pregnancy loss that occurs before a gestational sac has been found on ultrasound; a subclinical miscarriage may result in a heavier and longer menstrual bleed.
- **Clinical miscarriage.** A pregnancy loss after a gestational sac and perhaps a fetal heartbeat have been documented. Usually the woman has other symptoms of pregnancy, such as breast tenderness.
- **Threatened miscarriage.** The cervix is still closed, but there is spotting in early pregnancy and sometimes lower back pain or cramping.
- **Incomplete miscarriage/incomplete abortion.** Characterized by increased bleeding, cramping, and an open cervix. A miscarriage in which some tissue is left in the uterus. An incomplete abortion may require a D&C (dilation and curettage), a surgical procedure that removes remaining tissue from the uterus.
- **Inevitable miscarriage.** All non-viable pregnancies are an inevitable miscarriage.
- **Complete spontaneous abortion.** A miscarriage in which all of the products of conception have been expelled from the uterus.
- **Missed abortion.** The fetus dies, but remains in the uterus.
- **Ectopic pregnancy.** This term is used to describe a pregnancy in which the embryo implants outside the uterus, usually in the fallopian tube and occasionally in the pelvic cavity. Symptoms include β-human chorionic gonadotropin (β-hCG; a pregnancy hormone) levels that do not rise, possible abdominal pain, vaginal bleeding, and flulike symptoms. An ectopic pregnancy is diagnosed by a pelvic ultrasound that does not show a fecal sac in the uterus, or via laparoscopy. Treatment may include the surgical removal of the pregnancy from the tube. Every effort is made to save the affected tube. Methotrexate, a medication given to cancer patients, is also used to treat an ectopic pregnancy. This medication attacks tissues that are "foreign" or in the wrong place. Side effects are rare, but women receiving this treatment will have follow-up blood testing to monitor for any adverse effects.
- **Molar pregnancy.** Also called trophoblastic disease or hydatidiform mole, this unusual condition results in placental tissue growing rapidly and causing high β-hCG levels, but with no fetus present. Occurring in about 1 of 2,000

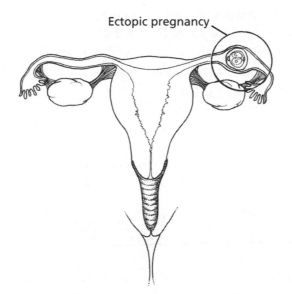

Ectopic pregnancy

pregnancies, the condition is diagnosed when the ultrasound shows no fetus and the tissue sent to the pathologist after a D&C shows trophoblastic disease. Women are often advised not to conceive for 6 to 12 months after a molar pregnancy and usually have blood levels for β-hCG drawn every 4 to 6 weeks until the levels drop to normal. There is a slight risk of cancer of the uterus (choriocarcinoma) in women whose β-hCG blood levels do not drop to normal after several months.

- **Recurrent or multiple miscarriage.** Clinically defined as the occurrence of three or more miscarriages, although many physicians use two or more.
- **Stillbirth.** The death of a fetus in utero after 20 weeks of gestation and before birth.

Pregnancy loss—no matter when it occurs—is the loss of a dreamed-for child. Later in this chapter, we will discuss the emotional impact of pregnancy loss and the healing process that follows. First, we will discuss the medical aspects of pregnancy loss.

## EXPERIENCING PREGNANCY LOSS

Some women experience symptoms before a miscarriage occurs, others do not. Some of the symptoms of a threatened miscarriage include vaginal spotting, (usually dark brown and changing to pink or red), cramping, and a decrease in breast tenderness or fullness. However, it is important not to panic if you have vaginal spotting, because women who spot often go on to carry a pregnancy to term. Breast tenderness can also fluctuate and may not necessarily mean that the pregnancy is in jeopardy.

When you see the physician, a pelvic examination and a transvaginal ultrasound will be done to determine whether the pregnancy is proceeding normally or is miscarrying. Ultrasound is more reliable the further along in the pregnancy—it is not reliable before 5 to 6 weeks from the last menstrual period. A pregnancy is dated from the first day of your last period.

---

### Voices

*"We were devastated by the loss of the pregnancy. We'd been trying for so long to get pregnant," admits Martin, who with his wife Kay had been trying for years to have a baby. They lost their IVF twins 4 weeks into the pregnancy. "But at the same time we were happy. We could get pregnant! As heartbreaking as it was, the miscarriage also gave us hope."*

---

## Threatened Miscarriage

Some physicians suggest frequent blood tests to monitor whether β-hCG hormone levels are rising normally. Others suggest bed rest, whereas others maintain a "wait and see attitude." This is a distressing time for most women. Every trip to the bathroom is filled with the dread of seeing more spotting.

A threatened miscarriage is anguishing because, in most cases, there is really not anything that you or your physician can do to prevent the loss of the pregnancy. Also, if you have heavy bleeding and cramping, it can be frightening. It is a difficult time for your partner as well; men feel especially helpless and isolated, and just as grief-stricken and afraid as their female partners.

## Confirmed Miscarriage

In some cases, the miscarriage can happen quickly and the fetal tissue will be expelled. If this happens before you get to a physician, try to save the tissue in a container. As difficult emotionally as this may be to do, preserving the tissue may help your physician determine the cause of your pregnancy loss.

If you have had a miscarriage, and the physical and ultrasound examinations confirm that all the tissue has been expelled, you may not need any further medical care. However, if the physician suspects that tissue remains in the uterus (an incomplete or missed abortion), a D&C may be ordered.

Your physician may do a karyotype, an analysis of the fetal tissue chromosomes. Karyotyping is only possible if the tissue is well formed and preserved. If the tissue is incompletely formed, it is likely that the chromosomal constitution will be abnormal and the miscarriage was inevitable. If the chromosomal makeup is normal, on the other hand, there is another reason for the miscarriage, which may or may not ever be known.

If you have Rh-negative blood type, and your partner is Rh-positive, you will need a drug, RhoGAM, to prevent a potentially harmful antibody from jeopardizing a future pregnancy.

After a miscarriage, repeat blood pregnancy tests are often done until the β-hCG level is less than 5 mIU/mL (milli-International Units per milliliter). If the β-hCG hormone level is not back to normal, it is possible that an ectopic pregnancy is present, and, if so, the physician will have to treat it medically or with surgery. If tissue passed from the uterus is confirmed to be fetal, this essentially eliminates concern about an ectopic pregnancy; however, in rare cases a woman can have both a uterine and an ectopic pregnancy.

### *Breakthroughs*

A recent study conducted by the National Institutes of Health is helping physicians learn more about the relationship between pregnancy loss and the timing of embryo implantation after ovulation. In the study, published in the *New England Journal of Medicine*, analysis of the hormone levels of 221 women with normal fertility who were attempting pregnancy revealed that implantation was most likely to succeed 8 to 10 days after ovulation. In addition, the later the embryo implantation occurred, the more likely the pregnancy to fail. Researchers believe there may be a communication that occurs between the embryo and the woman's body, perhaps through "messenger" proteins that give directions about where and when the embryo will implant in the uterine lining. This new information could help physicians to refine assisted reproductive technology (ART) procedures to improve success rates.

## CAUSES OF PREGNANCY LOSS

Physicians have determined that the causes of pregnancy loss fall into these categories:

- Genetic
- Age

- Structural
- Hormonal
- Infection
- Blood incompatibility
- Environmental
- Immune

## Genetic Abnormalities

In the majority of cases, pregnancy losses are caused by genetic abnormalities of the embryo or fetus itself, rather than genetic abnormalities in the maternal or paternal genetic make-up. At least 60 percent of miscarriages result from chromosomal abnormalities, usually occurring during cell division at the time of conception. Before fertilization, the sperm and egg cell each contain 23 chromosomes, which means that a fertilized egg should contain 46 chromosomes. Any disruption in the number or formation of the chromosomes can result in an abnormal fetus and may result in miscarriage.

The most common genetic abnormality found in spontaneous abortions is called trisomy and occurs when an extra copy of a chromosome is present. Down syndrome, or trisomy 21, is an example of a trisomy, caused by an extra chromosome 21. Another type of numerical chromosomal problem is polyploidy, which results when the embryo has an extra set or sets of chromosomes. In the case of triploidy, the embryo receives an extra 23 chromosomes, or 69 instead of the usual 46.

Another type of chromosomal abnormality is a structural one, in which one or more chromosomes either have a portion missing (deletion), or an extra portion added (insertion). One form of structural abnormality, translocation, occurs when one part of the chromosome attaches to another. Most chromosomal abnormalities occur randomly and spontaneously, and there is nothing that can be done to prevent the condition in the future. In just 3 to 5 percent of couples experiencing multiple miscarriages, a condition called balanced translocation of genes is responsible. In these cases, one partner carries the defective chromosome, and, unfortunately, nothing can be done to prevent the abnormality from occurring in an embryo the couple produces. The older pregnant woman is at increased risk for pregnancy loss because of age-related random chromosomal changes in her eggs that affect embryo viability.

## Structural (Anatomic) Abnormalities

Structural problems of the uterus may cause miscarriage. Uterine fibroids are noncancerous growths in the uterine wall that can cause infertility if they block the fallopian tubes or if their position affects the uterine lining. In these cases, the risk of pregnancy loss is higher, because embryo implantation may be affected. Sometimes a uterine septum, an abnormal structure that partially or totally divides the uterine cavity, can cause a miscarriage for two reasons: if the embryo implants on the septum, because circulation to the septum is poor; or if the septum prevents the uterine cavity from expanding during pregnancy.

Women whose mothers were given the drug diethylstilbestrol (DES) during their pregnancies may have a high number of uterine or other abnormalities, and some of these can contribute to miscarriage. Specifically, the T-shaped or small uterus, or cervical problems such as incompetent cervix, may contribute to higher rates of miscarriage and pregnancy loss in DES-exposed women.

If a structural problem is suspected, a hysterosalpingogram or sonohysterogram (ultrasound using saline solution to visualize the cavity of the uterus) will be ordered to evaluate the uterus and to rule out possible polyps, fibroids, or a septum. A hysteroscopy can be performed to correct these problems. Some women with uterine abnormalities can have successful pregnancies without treatment; others may need surgical repair.

An incompetent cervix may cause pregnancy loss because the cervical muscle is too weak to remain closed as the developing fetus puts pressure on the cervical opening. Miscarriage resulting from this problem occurs in the second trimester and is usually rapid and painless. An exam can be done before pregnancy to check for an incompetent cervix. If a pregnant woman has an incompetent cervix, sutures are placed in the cervical muscle at 13 to 17 weeks into the pregnancy to tighten the opening (cervical cerclage). To allow for a vaginal delivery, the stitches are removed when labor begins.

Many women wonder if a retroverted uterus, a uterus that is tilted backwards, can cause a miscarriage. About 30 percent of women have a retroverted uterus, and the condition is not usually a cause of miscarriage. If retroverted uterus is found, the physician may suggest sleeping on your stomach or doing some gentle exercises, such as the illustrated table pose, until 18 weeks of gestation to allow the uterus to move forward. Occasionally, a pessary, or soft plastic tube, is inserted into the vaginal canal to allow the uterus to gradually move to the correct forward position.

For more information on structural abnormalities and their potentially adverse impact on female fertility, see chapter 7, "The Female: Structural Problems, Age-Related Factors, and Treatment."

**TABLE POSE**

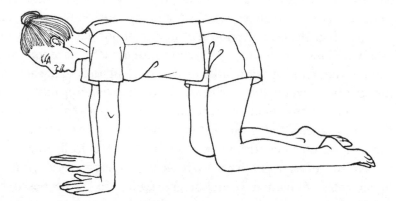

## Hormonal Abnormalities

Abnormal hormone levels could affect the uterine lining and prevent implantation and nourishment of the fertilized egg. Progesterone, produced during the luteal phase of the menstrual cycle and in early pregnancy, is the hormone that orchestrates the development of the uterine lining. If midluteal phase progesterone levels are low—less than 10 ng/mL (nanograms per milliliter) in a single sample or 30 ng/mL in three samples added together—the uterine lining may not develop enough to support the fertilized egg. Hormone levels alone are not sufficient to make the diagnosis, so an endometrial biopsy may be performed on cycle day 21 during a cycle in which you are not pregnant to see whether the lining is thick enough for the fertilized egg to implant. If there is a lag of two or more days in the development of the lining, treatment with hormones (clomiphene citrate, progesterone) may be started. See the discussion of luteal phase defect (LPD) in chapter 6, "The Female: Hormonal Disorders and Treatment," for more information.

Women with an abnormal level of thyroid hormone are at higher risk for miscarriage. Also, an elevated prolactin level can disrupt ovulatory patterns and sometimes affect the quality of the uterine lining. Hormone treatments can be given in these situations.

## Infections

Infections, such as German measles (rubella), herpes simplex, cytomegalovirus, and chlamydia, may cause pregnancy loss. These infections can cause pregnancy loss if the first infection occurs during pregnancy. They are not part of a recurrent miscarriage work-up.

If you are considering getting pregnant and are not sure you are immune to rubella, have a blood test. If you are not immune, you can be vaccinated and will have to postpone trying to get pregnant for 3 months. Recently, there have been outbreaks of rubella. If you were vaccinated against rubella after 1959, ask your physician whether there is any need to be revaccinated, especially if you are exposed to children who may have current infection. Contracting German measles during a pregnancy is dangerous to the fetus.

Toxoplasmosis and listeriosis infections may affect fetal development. Because cat feces carry the organism *Toxoplasma gondii*, which causes toxoplasmosis, pregnant women should not clean cat litter boxes.

A microorganism called *Ureaplasma urealyticum* may cause early pregnancy loss; however, it is also present in many fertile women. Cultures for this sexually transmitted organism taken from the vagina or penis (the organism can be present in both the female and male urogenital tracts) are expensive and require sophisticated laboratory equipment; some physicians do not feel this testing is needed. Many physicians simply treat both partners of a couple after a pregnancy loss with an antibiotic such as tetracycline or doxycycline, in case they do have this infection.

## Environmental Factors

Toxins may also result in pregnancy loss, or in fetal damage if a woman experiences regular exposure after 20 weeks of pregnancy. Chemicals such as solvents, insecticides, lead products, benzene, and mercury all seem to increase the chance of miscarriage. Studies indicate that the use of marijuana, tobacco, caffeine, and alcohol can affect fetal development and may cause pregnancy loss. See chapter 12, "Staying Healthy," for a full discussion on the lifestyle and environmental risks that can affect fertility or contribute to pregnancy loss.

## Immunologic Factors

Some research indicates that unexplained pregnancy losses may be attributed to immunologic factors, but this research is still in its early stages and treatment for such factors remains highly controversial. In rare cases, immune system cells can cause miscarriage by attacking the body's own cells (called autoimmune disorders) or attacking new but beneficial cells to the body, such as embryonic or placental cells (called allopathic disorders).

Here is an overview of what is known about immunology and miscarriage:

• *Antiphospholipid antibodies:* A rare condition, known to occur in less than 5 percent of couples with recurrent miscarriage, antiphospholipid antibodies (APA) is an autoimmune problem. If antibodies form against phospholipids, they could affect the ability of the blood to clot at the site of placental attachment. There are three primary types of APA: lupus anticoagulant (LA), anticardiolipin (aCL), and antiphosphatidyl serine (aPS). Pregnancy loss caused by these antibodies usually occurs after 10 weeks of gestation.

A few physicians recommend doing a panel of tests—seven tests in all—to determine the presence of APA. However, scientists have yet to confirm that these antibodies cause pregnancy loss, and the testing is expensive. Most clinics and physicians do recommend that the tests for elevated levels of LA, aCL, and aPS be performed. If levels are high, the tests are often repeated in 6 weeks, because false-positive results are common. (If the results are positive, it does *not* mean that you have the chronic disease, lupus erythematosus).

Treatment for APA includes 80 mg (milligrams) of aspirin (one baby aspirin) per day to reduce the risk of forming clots (both before and during pregnancy). Heparin, a blood thinner, may also be used; this drug can have some serious side effects that should be discussed not only with the prescribing physician, but also with an internist or primary care physician, and with the OB-Gyn who would follow you should you become pregnant.

### Voices

*"When I was 42, after having a miscarriage and several cycles of intrauterine insemination (IUI) and then in vitro fertilization (IVF)," Robyn, now 44 years old, recalls, "my husband and I were encouraged by our reproductive endocrinologist (RE) to try immunological testing. First they said I had antiphosholipids, so I went on heparin and tried another IVF, but the pregnancy didn't implant. We did more testing and the doctor now said I had elevated natural killer cells. So I was injected with my husband's white blood cells, month after month. At the end, we were out another $7,000 and my counts never moved. We stopped then, not knowing what to believe. It is hard for us; when we hear of some new treatment or test, we feel we should try it. It seems like there is always something new!"*

• *Blocking antibodies:* Failure to produce blocking antibodies does not appear to play a role in pregnancy loss. Forty percent of women who do not have the blocking antibodies have children without problems or pregnancy loss.

• *Embryo toxicity:* Cells make proteins called cytokines. Some cytokines stimulate the growth of cells, some inhibit growth; some cytokines may stimulate inflammatory response, whereas others inhibit the inflammatory response of cells. The embryo toxic factor-lymphocyte blood test (ETFL) is used to identify cytokines that kill embryos. There is no definitive treatment that is proven. Several therapies are under study to treat this condition, including intravenous immunoglobulin therapy (IVIg) and high doses of vaginal progesterone.

• *Antithyroid antibodies:* Approximately 23 to 35 percent of women with recurrent miscarriage have antithyroid antibodies, also known as thyroid peroxidase antibodies or TPA, compared with 10 to 17 percent of women with successful reproductive histories. This condition can put them at risk for thyroid dysfunction—especially hypothyroidism—which can contribute to miscarriage.

### Questions to Ask About
### Immunologic Therapy for Multiple Miscarriage

If you think you may be a candidate for immunologic treatment for miscarriage, consider these questions and points:

- Have you had a blood test to document that you do have high levels of one of the immunologic factors that may be associated with miscarriage?
- Because some of these tests can give false-positive results, discuss having a repeat test done.
- Heparin affects blood clotting time. If you are going to take heparin, tell your physician if you have hypertension, prolonged bleeding, bruise easily, or have stomach ulcers or ulcerative colitis.
- If you are taking heparin, ask your physician how often and what type of blood tests will be performed to monitor your blood clotting time.
- Aspirin can be irritating to your intestinal system, so tell your physician if you have a stomach ulcer or ulcerative colitis.
- Ask the physician whether heparin or aspirin will be continued if you get pregnant. If so, for how long into a pregnancy?
- Talk with an obstetrician about using either heparin or aspirin medications during the second or third trimester in pregnancy.
- Long-term use of heparin may cause osteoporosis. Discuss this with your physician and ask if you should be taking extra calcium.

### Questions to Ask About
### Intravenous Immunoglobulin Therapy (IVIg)

- Because immunoglobulin therapy uses blood products (150 donors are needed to make one vial), discuss the possible health risks to you from IVIg therapy.

- Discuss possible long-term effects from IVIg therapy on the woman's immune system.
- Discuss how many IVIg treatments will be needed. Ask about the timing and cost of each treatment. (Insurance will not cover this treatment as it is considered experimental.)

# HEALING AFTER PREGNANCY LOSS

Having a pregnancy loss is difficult and painful. Well-meaning friends and relatives may urge you to get on with your life, or attempt to console you with words that only intensify your pain. But healing takes time. You cannot just snap your fingers and get over your loss. Nor would you want to. As painful as it is, your pregnancy loss is an important experience in your life, and the only way you can move forward is to acknowledge your grief. Those who have never experienced pregnancy loss may find it hard to understand why you hurt. This is especially true if you have had the loss early in the pregnancy. In these cases, people may be trying to adjust to the news that you were pregnant, while at the same time struggling to absorb the fact that you lost the pregnancy.

### *The Best of Intentions, The Worst of Intentions*

You have a right to grieve and to discount insensitive remarks or attitudes. One of the most difficult things to hear when you lose a pregnancy is "It's for the best." People sometimes inadvertently say all the wrong things in their attempt to comfort you after a pregnancy loss. A few of the other most common and least favorite responses include "At least you know you can get pregnant;" "It was God's/Nature's way to take care of the problem;" and "Kids are a hassle anyway—you should be glad you don't have any." In your pain, it is difficult to accept such insensitivity in the context of helpfulness.

The people who love you want to help you feel better, and likely they share with you a feeling of deep sadness for your loss. The problem is, they often do not know how to express this properly and are unsure about what to say or how to act. Sometimes, all you can say in reply is, "This is a painful time for us; thank you for your concern." Other times, you can tell the people around you what you would most appreciate from them.

## Physical Concerns After a Pregnancy Loss

The loss of a pregnancy—whether it occurs at 6 weeks or at 19 weeks—often takes a surprising physical and emotional toll on a woman's body. After a miscarriage, you may continue to feel pregnant. Your abdomen may feel swollen, your breasts may be tender—but you know that the baby you were carrying is gone. (Vaginal spotting after a miscarriage is normal unless it becomes bright red or has a foul odor, in which case the physician should be notified. If a fever develops, or if your abdomen feels *very* tender, see your physician at once.) Your body had geared up hormonally for pregnancy, but must now go back to a nonpregnant state. When periods return, you may grieve the loss all over again.

On the recommendation of their physicians, many women have D&Cs after miscarriage, to be certain all tissue is removed to prevent infection and other complications. Although recovery from this surgery is usually quick, the stress of going through a medical procedure directly after such a loss may add to feelings of emotional distress and physical discomfort.

### Voices

*Regina is a 41-year-old woman who, with her husband Lou, is contemplating a second cycle of IVF. "From abortion to in vitro, I was a product of the times. I'd taken my fertility for granted when I'd had unwanted pregnancies in my youth, but now I wanted a pregnancy and it wouldn't take," Regina muses. "After my first IVF, I found myself pregnant with twins, two little heartbeats on the ultrasound. I was still scared to get too excited, but despite my fears I couldn't help myself. The ultrasound technician wasn't able to determine whether the twins were fraternal or identical, so another ultrasound was scheduled a couple of weeks later. Just shy of 12 weeks, at that second ultrasound procedure, it was determined that the cardiac activity had ceased in the twins; the embryos had died. I was scheduled to have a D&C. I was so anguished."*

Many women want to try to become pregnant again immediately after a pregnancy loss, as a way to reverse the setback or "replace" the lost child. Determination to succeed in becoming pregnant again substitutes for the normal grieving process. As few as 25 percent of women who experience miscarriage seek professional counseling after their loss. Allowing yourself time to grieve—and reaching out for the help of a therapist or RESOLVE support group—can help you work through all of the feelings, emotions, and questions that surface when miscarriage occurs.

From an emotional standpoint, many mental health professionals suggest that couples wait several months after a pregnancy loss to begin trying again.

But because of the woman's age or other treatment-related factors, a long wait may not be practical or advisable. After miscarriage, you will want to work closely with your healthcare team—including your RE, primary care physician or OB-Gyn, and therapist—to map out your options and establish the best time frame to continue your efforts to become pregnant. Many physicians suggest waiting two to three menstrual cycles, especially if you have had a D&C. The physician will want your β-hCG levels to decrease to normal (undetectable) levels so that they will not interfere with the quality of ovulation.

If you are suffering deep depression after a miscarriage, the short-term use of an antidepressant may be beneficial to help you cope through the time of grieving. Should an antidepressant be prescribed (for either partner of the couple, but especially for the woman), however, be sure to inform *all* members of your healthcare team, particularly your RE, that you are taking this type of medication. (See chapter 11, "Staying Centered," for information on exploring the emotions associated with infertility treatment, learning coping skills and stress-management techniques, and advice on seeking help from a therapist or counselor when it is needed.)

## Perspectives

Use your infertility journal as a healing tool to help move you through the emotional pain of going through a pregnancy loss. A miscarriage can unleash feelings of anguish, guilt, and remorse. Writing your thoughts down may help you to better process and deal with them. Both partners of a couple need to work together to avoid directing blame, either inwardly at themselves or outwardly toward each other. Perpetuating a cycle of "If only we hadn't" or "Next time we will" thinking can lead to undue stress and pressure. Indirect expressions of emotion in response to the miscarriage, such as bottling up emotions or excessive irritability or anger over small things, can be equally damaging. Nothing you did caused the pregnancy loss. Remember to be kind to yourself. Let the sorrow and grief out. Talk to your partner; share your feelings. Consult a therapist or counselor. Write in your journal and give yourself time to heal. You may also find at this time that you experience feelings of sadness about past losses in your life, such as the death of a parent. You may feel a little out of control and ask yourself why this has happened to you. The deep feelings of loss and grief may touch a wellspring of emotion inside you (the same is true for your partner, as well). Your infertility journal can be an outlet for channeling your grief and moving forward toward acceptance.

It is important to understand that you and your partner may not experience the pregnancy loss in the same way. Coping styles may be quite different. Many husbands feel it is their "job" to stay strong and "hold things together." The male partner may also feel left out to some extent, forced into a "helpless" position as the medical and emotional attention of the healthcare team focuses on the woman's recovery. If you find that you and your partner are at very different stages of processing your grief over a pregnancy loss and are having trouble communicating, consider seeking help from a therapist or counselor.

### Voices

*John remembers the sadness of losing the pregnancy and the terrible worry he had about his wife, Anne, as she was wheeled down the hall for emergency surgery. "All of a sudden, all I could think about was that Anne might die. I felt so alone when I looked down that hall at the operating room doors."*

*"My husband and I had gone through the infertility differently," shares Tess. "Chris was optimistic that modern technology would eventually find a way to help me sustain a pregnancy. While I gathered facts and figures and pursued statistics to figure out what the odds were and if something were worth pursuing realistically, he'd want to give me a big hug, telling me that everything would be all right when I didn't feel so sure it would be. We went for therapy to get all the emotions and conflicts out in front of us and it helped."*

## The Importance of Acceptance

Ritual is one way to honor your pregnancy loss and at the same time bring a sense of acceptance and closure to your emotional pain. One of the most familiar closure rituals in American culture is, in fact, the funeral, which allows family and friends to remember and honor a loved one. Some couples find a funeral to be an appropriate and comforting ritual for bringing closure to their loss, particularly if it is a late pregnancy loss. Even in early pregnancy loss, however, a small ceremony of recognition can be very helpful in allowing you to express your emotions. Such ceremonies give you permission to cry and grieve openly. Your remembrance ceremony might include close friends and relatives, or just you and your partner.

It is often helpful to include in your ritual something tangible that symbolizes the cycle of life. Many people find planting a special tree helps them find closure. As the tree grows and flourishes, it provides a living memorial. Some people use birdbaths or birdfeeders in a similar way. If these approaches are not practical in your circumstances or do not appeal to you, consider making a donation to an organization or charity in memory of your pregnancy loss. There are many ways you can honor your loss and at the same time allow you and your partner to move forward.

## Handling Reminders of Your Loss

There will be times when the pain of your loss resurfaces. Some you might expect, such as the return of your menstrual periods or the date your baby would have been born. Others might catch you by surprise, such as seeing children who are the same age your child would have been had your pregnancy progressed normally. It is both normal and healthy for you to experience sadness at these times. As a process of emotional healing, the intensity of your response will lessen over time. Rituals can also help.

Some people light candles at church or synagogue as a way both to acknowledge and honor the memory of what might have been. Others add to the original ritual, such as planting flowers around the tree they originally planted. Such remembrances tend to be more personal and more private than was your initial grieving process. Although family and friends may have been aware of your loss and provided sympathy and support, they may not remember relevant dates as you do. If you want support and comfort, let those who are close to you know that a difficult anniversary is approaching. Tell them what you would like them to do, whether simply to remember with you or to join you in a brief ritual.

### Posttraumatic Stress Disorder (PTSD) and Pregnancy Loss

Posttraumatic stress disorder (PTSD) occurs in a small percentage of people who experience pregnancy loss, especially when coupled with infertility. PTSD is simply the name for the condition that exists when your response to a traumatic event continues well beyond the typical grieving cycle. Symptoms tend to grow more severe over time, rather than less. A person with PTSD might find it so painful to be around children, for example, that she begins avoiding any environment in which such an encounter is possible. Extreme depression—the clinical condition in which ongoing feelings of helplessness, deep sadness, and listlessness interfere with everyday activities—is a key symptom of PTSD. If your feelings of sadness and depression continue for several months past a pregnancy loss or are affecting your ability to function normally day to day, consult a therapist for help. (See chapter 11, "Staying Centered.")

## Embracing the Future

The chances of having a successful pregnancy after a miscarriage are good—even after experiencing recurrent miscarriages. Research indicates that there is a 75 to 80 percent probability of having a successful pregnancy after two miscarriages, a 70 percent probability of success after three miscarriages, and a 60 percent probability of success after as many as four miscarriages.

## POSITIVE STEPS YOU CAN TAKE FROM CHAPTER 10

**Understand, as much as possible, the medical explanation and implications of your miscarriage.** As painful as losing a pregnancy may be, it is not an uncommon experience nor does it doom all (or any) future pregnancies. Try to get as much information as possible from your physician about the cause of your pregnancy loss—if it can be determined—and what your next step should be.

**Take the time to grieve for your losses.** Losing a cherished pregnancy involves dealing with feelings of grief, and it will take time for you to recover. Do not put yourself on a schedule.

**Look forward to the future with optimism.** Between the laws of nature and the advances in medical technology, chances are good that you can move on from your pregnancy loss to a successful pregnancy. If not, there are other options to consider for building your family. Communicate your feelings, your hopes, and your fears with your partner and with your physician.

# PART 3

# COPING WITH
# INFERTILITY

# 11 Staying Centered

Infertility can easily become the primary focus of your life. It does not start out that way, of course. Early in your journey, the world of options lies wide open ahead of you. Testing and treatment, although intrusive and disconcerting, have not yet invaded the inner sanctum of your well-being. *Next month*, you tell yourself, *we'll be pregnant*. As time passes, your hope diminishes and your world narrows. Life becomes an endless cycle of hormones and intimacy on demand. And before you know it, you cannot remember when life was anything else. Your quest for fertility demands—and receives—your complete dedication. As much as infertility treatment requires intense commitment, it is important to nurture other aspects of your life, too—namely, your relationship with your partner.

All relationships need care and attention if they are to flourish, and couples struggling with infertility are no different in this regard than couples who are not. There are, of course, no absolutes in how people cope and react to adversity. But it is not uncommon during a life crisis such as infertility for each person to withdraw into an area where he or she feels comfortable and less threatened. This could be work, hobbies, fitness, friends, church, or other social activities. Everyone has a way of retreating when the world becomes overwhelming. This is both normal and healthy—until it interferes with relationships or other aspects of living. It is easy to view other activities in your life as demanding your participation—additional work or pressing deadlines at the office, for example—instead of acknowledging that all those extra hours really may be just a way to avoid dealing with your concerns about your infertility and how it is affecting your relationship. Many experts suggest couples plan a special event for the end of a treatment cycle, preferably on the day you find out the results.

---

### Voices

*"When I'm with my wife, the infertility is always there and that is the top priority," says Glenn. "But I can go to work and just concentrate on that, and shut everything else out." Glenn and his wife, Louise, who went through 7 years of treatment before becoming pregnant through donor egg, became experts at riding the hope-disappointment cycle. Louise agrees, too, that distracting yourself from the pain can help a great deal. "Plan something really cool for the day after you're expecting the results of treatment—a special dinner out, a kayaking trip, a hike," she suggests. "That way, if you're pregnant and have to limit your activity, you're thrilled, but if you're not, you've got something really great to look forward to and that will help you start healing."*

---

## COPING DAY TO DAY

It can be difficult to keep infertility in perspective. Some days are easy, with opportunities to laugh and enjoy the day for what it brings. You can *almost* forget the infertility that usually dominates your thoughts and emotions. Other days, it seems everything around you is a reminder of your struggles. And sometimes coping is an hour by hour affair. Among the most common feelings related to infertility is that of being of out of control and helpless.

---

### Voices

*"I used one technique to stop what I called 'runaway negative thinking,'" explains Elaine, a 35-year-old single woman who spent 3 years trying to get pregnant. "When that thinking hits, you almost feel like you're losing your mind. I learned to control the negative thoughts by thinking out loud about what is immediate. 'I'm in my car. I'm driving 55 miles per hour. My hands are on the steering wheel.' I know it sounds dumb, but this technique really works and calms my thoughts tremendously."*

---

### Reducing Stress

There are many ways to lower the stress in your life. Those that work best are ones you can do anywhere, any time. Yoga, prayer, meditation, and exercise are often effective and can become part of your daily routine. Good nutrition, regular physical activity, and restful sleep are also important (more on these topics in chapter 12, "Staying Healthy").

## HOW INFERTILITY FEELS

Infertility is a life crisis, characterized by feeling that both your body and your life are out of control. Physically, there are many challenges to face as you navigate your course through infertility. Emotionally, you will feel like you are riding a roller coaster of hope and despair. As you come to terms with the losses infertility may bring, you will feel sadness and mourning. You grieve not just the biological child you are not making or the pregnancy you are not experiencing, but also the friendships you lose as your peers add second and third children to their families. You experience a loss of innocence as you realize the life you believed would treat you fairly has not done so. Infertility can feel like failure, especially if you have always gotten everything you have worked for—until now. If your sense of failure continues or grows with each month you are not pregnant, your grief and pain can intensify.

### *Secondary Infertility*

Couples who have a first child often intentionally wait to try for a second. Then to their surprise, the second child does not happen. More than 3 million Americans report experiencing secondary infertility. The problems can be the same as those that cause primary infertility, from ovulation and tubal problems in women to sperm problems in men, although age-related factors are more commonly found in secondary infertility. Testing and treatment are the same for either primary or secondary infertility.

Having one child does not mitigate the sadness and disappointment couples feel when confronting secondary infertility. Well-meaning friends and relatives suggest "being happy with what you have," advice that is both insensitive and inappropriate.

# COMING OUT OF THE INFERTILITY CLOSET

It is difficult to be open about infertility. But the self-imposed secrecy that tends to surround infertility is a major contributor to stress. Coming out in the open about your infertility can mean opening yourself to comments and criticisms from those who do not understand what you are experiencing.

### Voices

*"I made a very conscious decision, 2 or 3 years into our treatment, to be as vocal about what was happening with us as possible, because I believe it is ignorant people who make ignorant comments, and the only way to change that is to educate them," says Cindy. "To do that, one has to talk about the issues. The more we make infertility a mainstream issue, rather than keeping it to ourselves as if it were something to be ashamed of, the more we'll get things we want, such as better insurance coverage."*

*"It makes me angry that so many infertile women are ashamed about their condition, that they don't talk about it more," adds Lin. "The thing I've really enjoyed about being vocal about this is that I'll tell someone in the elevator, some stranger, who will almost inevitably say 'oh, I'm going through that too' or 'my sister is' or whatever. Always, they know somebody who's dealing with infertility. Most people don't realize how natural this is, how much it occurs in our communities."*

## Handling Negative Comments

Interestingly, although co-workers and relatives would not think to ask about your sex life, some seem to have little reluctance about telling you how you should start your family.

### Voices

*"I had people say to me, why don't you just adopt— it's probably a lot cheaper than in vitro fertilization (IVF)," says Brooke. "Why would someone want to put a price on us being parents?"*

*People do not usually intend to be cruel. Often, they feel their comments will help you feel better—which, of course, is not what happens. "Someone once said to me, oh, I have five kids and I'd be glad to give one up," says Kara. "She meant well, but it just wasn't the right thing to say."*

*Garrett asserts, "PLEASE STOP ALL THE MOTIVATIONAL STUFF. Everyone has a success story. Yes, at the beginning of this torturous process they helped a little. But there are very few people that have been through what Leah and I have been through. For people to say don't worry, it will happen . . . PLEASE! They have no idea of what they are talking about. Don't get me wrong, I believe it will happen for us, I just don't like it when people try to make us feel better about our infertility by giving us a pep talk."*

Many couples say it works best to share your circumstances only with people you know will be supportive. Unfortunately, people who make comments like the ones above typically consider themselves supportive! It usually does not accomplish anything to snap back—doing so only hurts the other person, and does not keep communication open. If the person is someone close to you, it sometimes helps to talk with him or her, privately, and explain why such comments, however well-intended, hurt you. If the person is an acquaintance or even a stranger, how you respond will depend on whether you have the energy to correct or educate him or her. Sometimes a simple "thank you for your concern" will end the encounter with minimal discomfort for all. Depending on your mood and the circumstances, you might want to invite the person to attend a RESOLVE meeting or to read RESOLVE educational materials to learn more about infertility. It sometimes becomes a matter of balancing your needs for understanding and emotional support with the general need to educate people about infertility.

It is also very important for you and your partner to agree on exactly who to tell and how much detail you want to share with family and friends. If one of you feels the details should stay private, it is essential for you both to honor that, remembering that something once told may be told again. When telling close friends or family members about what you are going through, also tell them what you need from them in the way of support and encouragement. Be specific—no one can read your mind! If you want your sister or your mother to call to see how this month's cycle is going, tell her. If not, just tell her you will keep her posted. By being specific, you help those who care about you to give you the support you need. You also make it easier to avoid being disappointed when you do not receive the responses you want.

## FAMILY AND FRIENDS

Some couples going through the ups and downs of infertility draw strength from family and friends. Others do not. The intimate nature of infertility can make it a difficult subject to discuss with those who do not know firsthand what you are experiencing. Still, it is important to find people with whom you can share your feelings. Sharing in this way both validates your emotions and relieves at least some of the stress, apprehension, and worry you feel. This, in turn, restores balance to your life.

## Voices

*Some couples find infertility builds relationships with family, especially parents and in-laws, that otherwise would not evolve. "We crossed some bridges with my folks, and we all grew a lot in the process," says Dana. "My father read an article in the local paper about a minister who shared her infertility struggle with her congregation. That opened his eyes to what Charles and I were going through. He opened the dialogue by showing me the article and asking questions. It was interesting. All of a sudden you find yourself able to talk about these very personal things with your parents and your in-laws."*

*Some couples share certain aspects of their experiences and feelings with some friends, and other aspects with other friends. "I can't think of anyone who knows all the facts," says Sharissa. "I have RESOLVE friends who know about the infertility. I have close friends who know more about the sadness and depression. I never felt that I was understood like I wanted to be or really heard, either, by most of our friends and family."*

Many families struggle with how to support the couple experiencing infertility. Parents who want to be grandparents may feel the couple is not trying hard enough, or just needs to relax (everyone's least favorite piece of advice). Most couples experiencing infertility appreciate their parents' support and interest, but not their advice. An appreciative comment to your parents, along with a tactful reminder that you have good professional advice from your medical team, infertility counselor or attorney, and good support from your peers within RESOLVE, may help.

Some people find themselves cultivating new friends from infertility support groups, other people who are experiencing similar events and emotions. The bonds that form in such friendships can be deep and enduring. These friends understand and share the highs and lows, the laughter and the tears, in ways that fertile friends cannot. Some such friendships last a lifetime, whereas others fade away as couples resolve their infertility through adoption, pregnancy, or choosing to remain childfree.

> ### *Voices*
>
> *"Dealing with family and friends has been hard," Amanda acknowledges. "People just don't understand how to deal with it. We have some friends that have done really well, and others that just never got it. People just don't understand that every month when you get your period, you're experiencing a death. They already have their kids, and they can't put themselves in your shoes."*

## LIVING IN A FERTILE WORLD

When you are experiencing infertility, holidays can be particularly difficult in such a child-focused culture. Birthdays, Mother's Day and Father's Day, Christmas, Hanukkah, Passover, Easter, and even Halloween can be painful for those whose lives are defined by infertility. The world is a fertile place, as it must be if humankind is to survive. As hard as it can be, do not take it personally. People with children do not mean to flaunt their fertility when they flop into the booth beside yours in a restaurant, their boisterous offspring in tow. It just feels especially sensitive to you when you would like to be in their places.

> ### *Voices*
>
> *"It's both funny and a tragedy that couples without children are discriminated against during holidays," says Ian. "We are always the ones asked to stay late, work overtime, work through the holidays. Certainly we don't begrudge our co-workers with tiny toddlers the opportunity for another photo memory. But it seems unfair that no one considers my wife and me to be a family that also celebrates special times. It's very significant that our culture dictates that children are the focus of holidays. I hated that each year my wife and I would throw ourselves more and more into work and our careers right about the approach of Halloween, continuing straight through the New Year."*

Some couples establish holiday plans for themselves and announce them well in advance, such as a ski vacation or a tropical cruise. It is totally appropriate for you to protect yourself during difficult times of celebration. You do not have to go to a baby shower if it will take you hours to steel yourself for the experience and a day to recover from it. Of course the others will miss you, but you are just one of many who received invitations. You can send a nice card with a gift certificate to show that you care.

Sometimes the most difficult times are not traditional holidays so much as personal anniversaries, such as the anniversary of the death of one of your parents. The dates of infertility losses are also painful—failed IVFs, due dates that came and went, miscarried pregnancies. Some people use rituals, such as lighting a candle at home, synagogue, or church, or pausing in the day's activities for a moment of silence. Others plan special activities to provide comfort, such as dinner at a favorite restaurant or a weekend retreat.

> ### *Voices*
>
> *"The hardest times for me were the anniversary of my father's death," says Joanne. "My father always wanted to be a grandfather, and he was so sad for me that I wasn't able to become a mother. Each year, I dread the day he died because I feel like I let him down."*

Here are some tips for coping during the holidays:

- Find new ways for you and your partner to celebrate. Do not feel obligated to traditions from the past. Start some traditions of your own.
- Keep your visits with family and friends short, and avoid times that would be particularly painful. Instead of watching your nieces and nephews open their holiday gifts, for example, arrive later. Or get to a gathering in time for dessert, but miss the main meal.
- Use gift certificates or shop by catalog to avoid children-filled stores.
- Do something special just for you. Get a massage, for example, or have a facial.
- Define your holidays with activities that feel right for you and your partner rather than by "shoulds" to make others happy.

## INFERTILITY AND THE WORKPLACE

For many people work is a place where they must both hide their infertility and endure the fertility of those around them. Women are particularly affected, since they are the ones who undergo ovulatory stimulation and have to deal with medical appointments that can mean hours and even days away from work. Although the Family and Medical Leave Act (FMLA) requires many employers to allow both men and women to take unpaid leave for pregnancy and related matters without worry about losing their jobs, doing so is often not practical or is cost-prohibitive in terms of lost wages and benefits. As well, smaller employers—which account for nearly half of the nation's employment—are not bound by the FMLA. And although the FMLA may assure you can return to your job, taking extended periods of time off work can derail your career track.

Telling your boss about your infertility is a personal decision that you will have to weigh in terms of costs and benefits. Since it is obvious that they are out of the office for a reason, some people choose to disclose only that they are undergoing medical testing and treatment for non–life-threatening problems. This clarification is important because without it your boss or co-workers could speculate that you have cancer or another terminal illness.

### Voices

*"I can still remember calling my doctor in tears, begging him to give me another excuse I could tell my co-workers for being out of work for 6 weeks following surgery,"* says Marjorie. *"I was in a typical male-dominated, glass ceiling type of company and I couldn't say I was infertile and taking time off work to deal with it. If they knew I were trying to have a baby, I could forget any career aspirations, just kiss it all good-bye. I lied to everybody about why I was going in for surgery, and then I was really quiet about everything I was going through for the next few years."*

*Perri resolved her situation at work by leaving the company and taking 6 months off to reassess her ambitions and goals. "When I started working again, I made the conscious decision that I was going to be very vocal and open about what I was doing,"* Perri says. *"It felt so good not to have to lie to my boss. I'm the president of my own company now, and I really only work part time."*

## REDUCING ISOLATION

Despite your need occasionally to envelop yourself in other activities, it is especially important to remain connected with each other, no matter how bumpy the road becomes. This can be especially challenging for men, who often feel pressure to suppress their emotions and are not sure what to do to be supportive. Instead of talking about their feelings with their partners, they withdraw.

### Voices

*"Men are never supposed to cry,"* says Roger, who with his wife Anita battled infertility for 6 years before the birth of their son. *"Guys aren't supposed to show emotion because showing emotion is showing weakness. But that doesn't mean the emotion isn't there. I felt it just as deeply as Nita did. Every moment of sadness. Every moment of joy."*

Consider joining a support group where you can talk with others experiencing the same emotions and concerns as you. You can also read books by people who have walked the infertility road and want to share their experiences with others. It is reassuring to know you are not alone, and that your emotional reactions are normal.

A support group is a group of people in a similar life situation who come together in a confidential setting to share feelings, concerns, information, and creative ways to cope with or solve their problems. In a support group, members seek help from, and give help to, each other. Members of an infertility support group may share experiences and information about medical treatments, talking with family and friends about infertility, adoption, surrogacy and donor issues, and other aspects of this difficult journey. With the help of an experienced leader, the group can work through feelings of grief, anger, and depression while moving to resolution.

You might find a support group helpful if:

- You want to learn more about infertility and to maximize or strengthen your coping mechanisms.
- You feel lonely and isolated, and that there is no one you can talk to about your infertility who understands.
- Your infertility is affecting other aspects of your life, including friendships, work or career, and your relationship with your spouse or partner.
- You are having trouble navigating through medical treatment options or deciding when enough is enough.

Support groups are not intended to replace counseling or therapy. What you share with the group is up to you. Support groups typically end after 10 or 12 meetings.

## KEEPING THE FAITH

Spirituality—no matter what the belief system—is often the element that pulls people through times of extraordinary challenge. Believing in a higher being can relieve the stress and offer comfort.

### Voices

*"When I was 4 months pregnant, I wrote an article for my church bulletin about how the whole process of infertility had killed my faith in God," recalls Phyllis. "I was so*

*angry! But now I truly believe this child was all His. We had nothing to do with it. Somehow, having someone else to share the blame with really helped."*

Many studies show that people with strong spiritual beliefs and support systems heal more quickly from injuries and illnesses, and are more likely to overcome health-related adversity. Some people find prayer a powerful means of both reducing stress and restoring hope. Others find ways to personalize traditional religious beliefs, even to the extent of "bending the rules" to accommodate the treatments they need. Sometimes what used to feel comfortable and helpful no longer does. Many couples find the family orientation of churches and religious services fail to meet their needs. They feel left out. For some individuals and couples, the infertility treatment most likely to make them parents is in direct opposition to the tenets of their religion.

### Voices

*"My husband and I are deeply spiritual people although we could not find a home within structured religion," says Drew. "For many years we sought guidance through ministers, preachers, and churches. But we always had the feeling that the infertile couple is not welcome in the eyes of the church community. Certainly the high tech part of our medical procedures were judged and disapproved. So we followed our hearts and created our own religion."*

*"We are Roman Catholic, and much of the treatment we have been through is not accepted by the Catholic Church," says Joyce. "I try not to let it bother me too much because personally I feel I am doing nothing wrong. I truly believe that God wants us to be parents, no matter how it ends up happening."*

People often turn to religion for answers to difficult questions. It can be frightening when your faith feels weakened by the infertility experience. Feeling angry with or betrayed by the spiritual being or force in which you believe can be devastating. Some people find they can no longer pray or attend services. The whole question of "why me" is unanswerable. Infertility *is* unfair. Your task is to find the inner strength to survive and even thrive despite your challenges. Your faith and your belief system, if you can connect or reconnect with it, can help you shift from asking "why me" to "how can I cope."

### Voices

*"I once did a call-in talk show about infertility, and afterwards my RESOLVE chapter asked for a list of the questions people called in, thinking we could use this to iden-*

*tify needs," says Megan. "One caller said 'you should just accept the fact that God has tied your tubes.' As I've matured, I've come up with a response for this—I relate a joke.*

*"There was a man who kept saying God would provide. Then there came a flood. As the man sat trapped on his roof, a rowboat came by, then a motor boat, and finally a helicopter. Still the man waited for God to take care of him, and the water got higher and higher. The man drowned. When he arrived at the Pearly Gates, he asked St. Peter what had happened. 'I kept waiting for God to save me, but he never did.'*

*"St. Peter says to the man, 'Who do you think sent the rowboat, the motorboat, and the helicopter?' Overcoming infertility can be a similar situation."*

## SEEKING PROFESSIONAL COUNSELING

Infertility is a stressful event in your life, and it is normal to feel a wide range of emotions while dealing with diagnosis and treatment. Although often you can manage these feelings by talking with your partner and with friends who understand what you are going through, there are certain indications that professional counseling could be beneficial. These include the following:

- Signs of depression:
  - Persistent feelings of sadness, guilt, or worthlessness.
  - Dramatic changes in your appetite or sleeping habits (eating and sleeping more or less than usual).
  - Loss of interest in usual activities and relationships; social isolation.
  - Thoughts about suicide or death.
- Agitation and anxiety.
- Significant mood swings.
- Constant preoccupation with infertility.
- Increased use of alcohol or drugs.
- Being stuck in one feeling, such as rage, envy, guilt, or a sense of being out of control.
- Being bothered by old issues that you thought were resolved, such as your parents' divorce or the death of someone you loved.

If you are considering other family-building options, such as donor egg/sperm, surrogacy, or adoption, an experienced counselor can help you sort out the issues involved. Counseling can help you and your partner maintain a healthy relationship, and even deepen the one you had together before becoming parents became your primary focus.

### *Voices*

*Sometimes the pressure of dealing with the many challenges of the infertility experience is more than you can handle. The outside perspective of a professional counselor can help you gain insight into your situation and your feelings, and give you additional tools for handling both. "I was so anguished, so sad, I was inconsolable," says Deana, who conceived and then lost twins after 3 years of trying to become pregnant. "I just went about my routine with the motions but not the emotions; I was so numb. I gave myself a few months off from infertility treatment. I sought out a mental health counselor and went for therapy."*

When choosing a mental health professional, look for one with experience in dealing with infertility issues. Qualified infertility counselors may be psychiatrists, psychologists, social workers, psychiatric nurses, marriage and family counselors, or clergy. In addition to professional credentials, the therapist or counselor should have experience and training in addressing the unique issues that arise with infertility counseling. Your physician may have a referral network, or your local RESOLVE chapter can be contacted for good counseling resources. Organizations such as the American Society for Reproductive Medicine's Mental Health Professional Group, the National Association of Social Workers, and the American Psychological Association also have lists of qualified mental health professionals from which you can choose. (See the Resources in the appendix of this book for additional information.)

Once you have several referrals, evaluate your needs and review your options. What are the specific issues and areas you would like to address in counseling? What resources are available through your job, such as an employee assistance program (EAP)? Are you comfortable using such a service? What does your insurance policy cover? Does the therapist you are considering accept your insurance or offer a payment plan? Before choosing a therapist, interview at least two and ask each the following questions:

- What type of degree did you earn and from what school was the degree awarded? Is the school accredited?
- What was the length and specific area of concentration of your clinical training? To what professional organizations do you belong?
- When did you establish your practice? What is your training and experience in infertility counseling?
- What percentage of your practice deals with reproductive loss (or infertility) issues?

- What treatment modalities (approaches) do you use? Do you prescribe medication, or do you work with someone who can prescribe? Are the medications you/they prescribe approved for use by individuals trying to become pregnant or during pregnancy?
- How many sessions would there be, and how often would they occur? How long would each session be? What is your policy about canceled or missed appointments?
- Will you accept phone calls from me, and is there a fee?
- Under what circumstances would you discuss my case with other medical professionals?

If the answers to these questions are satisfactory and working with the therapist fits into your schedule and financial plan, consider how you, your partner, and your therapist will work together. After your first session, ask yourself the following questions:

- Do I/we feel comfortable with this person? Could I trust him or her with my feelings?
- Do I feel respected and understood? Was I treated as a human being or as a "sick person"?
- Do I feel this person understands infertility issues?
- Did the therapist answer questions to my satisfaction? Is the therapist honest and direct?
- Do I already feel helped and hopeful?

If you answer any of these questions in the negative, consider discussing the problem with the therapist or make an appointment to see someone else. If you are already in therapy, and you or your partner experiences any of the following, consider changing your therapist:

- You feel uncomfortable emotionally or physically in the presence of the therapist.
- You dread your appointments or feel you are getting worse.
- You feel you are getting nowhere or that you are able to manipulate the sessions by avoiding the hard issues.
- You sense that the pain you feel about infertility experience is being minimized.
- You feel you are educating the therapist about infertility.

Admitting that you need help coping with your feelings and your decision making is often as hard as admitting that you are having trouble having a baby. But by doing so, you will be on your way to meeting some of the challenges you face.

## POSITIVE STEPS YOU CAN TAKE FROM CHAPTER 11

**Feeling consumed, physically and emotionally, from the infertility experience is normal.** Reducing stress through exercise, meditation, or hobbies and reducing isolation through support group connection can help you feel more in control and centered.

**Most friends and family members offer comments meant to comfort; their insensitivity is usually due to being uninformed about this experience.** Try to be prepared to handle insensitive comments and stressful family or social encounters. If you are able, offer suggestions for improving your interactions while you are moving through the crisis or educational materials on its depth and meaning to you.

**The infertility experience may pose one of the biggest challenges to your life plan or faith that you have ever faced.** It is common for couples and individuals to seek spiritual guidance or help from qualified mental health professionals. Consider these avenues if you are feeling overwhelmed.

# 12 Staying Healthy

When you are trying to conceive, it is wise to be in the best health possible. For most people, this means eating a nutritious diet and incorporating regular exercise into your daily activities.

## WHY IT IS IMPORTANT TO TAKE CARE OF YOUR HEALTH

Keeping yourself in good physical condition is a good idea whether you are trying to conceive or not. A fit body has the resources it needs to stay healthy. Many health experts believe Americans could virtually eliminate their risks for heart disease, the country's leading cause of death, through regular exercise and nutritious eating habits to keep body weight and cholesterol measures at recommended levels. For example, thousands of people are able to regulate conditions such as mild to moderate hypertension (high blood pressure) and type 2 diabetes (non–insulin-dependent) through exercise, diet, and weight control.

You would not set out to drive from San Francisco to Boston in a car that was in unsound mechanical condition. By the same token, you do not want to embark on this journey with a body that is not fit. Most people slide into unhealthy habits unintentionally. With more to do and less time to do it, life becomes more complicated and time becomes more scarce. Physical activities, especially team and organized events, become luxuries to be squeezed in rather than essentials to plan around. The convenience of fast foods, from take-out to take home and prepare in just minutes, can lead to nutritional compromises.

## Improper Body Weight

Women who are significantly underweight or overweight may have difficulty getting pregnant. Low weight can lead to an alteration in the gonadotropin-releasing hormone (GnRH) and follicle-stimulating hormone–luteinizing hormone (FSH/LH) signals that the brain sends to the ovaries in women and testes in men. If a woman is significantly underweight, she may not ovulate (a condition known as *anovulation*), or the lining of her uterus may not be ready to receive a fertilized egg because of inadequate ovarian hormone production. In men, being underweight may lead to decreased sperm function or sperm count. Being overweight or obese also can affect the hormonal signals to the ovaries or testes. Increased weight may increase insulin levels in women and disturb estrogen levels, which in turn may cause the ovaries to overproduce male hormones and stop releasing eggs. If you or your partner are significantly underweight or overweight, or have recently gained or lost a significant amount of weight, talk to your physician.

- Eat a balanced diet that allows you to maintain a healthy weight. Consult the desired height/weight charts for women and men, compiled by the Metropolitan Life Insurance Company for its *Statistical Bulletin*, that appear on page 235. Weights in the charts are based on wearing indoor clothes and 1-inch heels.
- Before you try to lose or gain weight, talk to your physician about how your plan may affect your fertility.

## Eating Well

Good nutrition is essential for your body to function. You need a balanced intake of proteins, carbohydrates, fats, fiber, vitamins, and minerals. These nutrients come from the foods you eat—dairy products, vegetables and fruits, meats, fish, nuts, and grains (breads, cereals, rice, pasta). The U.S. Food and Drug Administration (FDA) developed a food pyramid in 1992 to revise traditional thinking about the basic four food groups (see page 236). The food pyramid outlines recommended servings, from among the six categories of food products, for healthy eating. You cannot go wrong by following these recommendations, which are light on fats, sweets, and meats and heavy on fruits, vegetables, and grains.

## DESIRED WEIGHTS OF WOMEN AGED 25 AND OVER

| Height (in inches) | Small Frame (in pounds) | Medium Frame (in pounds) | Large Frame (in pounds) |
|---|---|---|---|
| 58 | 102–111 | 109–121 | 118–131 |
| 59 | 103–113 | 111–123 | 120–134 |
| 60 | 104–115 | 113–126 | 122–137 |
| 61 | 106–118 | 115–129 | 125–140 |
| 62 | 108–121 | 118–132 | 128–143 |
| 63 | 111–124 | 121–135 | 131–147 |
| 64 | 114–127 | 124–138 | 134–151 |
| 65 | 117–130 | 127–141 | 137–155 |
| 66 | 120–133 | 130–144 | 140–159 |
| 67 | 123–136 | 133–147 | 143–163 |
| 68 | 126–139 | 136–150 | 146–167 |
| 69 | 129–142 | 139–153 | 149–170 |
| 70 | 132–145 | 142–156 | 152–173 |
| 71 | 135–148 | 145–159 | 155–176 |
| 72 | 138–151 | 148–162 | 158–179 |

## DESIRED WEIGHTS OF MEN AGED 25 AND OVER

| Height (in inches) | Small Frame (in pounds) | Medium Frame (in pounds) | Large Frame (in pounds) |
|---|---|---|---|
| 62 | 128–134 | 131–141 | 138–150 |
| 63 | 130–136 | 133–143 | 140–153 |
| 64 | 132–138 | 135–145 | 142–156 |
| 65 | 134–140 | 137–148 | 144–160 |
| 66 | 136–142 | 139–151 | 146–164 |
| 67 | 138–145 | 142–154 | 149–168 |
| 68 | 140–148 | 145–157 | 152–172 |
| 69 | 142–151 | 148–160 | 155–176 |
| 70 | 144–154 | 151–163 | 158–180 |
| 71 | 146–157 | 154–166 | 161–184 |
| 72 | 149–160 | 157–170 | 164–188 |
| 73 | 152–164 | 160–174 | 168–192 |
| 74 | 155–168 | 164–178 | 172–197 |
| 75 | 158–172 | 167–182 | 176–202 |
| 76 | 162–176 | 171–187 | 181–207 |

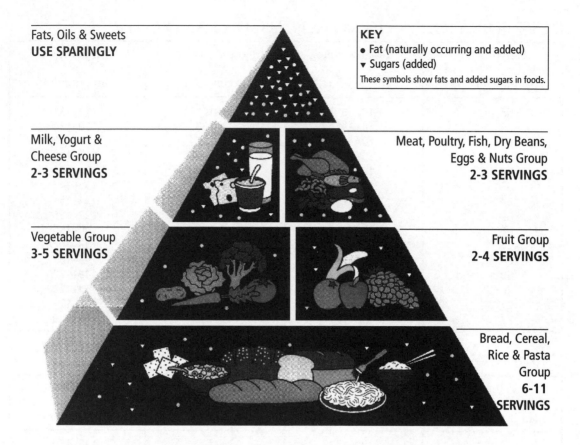

Fats, Oils & Sweets
**USE SPARINGLY**

**KEY**
- • Fat (naturally occurring and added)
- ▼ Sugars (added)

These symbols show fats and added sugars in foods.

Milk, Yogurt &
Cheese Group
**2-3 SERVINGS**

Meat, Poultry, Fish, Dry Beans,
Eggs & Nuts Group
**2-3 SERVINGS**

Vegetable Group
**3-5 SERVINGS**

Fruit Group
**2-4 SERVINGS**

Bread, Cereal,
Rice & Pasta
Group
**6-11
SERVINGS**

Here are a few tips to help you better balance your food intake with your body's needs.

- **Evaluate your eating habits.** Keep a food diary for a week. Write down what and how much you eat and drink (including water). For items you eat or drink at other than regular meal times, jot a few comments about why you ate or drank. Do not make any efforts to change just yet—this is a fact-finding mission. Be honest; you do not have to show your food diary to anyone else.

- **Determine your nutritional needs.** Most people eat more than they should from the food groups they should limit. The federal government has established average daily calorie amounts for adults—from 1,500 to 2,500 calories a day, depending on your body size and activity level. Although individual needs vary, the average person requires 15 calories for every pound of body weight to maintain that weight (your weight $\times$ 15 = your daily calorie needs). A nutritionist can help you determine your daily needs.

- **Modify your eating habits.** After you have a week's worth of documented intake, take a look at the patterns that emerge. Compare what and how much you eat with the food pyramid and the recommended calorie intake you need to stay at your ideal body weight. Again, a nutritionist can help you design a nutritional plan to lose, gain, or maintain weight.

- **Make changes slowly.** Do not set out to completely remake yourself. The most effective changes are those you make gradually and consistently. Moderation, not deprivation, is the key to succeeding in making permanent nutritional changes. Cut back on the amounts of less-nutritious foods that you eat, and replace them with servings of more-nutritious foods. Let your taste buds and your body adjust to one change before adding another.

- **Be patient, and treat yourself with kindness.** You did not get to where you are overnight, and you will not get to where you want to be overnight, either. Slow but steady weight loss or gain is the most effective route to your goal.

## What about Vitamins?

**• Folic Acid**

Folic acid, a B vitamin, plays a critical role in preventing neural tube defects, disorders in which the spinal cord tube fails to close normally in a developing fetus. Common neural tube defects include spina bifida, in which part of the spinal cord remains outside the body at birth, and anencephaly, in which the brain does not develop at all. Such defects occur in about one in every 1,000 births in the United States. Folic acid taken before conception has been shown to reduce their incidence.

The U.S. Public Health Service recommends that women take 0.4 mg (milligrams) of folic acid daily during their reproductive years. Although it is found mainly in leafy green vegetables, beans, asparagus, citrus fruit, whole grain foods, and liver, it is difficult to consume sufficient amounts of folic acid through diet alone. Check with your physician or a nutritionist about proper supplementation.

> • Iron
>
> Iron deficiency can increase the risk of miscarriage, premature delivery, and low-birth-weight infants. The need for iron increases with pregnancy, and it is important to build adequate stores of iron in the body before conception. A complete multivitamin plus minerals formulation usually provides this needed nutrient. Again, check with your physician about individual need for iron supplementation. Too much iron can be unhealthy.

## Regular Exercise

For optimal health, adults should get at least 30 minutes of moderate aerobic exercise each day—enough to get the heart pumping and the lungs expanding—as well as more intense aerobic activity of 1 hour or more, 2 or 3 days a week. This is not as overwhelming as it might sound. A brisk, 15-minute walk at lunch and again in the evening easily gives the recommended minimum 30 minutes. And it is not usually difficult to stretch those 30 minutes to 45 or even 60 minutes.

Before either you or your partner embarks on a rigorous new fitness regimen, talk to your physician about how your activity may affect your plans to get pregnant. This is especially important if your current lifestyle is relatively sedentary. Here are some tips to get your exercise program off to a good start.

- **Make exercise part of your daily routine.** Set aside a block of time each day (at least 30 minutes a day, 3 or 4 days each week) that is your exercise time. Try to let nothing interfere with this time. Invite others, including your partner, to join you in your activities if you like.
- **Do what you like.** Exercise, although it is work for your body, should be fun. If you like swimming better than walking, then swim. What matters is that you find something you like, and you do it.
- **Vary your routine.** As much as you like a particular activity, it will lose its enchantment if you do it all the time. Try new activities, just to keep things interesting. Varying your activities also helps you cross-train muscle groups for better overall fitness.
- **Find ways to be active.** Look for ways during the day to engage in physical activity, however brief your opportunities are. Take the stairs instead of the elevator, park at the back of the lot instead of near the front, walk or ride your bicycle to work one day a week, or get off the bus one stop early. Your day contains endless opportunities to give your body little workouts that add up to big gains in fitness and well-being.

• **Pay attention to your body.** If something hurts, stop to assess the problem. Are you using different muscle groups, or have you injured yourself? Pay no attention to the old adage, "no pain, no gain." It is entirely off the mark. Pain is your body's way of getting your attention to tell you something is not quite right. It is up to you to figure out what, and what adjustments to make. Do not give up because you experience some discomfort, but do not push yourself when pain is a problem.

Too much of a good thing can be as harmful as too little. Although regular and even strenuous exercise is a clear benefit for your health, extreme exercise can create other problems. Too much exercise is difficult to define because it varies among individuals, but it can cause reduced sperm production in men and the cessation of ovulation in women. If either of these conditions could be a factor for you, take a close look at the amount of exercise in your life. If you think you could be exercising too much, discuss your concerns with your physician. And men who use anabolic or androgenic steroids to enhance weight-training regimens may also be contributing to a drastic drop in sperm count, according to a recent British study. Although sperm counts usually rise again when steroid use stops, this is not always the case.

## THE ROLE OF STRESS

Regular physical activity also relieves stress, which is a part of everyone's life to some extent. Stress may feel more of a part of *your* life now than ever before. Many contemporary work environments emphasize getting more done with fewer resources. As efficiency experts have wryly observed, the now omnipresent computer has not really saved any of us time. Although this electronic marvel has revolutionized the way we live, it has done so by making it possible to do more in less time. The outcome is more work—and few can escape the effects. Today's adults work harder, and often longer, than their parents did.

No doubt you have often heard the well-intended advice, "just relax"—your stress level may skyrocket just seeing the words again. Although relaxation is not, of course, the cure for infertility, there is a grain of truth buried in the platitude. High stress levels affect many bodily functions and are known to contribute to various health conditions—from migraines to back pain and heart disease. Excess stress keeps your body in a continual "fight or flight" mode. This remnant from a time when the day's primary challenge was making it from sun-

# RELAXATION, MEDITATION, AND DEEP BREATHING

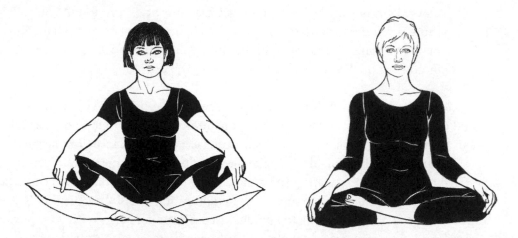

*Relax in a comfortable seated position, supported by pillows if necessary. Take 10 full, deep breaths and concentrate your attention on each inhale and exhale. Relax in meditation for 20 minutes. Allow your thoughts to pass through your mind and let them go without attachment or judgment. A regular meditation practice can help you relax, focus, and reduce the stress of infertility.*

*The action of the diaphragm muscle moves the breath into and out of the lungs. Deep breathing exercises bring oxygen to the lungs, which nourishes the blood and stimulates the brain. To feel the diaphragm moving, place your hand on your abdomen and take a full, deep breath in, releasing it slowly on a count of 10.*

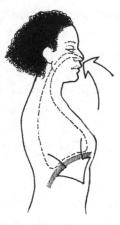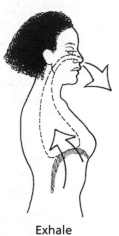

Inhale                    Exhale

rise to sunset without becoming some prehistoric creature's meal keeps your body alert—adrenaline flows, blood pressure rises, breathing and heart rate quicken, muscles tense. Today's stressors may not produce all these physical changes because, unlike the close encounter with a sabertooth tiger that shocked a primitive ancestor into action, stress just accumulates. After a while, your state of heightened awareness (which is what stress creates) feels normal—to your mind. But your body views the situation as one of sustained risk. One result of continued heightened levels of stress may be irregular ovulation, perhaps a throwback to a time when it would not be safe to reproduce.

The answer is not just a weekend away from it all in a fancy hotel, with room service and not a care in the world for 48 hours. Although certainly indulging yourself now and again can be relaxing, a more effective long-term approach is to reduce and control the stress in your everyday life. This gives your body a chance to rest, recycle, and recover. Most people cannot totally eliminate stress from their lives—and even if you could, you probably would not want to. Stress, in moderation, provides the incentive and stimulation for you to enjoy life. What stress can you eliminate or change? Often, more than you realize. The key is to identify what causes stress in your life. Then you can decide whether you can, or want to, change the causes. Do you have a demanding, high-stress job? Can you do the same job in a less stressful way, or in a less stressful setting? Do you like the job enough to make the stress worthwhile? Of course, not all stress is job-related. Financial challenges also generate stress, especially when you add in the costs of infertility treatment. Do you put a down payment on the house of your dreams, or schedule another IVF cycle? Family pressures can cause problems, too, from parents and in-laws who can't wait to have grandchildren to siblings who can't understand why this is such a big deal for you. If "high stress" defines your life, consider doing a decision tree to help you determine how to make the changes you want to make.

The emphasis in this chapter on the physical aspects of stress does not mean stress is purely physical, or that stress alone causes infertility. Stress has a huge emotional component, as we discuss in chapter 11, "Staying Centered." In reality, it is nearly impossible to separate the dimensions of life into "physical" and "nonphysical." One interplays with the other. Stress can contribute to infertility, both in terms of the physical changes it creates in your body and in the way it makes you feel.

Stress can be a factor in male impotence, for example, just as it can interfere with the intricate series of biochemical and physiological events that constitute the reproductive cycle in the female body. Because stress represents an integration of mind (how you feel) and body, activities that calm both can be very effective in reducing the harmful effects of stress. These might include yoga, tai chi, dance, meditation, and visualization. Regular exercise is one of the best ways to control stress. Running, bicycling, swimming, a good game of racquetball—these are just a few of the activities that let your body put to good use the "fight or flight" energy it has accumulated through the stressful events of your daily life. Reducing stress does not mean that you will become fertile; rather, the infertility may become more manageable and you better able to cope.

> ### *Voices*
>
> *Marianne, who had been diagnosed with a severe case of endometriosis, tried QiGong, a Chinese movement/meditation practice. "It was helpful, but I had the fantasy that it would get rid of my endo. When it didn't, and I needed surgery again, I never went back to it."*
>
> *The strong desire to look for a magical solution to your infertility problem can create unrealistic expectations—and possibly cause more stress. Cultivate stress-management techniques with the goal of promoting general health and well-being, which will help you stay centered through the crisis times.*

## LIFESTYLE RISKS THAT COULD AFFECT FERTILITY

Certain lifestyle factors can have a significant effect on your ability to conceive. Others can leave lasting or even permanent damage in their wake. You can mitigate some by changing your personal habits.

### Sexually Transmitted Diseases

The rise of sexually transmitted diseases (STDs) may explain much of the rise in infertility seen in both men and women during the late twentieth century. A 1998 study by the Johns Hopkins University School of Medicine reported that the overall rate of chlamydia infection among young female army recruits was 9.2 percent, which means that nearly 1 in 10 of these young women may later encounter fertility problems. A 1998 study in *Fertility and Sterility* found that more ectopic pregnancies (nonviable pregnancies that implant outside the uterus) than previously thought may be caused by chlamydial infections. One of the oldest known STDs, gonorrhea, remains the top infectious disease in the world despite the ease of treating it with antibiotics. A particular threat to women because they may not show symptoms, gonorrhea can leave devastating scarring that destroys fallopian tubes. Untreated, STDs of all kinds can cause a variety of problems in the reproductive tracts of men and women. Although the best cure is prevention, early treatment is essential. Both partners should receive treatment even if only one is diagnosed with an STD.

## Cigarette Smoking

A 1994 study in *Fertility and Sterility* showed that the sperm counts of three male smokers were more than 10 percent lower than those of nonsmokers. After quitting, the three men had sperm counts 50 to 800 percent higher just months later. Although the reasons for this are not entirely clear, scientists do know that cigarette smoke causes carbon monoxide to replace oxygen in the red blood cells, reducing the level of oxygen and related nutrients other cells receive. As well, cigarette smoke delivers more than 4,000 chemicals into your lungs and bloodstream. Aside from the 43 known to cause cancer, dozens or even hundreds could have detrimental effects. Another study showed that male smokers are more likely to produce sperm with an extra Y chromosome (which may be linked to impaired mental and psychological development), as well as "round-headed" sperm, which have been linked to infertility.

### Voices

*Barbra and her husband, Jack, are looking into donor egg after several failed IVF cycles. Barbra says, "Unfortunately, I smoke, and the stress made me smoke even more. However, every time I went through a cycle I quit, then when it failed, I started right back up again. My advice to other couples: Stay away from negative vices—even to relieve stress."*

In women, smoking may increase the risk of miscarriage, premature birth, and low-birth-weight babies by having a long-lasting toxic effect on ovarian function. In addition, one study indicates that women who smoke while undergoing infertility treatment could substantially reduce their chances of becoming pregnant. The longer a woman smokes, the fewer eggs and embryos she produces. According to this study, women undergoing IVF who have a history of smoking one pack a day for 10 years produce 2.5 fewer eggs and 2.0 fewer embryos per cycle than nonsmokers undergoing IVF.

Tobacco, regardless of its form, delivers the highly addictive drug nicotine into your system. Nicotine affects your brain and the chemicals it produces, altering the biochemical balance of your body for the duration of its presence (about 20 minutes after its absorption). Even the nicotine in smoking-cessation products has the same effect. Although this might be a worthwhile trade-off in the short term, it is important to realize the potential effects. If you smoke, quit as soon as possible, for your own health as well as to increase your chances of conceiving and bearing a healthy baby.

### Perspectives

Make a list in your journal of any lifestyle factors that could be inhibiting your, or your partner's, ability to conceive. Look carefully around your home and workplace for potential toxins, and remove them, if possible. Make an agreement to work with your partner as a team to cut back on or eliminate smoking, caffeine, alcohol, or whatever habit you may need to break. Be determined, but supportive; avoid nagging or negative statements if your partner is struggling, and instead, reinforce the strong desire you share to reach your goal of beginning a family. If your workplace brings you into regular contact with environmental hazards or toxins, speak to your boss or to someone in human resources about what you can do to minimize exposure, at least for a limited time while you are trying to conceive. In men, consider the 3-month production time for sperm as a time of cleansing; sperm that are mature now show the effects of your lifestyle 3 months ago.

## Alcohol Consumption

Alcohol has potentially serious consequences for couples attempting to conceive and for the child they could create. Fetal alcohol syndrome (FAS) is the number one preventable birth defect in the United States. Although intense publicity has done much to increase awareness about FAS, many people still believe it is a risk relegated to problem drinkers. It is not. Although the more you drink, the higher the risk, there is no known safe level of alcohol consumption. Studies suggest FAS and its less-severe counterpart FAE (fetal alcohol effects) can occur in a child conceived during a "binge"—an episode of heavy drinking over a short period.

Alcohol consumption can decrease sperm production in men. Preliminary research from the U.S. Health Care Financing Administration also suggests the probability of conception is reduced by more than 50 percent during menstrual cycles in which women reported ingesting any alcohol. Alcohol consumption during pregnancy can also cause health problems for the woman. If you are trying to conceive, it is best to reduce or, better yet, eliminate alcohol from your lifestyle.

Changing or eliminating habits such as drinking even moderate amounts of alcohol or smoking tobacco can be desperately hard. Both addiction and ingrained social habit may play roles in these behaviors. Try cutting back gradually, get support if you need it, and keep in mind your worthy goals of better health and fertility.

## Caffeine

The possible interaction between caffeine and fertility is much less clear than the connections with smoking or with drinking alcohol. Study findings are often contradictory. In one study of 2,500 pregnancies, women who drank three or more cups of coffee a day had more than twice the risk of delaying conception by more than 1 year. In general, the more caffeine consumed, the lower the probability of pregnancy. Researchers are not sure of the reasons for this. Some speculate that caffeine can cause chromosomal abnormalities or damage to DNA. It is also possible that caffeine-containing beverages replace more nutritious foods and drinks in the diet, resulting in miniscule but essential deficiencies that prevent conception. Yet another study hints that drinking caffeine-containing tea could actually *improve* your chances of getting pregnant. In this study, women who drank more than a half-cup of caffeine-containing tea every day nearly doubled their odds of conceiving compared with those who did not drink tea. This study's researchers believe the polyphenolic compounds in tea may promote fertility by inhibiting chromosomal abnormalities. They also caution that the study examined only women who drink tea, not those who drink coffee or cola soft drinks. It may be that tea drinkers simply lead better lifestyles all around by eating less fat, exercising more regularly, and smoking less, compared with their coffee-drinking counterparts.

It does seem clear that once you are pregnant, limiting caffeine intake is the best choice. In a study of nearly 3,000 women in their first trimester of pregnancy, those who reported drinking three or more cups of caffeine-containing coffee or tea each day had greater than twice the risk of miscarriage as women who abstained during pregnancy. Just over 9 percent of 143 women who reported consuming more than 300 mg of caffeine daily had a miscarriage, compared with only 4.8 percent of the 1,144 pregnant women who said they drank no caffeine-containing beverages.

### How Much Caffeine is Too Much?

To be on the safe side, limit the amount of caffeine you consume each day to less than 100 mg. How much caffeine is present in coffee, tea, or soft drinks? It adds up faster than you might suspect:

one 6-ounce cup of brewed coffee     120 to 140 mg

| one 2-ounce cup of espresso | 60 to 90 mg |
| one 6-ounce cup of instant coffee | 60 mg |
| one 6-ounce cup of black tea | 25 to 110 mg (depending on how strongly brewed) |
| one 12-ounce soft drink | 35 to 45 mg (varies brand to brand) |
| one 6-ounce cup of green tea | 8 to 30 mg (depending on how strongly brewed) |
| one 6-ounce cup of decaffeinated coffee | 3 mg |

## Drug Use

Unregulated and illicit ("recreational") drugs typically contain unknown substances that can be as harmless as powdered sugar or as dangerous as pesticides. The effects of these substances can at best be unpleasant and at worst cause great harm or even death to you or your fetus. In addition to posing the risk of immediate cardiac death, cocaine has been linked to placental abruption and preterm labor in women. Marijuana use is linked with hyperprolactinemia (a condition characterized by concentrations of the hormone prolactin that are persistently too high) and ovulatory dysfunction. Drugs such as marijuana, anabolic steroids, and others may affect sperm counts in men.

Even regulated medications, prescription or over-the-counter (OTC), can affect fertility. If you are taking medication to regulate your thyroid, make sure that you have your thyroid blood levels checked regularly and your medication adjusted accordingly. Some medications used to treat ulcers, psoriasis, and high blood pressure can affect a man's sperm count and sex drive. Certain antibiotics, such as nitrofurazone, nitrofurantoin, and even erythromycin, can have short-term adverse effects on sperm count and motility. Chemotherapy drugs and radiation therapy are also known to have an adverse effect on fertility in both men and women. Discuss any possible effects on fertility with your physician or pharmacist before beginning any new prescription. Often there are alternatives that are just as effective without the fertility consequences.

### *Boxers or Briefs?*

A 1998 study by the State University of New York at Stony Brook may shed some new light on this old dilemma. Previous thinking held that briefs may contribute to higher scrotal temperatures, which can adversely affect sperm production. Semen samples from 97 men in this study revealed that underwear type had no particular effect on sperm count, concentration, or motility. Switching from one to the other did not have a significant effect either. Excessive exercise, long, hot tub baths, soaking in Jacuzzis, or sitting in saunas may affect men's fertility and should be avoided.

## Use of Lubricants During Sexual Intercourse

A number of products used for lubrication during intercourse, such as petroleum jelly or vaginal creams, have been shown to affect sperm function. If you use a lubricant during sexual relations, check with your physician or pharmacist about its potential effects on your fertility.

## Exposure to Toxic Chemicals

In some cases, environmental or occupational exposure to chemicals or toxins may affect your ability to conceive. The U.S. Environmental Protection Agency (EPA) announced in August 1998 that it would conduct large-scale screening of more than 15,000 chemicals for links to cancers and deformities in humans. The chemical screening will concentrate on developing a "suspect list" of chemicals thought to behave like estrogen and other hormones that affect the development of female and male reproductive tracts. Although there remains considerable controversy about the effect of toxins on fertility, if you are having trouble conceiving, you should consider whether or not you or your partner have been exposed to the following:

- **Lead.** Exposure to lead has been shown to have an impact on fertility in humans.
- **Ethylene Oxide.** Exposure to ethylene oxide, a chemical used in the sterilization of surgical instruments and in the manufacture of certain pesticides, may cause birth defects in early pregnancy. It also has the potential to cause early miscarriage.
- **Pesticide and Herbicide Exposure.** Handling the toxins found in pesticides and herbicides might cause ovarian problems in women, possibly leading to early menopause. Studies also show that men exposed to the pesticide chlordane experienced lower sperm counts and obvious damage to the quality of the sperm-producing part of the testicles (called the seminiferous tubules). A 1997 study published in *The American Journal of Industrial Medicine* reveals that, as has been shown for men, women in agricultural occupations show an increased incidence of infertility. These women had a 4 to 16 times greater risk of ovulatory or tubal problems.
- **Other Toxins.** Individuals working with paints, varnishes, dry-cleaning

chemicals, and certain substances found in the chemical and waste-materials industries and in paper manufacturing tend to have a higher risk of reproductive problems, including miscarriage.

## KEEP YOUR HEALTHCARE TEAM INFORMED

Be sure to keep your healthcare team informed about past and current health problems, exposure to toxins, and any recent changes that could affect your health, such as starting an exercise program or altering your diet. This information could lead your physician to reevaluate or revise your treatment plan.

### POSITIVE STEPS YOU CAN TAKE FROM CHAPTER 12

**Establish good nutritional and exercise habits.** Healthy habits will help you manage the stress of the infertility experience and may help you to conceive. Making small and gradual improvements to your daily exercise routines and improving your diet, if necessary, will result in better general and reproductive health.

**Revise current lifestyle habits.** Stopping smoking and avoiding or limiting alcohol could improve your chances of conceiving.

**Avoid possible toxins.** Removing environmental hazards from your home or workplace also could improve your chances of having a baby.

# 13 Enhancing Your Relationship: Sexuality, Intimacy, and Infertility

aking love. The union of two bodies, the melding of two souls. It is the essence of romantic love in American culture, the hallmark of adult partnerships. When becoming pregnant becomes your overriding goal, however, even the most passionate relationship can turn mechanical. Making love becomes having sex to make a baby. Often, that holds no attraction for a couple who *has* to do it.

---

### *Voices*

*"Infertility places a strain on your marriage that will also strain your sex life," says Gemma. "Charting your ovulation and having sex at the 'right' times, whether you are in the mood or not, for months on end tends to change your perspective on sex."*

---

Intimacy is a complex series of emotions and feelings that often are intertwined, in humans, with sexuality. The word *intimate* comes from a Latin word that means *innermost*. To have an intimate relationship with another person is to share one's innermost self. In contemporary culture, however, intimacy and sexuality are often viewed as one and the same, which is not entirely accurate. Although, of course, sexual relationships are most satisfying when they involve intimacy, sex does not require intimacy, and intimacy can exist without sex. This is never more clear than when infertility enters a relationship.

## THE NATURE OF SEXUALITY

There are a number of ways to define sexuality. Implicit in most is a connection to reproduction. Scientists define sexuality as the biological drive to reproduce, a physical phenomenon shaped and directed by forces as old as life itself. Sociologists look at sexuality as a process of social interaction with the goal of creating a family. Psychologists perceive sexuality as an expression of communication involving both self and others. Sexuality is one of the earliest defining characteristics of a newborn—is it a boy or a girl?

Among humans, sexuality has become highly socialized and ritualized. In some respects, this makes sexuality in infertility all the more challenging. With public displays of commitment such as weddings, couples put forth their intentions for all to see. Infertile couples, however, are unable to demonstrate the socially desired (and even expected) results from their sexual union, a child. As months, and even years go by, the couple may feel isolated and embarrassed as these expectations go unfulfilled. Little wonder that sex may become a problem, even dreaded, during infertility.

If necessary, couples have the capacity to engage in sex that is purely mechanical. While you and your medical team are monitoring the frequency and timing of sexual activity during infertility treatment, it is hard for sex to be anything but mechanical.

### Voices

*"It was very hard to make love to my husband, Cody, because I was so sad the end result would not create a child," says Lauren. "Emotionally it took a long time to separate the two issues. We were able to work through it, but sometimes I still think about it."*

*Sierra and Daryl experienced similar difficulties. "I couldn't believe my wife couldn't let go of her emotional pain long enough to have sex and pleasure with me," Daryl says. "I still loved her but she didn't think I did. It was like she no longer found me sexy, and I felt really awful about the whole thing. I didn't know what to do, I just knew it was a bad scene." Sierra and Daryl eventually worked through their sexual estrangement to come back together as a couple again, although it was not easy. "When we had failed to build the big family we wanted after 10 years of marriage, I quit thinking it would ever happen for us," Daryl says. "I lost my positive faith. I remember feeling very out of control, wanting to plan and figure out what it all meant but not knowing which step to take next. Eventually we just got comfortable with the infertility and it became our identity. We knew we were in it together for the long haul, which made it easier to be close and to trust one another again."*

*Nona and James also relied on the strength and long-term commitment of their relationship to carry them through. "The sex-on-demand was difficult, but not as bad as it could have been because we both thankfully enjoy the activity," says Nona. "Jim and I had been together as a couple for 8 years before we knew we were infertile, so we had a pretty solid base."*

## LOSS OF INTIMACY

One common frustration for many couples dealing with fertility issues is the number of well-meaning but misguided friends and relatives who say, "just relax, you'll get pregnant when you stop trying so hard." The implication is, of course, that the lack of conception is somehow their fault. Couples get the message that if they could just relax and get back the feelings then they could reverse the infertility. As time goes by without conception, the feelings of failure and loss of intimacy may grow.

### *Voices*

*"It has now been over a year that Antonio and I have been trying to conceive," says Joelle. "Sex has become not the joy of sex, but the job of sex. It was taken out of the bedroom and into the cold, sterile environment of the clinics."*

*Although most of the emphasis on sexuality and intimacy focuses on married and opposite-sex couples, the stress of infertility strains same-sex relationships as well. "We're a bit different in that sex is not how we will get a baby," says Clarisse, who is pregnant as the result of an IVF using her partner Diane's egg and donor sperm from a sperm bank. "Nevertheless, our sex life has suffered tremendously. Between the drugs, the shots, and the pervasive sense of failure on both our parts, the question of sex was very difficult."*

*Rhonda and Zack have been grappling with infertility for 5 years. "There was never a question that we loved one another or wanted to stay together," says Rhonda. "But I wanted to go the fertility treatment route to start a family, and he wanted to go the career route first so he had a way to support a family. All 5 years, we fought about it all the time. He didn't accept the restrictions and demands of fertility treatment. I was so angry I couldn't even talk to him, let alone feel intimate with him." Although Rhonda is now pregnant as the result of IVF, she is seeing a counselor to help her sort through the mix of feelings she has about her infertility and her husband's reactions. She feels she and her husband have made good progress in working through their intimacy difficulties. "You really need the support of your mate," Rhonda says. "There are many emotional aspects, and for us this has been difficult to resolve. You can't really discuss it with most of your friends."*

# WHEN THE PROBLEMS ARE PHYSICAL

Most intimacy problems have emotional components. Couples blame themselves or each other, or have different ideas about how to resolve their situation. The strain on their relationship shows in many ways, including their sex lives. Occasionally, however, sexual problems are physical. If not identified and corrected, these problems will soon affect intimacy. Sexual difficulties such as impotence (an inability to achieve erection) can be due to physical or emotional causes, related to or independent of infertility. They can consume, and even destroy, a relationship. It can be especially challenging to deal with sexual problems when you are already dealing with infertility.

Performance anxiety, caused by the pressure to have sexual intercourse when the woman's ovulation patterns dictate, rather than when desire arises, can cause episodes of impotence in men. It can also be difficult for some men to perform sexually when the infertility problem lies at least in part with them.

### Voices

*"Our sex life turned pretty much to mush shortly after our first diagnosis," Whitney says. "I think part of the excitement was the mystery of knowing you could be creating a new life. When suddenly that became impossible to do, our lovemaking took on an air of sadness for me. Several times I would just cry, which caused periods of impotence for my husband."*

New drugs that help men maintain an erection are now available, but they do not ensure that there will be an ejaculation with adequate sperm. If a man has problems producing sperm on the day of an intrauterine insemination (IUI) or in vitro fertilization (IVF) treatment, the couple may consider freezing a semen sample in advance that could be thawed and used as a backup.

Some drugs used in the treatment of infertility may affect libido and/or sexual pleasure. For example, the gonadotropin-releasing hormone (GnRH) agonists may cause vaginal dryness, and clomiphene citrate may dry up cervical secretions and make intercourse uncomfortable. Sometimes the need to have sexual intercourse at specific times and days in the month may make foreplay a challenge, which can result in painful intercourse when the woman is not quite ready. If lubrication is a problem during intercourse, the raw white of an egg or a special vaginal lubricant product can be used. Be sure to check the label of the product for its effect on sperm, and do not use KY Jelly, a Vaseline petroleum product, or saliva, as these can adversely affect sperm.

# RESTORING INTIMACY TO YOUR RELATIONSHIP

Remember when your relationship was young, and everything you did together felt intimate? Even the way you looked at each other spoke volumes about your feelings for one another. Sex, of course, was the ultimate intimacy. But it was not the only time you had such feelings of closeness. Rediscovering those feelings and having spontaneous sex, on your own schedule, might be just what the doctor should order.

---

### Voices

*"Intimacy? Forget it!" says Fred. "Having sex because you have to is no fun. It gives sex a bad name. Don't get me wrong, I love my wife and love having sex with her. I just like to do it on our schedule, not the doctor's."*

---

It is easy to lose sight of the closeness you once had when your only focus is on baby-making. Why not plan a vacation for yourselves, even if only a weekend at the local Holiday Inn? Turn your attention to each other. It won't be easy, and you may feel anxious about losing precious time if it is not devoted to watching the calendar and reading ovulation predictor kit results. You may find it time well spent, however, if you are able to renew your relationship and energy for continuing treatment or decision making.

This is not the "go away, relax, you're just too uptight" lecture. This is a suggestion to spend some time rediscovering each other. Try not to think about making babies, or even making love. You might feel awkward at first, uncertain how you should act and talk to one another. Just let whatever unfolds, unfold. Don't make any plans. Order room service and watch movies, go to an art museum, or take a walk. Sex is *not* your mission. If it happens, fine. If it is wonderful, great! But if all you do is fall asleep wrapped in each other's arms, your weekend away has been a success. And if you find it too difficult to get away for a weekend because of work schedules or finances, be creative.

Plan ways in which you can be close and intimate without feeling the pressure of sexual intercourse:

- Give each other a massage.
- Make a list of three things you love most in your partner and leave it on the refrigerator door.
- Tell your partner several things he or she has done that has made life a little easier during this difficult time.

What did you and your partner do when your relationship was new and infertility was the furthest thing from your mind? Can you re-create, at least by suggestion, the image of a favorite date or activity? What you do doesn't matter so much as that you do it. Your only mission is to find each other again.

### Voices

*"No sex does not by any means mean no intimacy,"* Michiko *says about the times when sex was a problem for her and her husband Asa. "We joked a lot about it. We are the most affectionate couple we know. Even our friends comment on it. We cuddle a lot and we kiss a lot and we touch even if we aren't being very sexual. We hold hands on the street and touch under the table at dinner. We love each other very much, and we have learned there are many ways we can get that message across that don't depend on sex."*

## OTHER MARITAL ISSUES

Sometimes one partner feels the pressing desire to start a family, even if it requires treatment or alternative family building, while the other may feel more ambivalent about starting to try to have children. Men may feel that having children would be wonderful, if it happens easily, but may be reluctant or unwilling to undergo infertility treatment or consider other options. For many men, the hardest part of the infertility experience is the sadness and distress that they see in their partners. Men often want to fix things and to make things better, and this may be one time when they cannot.

Often, it is the woman who first feels the deep sense of loss, grief, and mourning. It may take several months for the man to get in touch with his feelings of loss regarding their infertility. It is hard for a couple if they are at different places emotionally. The best advice is to listen to each other and not try to fix the situation or pressure your partner to feel like you do.

### Perspectives

A woman not only feels the loss of not having a baby, a pregnancy, birthing, and nursing, she may also feel out of step with all her friends who are having babies easily. Infertility can make a woman feel badly about her body and her femininity, as well. Women also feel out of control of their life plan when struggling with infertility.

A man not only feels the loss of a biological child and the loss of the genetic line, he may miss having the pregnancy and birthing experience with his partner, as well. The man is the partner who often tries to keep a positive viewpoint and may have a hopeful attitude that "science will come through for us." Many men do not easily show emotions or vulnerable feelings. Men who are diagnosed with a male factor problem may feel like it is an assault to their manhood.

Your infertility journal can be a useful tool in helping you express thoughts and feelings you may find it hard to share with others, even your intimate partner. Writing things down may even bring to the surface feelings you had not been able to face previously, or deal with consciously. In the same way that support groups, such as RESOLVE groups, offer a safe place to work things out, your journal can serve the same purpose. When you feel comfortable, share your thoughts and feelings with your partner.

Joining a RESOLVE support group can be very helpful in reducing the isolation couples often feel and also in reassuring them that their emotional responses to the infertility experience are normal. It is important to have a support network that you can turn to when you need an emotional boost. Some people find it easier and more effective to get this support from others in similar situations and form relationships easily with those they meet at RESOLVE and other group meetings. It can be a relief to meet people who are going through the same things you are, who are also working through their options and dealing with the strain that infertility can put on an intimate relationship.

It is also important to maintain friendships with work colleagues or neighbors who may or may not know about the infertility. Although it helps to talk through your frustrations, concerns, and fears related to infertility, it is also important to have contacts with whom you can chat about things that do not really matter—the weather, the traffic, the new boss. These conversations help you maintain perspective and remind you that there is a world beyond infertility, even if it does not feel that way to you.

### Voices

*"Nat felt a lot of pressure that once I got pregnant and we were starting a family, he'd have to really start to provide," says Aliza, whose husband, Nathan, has his own business. "He felt a lot of financial pressure. He could have forever said, 'not yet, not yet . . .'" But it was not easy for Nathan to talk about his concerns, which further frustrated Aliza. "I'd try to talk to him but he'd completely shut me off," she says. "I didn't get anywhere. He'd just brush it aside and tell me to relax."*

*Responds Nathan, "That was my response then. The 'men are from Mars, women are from Venus' thing didn't make sense to me then. It sure does now. I do think Ali wanted a child more than I did. I was busy. It wasn't the main thing on my mind."*

*Aliza and Nathan became active members of their local RESOLVE chapter. Over time, Aliza recalls, she was able to become less intense about having a child, and Nathan was able to feel more comfortable about having children if that was how things were to work out for them. After 5 years of unsuccessful treatment, they have resolved childfree. Aliza leads a support group for couples who have made a similar decision.*

# NURTURING YOUR INDIVIDUAL NEEDS

It is easy to overlook yourself as an individual when much of your life focuses on how the two of you as a couple can bring another life into the world. It is also important to reconnect with yourself once in a while, to indulge in pleasures that validate your sense of self. If you like to read, stay up late on a Friday or Saturday night and lose yourself in a good novel, or watch an old movie on cable. Take the dog for a long walk on the beach. Go shopping, if that is something you enjoy.

Men often find that focusing on their jobs is a way to find distraction from the pressures of infertility treatments. (Women can also fall into this pattern.) But men, too, should feel that they can indulge themselves during this stressful time. A midweek afternoon of golf, an evening bicycle ride, or even tickets to a Saturday baseball game with a couple of friends can provide a much-needed break.

# IMPROVING COMMUNICATION

Infertility is not something that flits around the edges of your life, like a nagging cold. It strikes at the core of your emotions, becoming all consuming. Few waking hours pass without mention, or at least thought, of what will happen next.

### A Voice on the 20-Minute Rule

"Sometimes I thought we would go nuts just discussing the issue of infertility to death," says Doug. "Once we found the RESOLVE golden rule of the 20-minute limit, then my wife felt she was heard. I felt I was not trapped in an endless discussion, and talk of infertility was banned for the rest of the day. That helped me to get through the years of infertility."

The 20-minute rule is simple: Conversation about infertility is limited to 20 minutes a day. Set a timer. Each partner takes 10 uninterrupted minutes to say whatever is important to him or her, to raise new issues, or to explore feelings. When the timer goes off, the time's up. The 20-minute rule can help keep endless conversations about infertility from dominating your life.

It also helps to keep discussions about infertility out of the bedroom. This frees the bedroom for intimate interactions not connected with infertility, giving your relationship a "safe" haven.

Sometimes a man's indifference to discussing infertility issues is simple frustration. Other times, it hides underlying concerns, such as feeling helpless to help.

### Voices

*"I know my wife had other outlets for discussing her infertility issues, which was good because I didn't want to discuss it very much," says Judson. "It just seemed very fruitless for us, and I felt like I couldn't fix the problem."*

Talking through each person's feelings and needs is an important aspect of open communication. It is important to share what you are feeling with your partner, but it is also important to be clear about what you need from your partner. No one can read another's mind; it is helpful if you state clearly what helps. Here are some examples of clearly stated needs:

- "I want you to go with me to the ultrasound."
- "I don't want us to stay a long time at your sister's shower."
- "I need you just to hold me and let me be sad; don't try to make me feel better."

## SEEKING PROFESSIONAL COUNSELING

The tests, the treatments, the expenses, the tentative exhilaration at an apparent success and the depression at its failure, the feeling that you are no longer in control of your lives—these are all factors that pressure a relationship. Sometimes the roller-coaster ride of infertility brings to the surface other problems, too, that otherwise might have remained underground in your relationship.

### Voices

*"I not only needed to talk with a psychologist about the anxiety of infertility, but about my husband and our marriage and how these were gyrating at different revolutions in different spheres," says Laila.*

It can be difficult to know whether you could benefit from couples counseling. In general, you should think about seeing a counselor or therapist if:

- You and your partner disagree or fight frequently.
- Sex has become an unpleasant chore.
- You and your partner have widely different priorities about families and children.
- You cannot talk about infertility or other options with each other.
- You are saying hurtful things to each other.
- One or both of you are distancing yourself from the other (working excessively, for example).
- You are using alcohol or drugs to dull the pain.
- One or both of you has some of the signs of depression (see chapter 11, "Staying Centered").

Of course, most couples dealing with infertility go through these kinds of issues periodically. When they dominate your life, however, it is time to confront them. That is usually most effective when there is a neutral third party who can help you sort things out and balance your needs and priorities. There are many kinds of therapists in practice. What is most important is that you select a therapist who is very familiar with infertility issues and treatments, and has experience in treating clients (individuals and couples) who are coping with infertility. If the problem is a specific sexual problem that may be unrelated to the infertility, referral to a sex therapist would be appropriate if the other therapist is not experienced in treating these problems. Chapter 11, "Staying Centered," offers suggestions for how to choose a therapist or counselor.

It can be difficult to have what are typically private acts suddenly become topics of public discussion, as often happens with infertility. Reproductive specialists know sexual issues and problems are common when dealing with infertility. Even if it is uncomfortable for you, it is important to talk with your healthcare team about your concerns and any problems. Often, just discussing the matter can put your mind at ease. If your physician feels you would benefit from counseling or other treatment for your issues, he or she can make a referral to an appropriate and qualified specialist.

## POSITIVE STEPS YOU CAN TAKE FROM CHAPTER 13

**Know that you and your partner are not alone.** Problems with sexuality and intimacy over the course of the infertility experience are pervasive, and the problems can worsen with time. Understanding that these are the normal consequences of this stressful experience can help you feel less panicked and isolated.

**Recognize that intimacy can exist apart from sexuality.** Try to nourish intimacy with mutual kindnesses and the occasional mental, even physical, break from the rigors of your infertility journey.

**Consider seeking peer support.** Joining a support group can give you and your partner a break from the intensity of infertility issues and feelings of isolation. You might want to consider professional counseling if specific aspects of the crisis begin to dominate your life.

# 14 Creating a Financial Game Plan and Getting Through the Insurance Maze

When your mind is on building a family, the last thing you are thinking about is money. But once you start exploring your treatment options, you will quickly find that your choices come with price tags—and some with sticker shock. Only about one fourth of all health plans cover infertility services, and most of those pay for only the basics. When it comes to assisted reproductive technology (ART) procedures, such as in vitro fertilization (IVF) and gamete intrafallopian transfer (GIFT), you may be mostly on your own. Unless you have a bottomless checking account, it is time to stop and take stock of your resources.

## HEALTH INSURANCE

"Don't sweat the small stuff" is a wonderful life philosophy. When it comes to your health insurance, however, it is the small stuff that matters most. It often seems like there are more exceptions than rules when it comes to figuring out what services your plan covers. What should be easy to understand becomes confusing and complicated, clouded in industry jargon that nearly qualifies as a foreign language.

Most people already have a health plan when they decide to seek treatment for infertility. It often comes as a shock to discover that most health insurance coverage does not cover much in the way of infertility services. Some states require insurers to offer or cover certain services; most do not. If you do not live in a state where infertility insurance coverage is mandated by law, it is unlikely you can purchase additional coverage just for infertility. However, a careful reading of your existing health insurance policy may reveal some coverage for infertility treatment, even if it is not comprehensive. Also, there is nothing to stop an enlightened employer from negotiating infertility benefits with an insurance company and offering them to employees, even in states where coverage is not mandated.

Most people have insurance coverage through their employer, union, or a professional association, although some have individual plans. It is important to find out how your health plan works and what services it covers *before* you travel too far down the infertility diagnosis and treatment road.

## Kinds of Healthcare Coverage

The first step in assessing your health insurance is to determine what kind of insurance coverage you have. Common plan types include the following:

• **Fee-for-service.** Usually the most expensive kind of plan, fee-for-service offers the greatest choice. You can choose virtually any physician and your insurance will pay the determined amount. Most plans require you to pay a portion of each expense, either as a percentage, a flat rate copayment, a deductible, or a combination. Some plans pay a flat rate for each type of service, and you pay any balances.

• **PPO—Preferred (or Participating) Provider Organization.** In a PPO, your insurance company requires you to select from among a list of physicians with whom it has negotiated agreements. These physicians are in private or group practices in the community. Generally, physicians participating in PPOs agree to accept a reduced payment in exchange for an increased volume of patients (those that the insurance plan funnels their way). Many PPOs also require you to pay a portion of your expenses through copayments or deductibles. Most PPO plans will pay a substantially reduced amount for care provided by a physician who is not part of the PPO.

• **HMO—Health Maintenance Organization.** HMOs are the most restrictive in terms of provider selection, although they sometimes offer the broadest range of benefits, particularly in preventive care. An HMO can be either staff model (the company owns its facilities and employs its physicians) or network (similar to a PPO). You must receive your care from physicians who are part of the HMO. Most HMOs will not pay for care provided by non-HMO physicians. With an HMO, you may also have copayments and deductibles, although they are usually smaller than with other kinds of health plans.

• **Self-insured.** Large employers have the option to self-insure. This means they act as their own insurance companies—they collect premiums, pay claims, and make coverage decisions. Self-insured plans follow federal, rather than state, regulations. Often, self-insured companies hire an outside firm to administer the plan, although an internal department can handle this responsibility as well. Self-insured plans can function like fee-for-service, PPO, or HMO plans, depending on how companies choose to set them up. This means you may or may not have restrictions on which physicians you can see, and your out-of-pocket expenses (what you have to pay for yourself) will vary. **The most important aspect of self-insured plans from the perspective of infertility care, however, is that they are generally exempt from state mandates.**

Each plan type has advantages and disadvantages. If choices are available to you, as they often are when you obtain your healthcare insurance through an employer, consider both the plan type and the benefits carefully. An HMO might cover diagnostic testing for infertility, for example, although only when provided through its physicians and facilities. Smaller HMOs in particular may not have reproductive endocrinologists and other high-level specialists available, relying instead on OB-Gyns with special training in infertility issues. A fee-for-service plan, which generally allows the widest choice of providers, may have more restricted benefits.

## Subscriber and Dependent Benefits

Although most health plans offer the same benefits for everyone covered, some offer different benefits for the subscriber and for dependents. (You are the subscriber if the plan is in your name, such as when your health insurance is through your employer.) Generally, the subscriber has the better benefits when this is the case. Dependents (spouses and children, and occasionally domestic partners) may have less comprehensive routine benefits, such as adult physical examinations every 2 years instead of annually. This becomes especially important for infertility diagnosis and treatment matters, because many health plans that offer any coverage for them consider these to be preventive services. A less common variation on the split benefits theme is for dependents to have the same benefits but pay higher copayments and deductibles.

## What Is Covered and What Is Not

In theory, all healthcare services are covered unless your health plan specifically excludes them. This theory has been the basis for a number of successful legal challenges resulting in overturning a health plan's denial of coverage for infertility services as well as for other healthcare services. In practice, most infertility services end up excluded by inference—insurance companies classify them as "experimental," "not standard practice," or "not medically necessary." Insurers insist these catch-all exclusions are intended to help protect people from risky or ineffective procedures. Industry critics counter that excluded services are often expensive and useful for a few rather than the many. Reality no doubt lives somewhere in the middle.

What matters most for you is that you know what *your* plan covers and excludes. Most people have no more than a passing familiarity with their healthcare benefits because the only documentation they have ever seen is their benefits brochure. Although your benefits brochure is usually attractive and easy to read, it only presents a summary of your benefits and an overview of how to use them. In most states, regulations govern the content and sometimes the presentation of benefits booklets and brochures. So the information is accurate. However, it is not complete. (Check the fine print—there is usually a disclaimer that says the benefits brochure is not a contract and is therefore not binding, or some such similar language.) And although the benefits brochure is a handy guide for your reference, it also has a secondary mission—it is a marketing tool for your health plan. Learning the details of your health plan can take some digging and effort, but it is well worth it. These steps can give you a good start:

• **Get a copy of your health plan contract.** To really know what services your plan pays for and rejects, you need a copy of the health plan contract. If you have an individual plan (you bought it yourself, not through an employer), you had to sign a contract to get coverage and should have a copy. If your health insurance is through your employer, your employer has the contract. Someone in your benefits or human resources department should be able to provide you with a copy. If you are unable to obtain a copy of your health insurance contract, try requesting one directly from your health plan. If you still strike out, contact your state's insurance commissioner. All states have regulations requiring insurers to file copies of contracts and rates.

• **Identify covered services.** Don't let the "legalese" scare you off. Contract language has become far more "human" than it used to be. Just take your time as you make your way through the contract. On a separate sheet of paper, list what your contract specifies as covered services. These often fall under basic categories, such as "Inpatient," "Physician's Visits," "Maternity," or "Preventive Services." Note whether there are different benefits for subscribers and dependents.

• **Identify limitations and restrictions.** Many health plans have limitations or restrictions on benefits. If your plan is a PPO, for example, it may pay a significantly lower rate to a non-PPO physician (leaving you to pay the balance). An HMO requires you to see physicians and use facilities within its network. Other limitations might include dollar or frequency caps on certain services (for example, one adult physical examination per year, or up to $150 for vision benefits). Many health plans require you to pay a copayment, deductible, or percentage of certain, or even all, health services. Plans that cover limited infertility services often consider them preventive services, so any restrictions that apply to preventive services would also apply to infertility diagnosis and treatment. Plans also may limit the number of times they will pay for the same service (a plan may cover four sperm washings, for example, then refuse to pay for any more). On your separate sheet of paper, list all the limitations and restrictions your contract stipulates.

• **Identify exclusions.** Every health plan excludes coverage for certain services—care and items for which the health plan will not pay. (This does not mean you cannot have these services, just that your health insurance will not pay for them.) Many exclusions are fairly standard, such as those denying payment for dental work (a separate dental plan, if you have one, covers dental benefits). Some exclusions are specific, whereas others are more general. Many health plans specifically exclude most ART services, such as IVF. List the exclusions that *could* apply to infertility services (including those alluding to experimental procedures).

• **Identify waiting periods and preexisting condition limitations.** Some health plans require you to wait a certain amount of time before receiving care for preexisting conditions (health conditions you have before you enroll in the plan). Under a federal law passed in 1996, called the Health Insurance Portability and Accountability Act (HIPAA), health plans cannot exclude coverage for a preexisting condition for more than 12 months. This applies only to conditions that are covered under the plan. If you had insurance coverage for at least 12 months before joining a new plan, there can be no waiting period for benefits covered under the new plan. If you had coverage for less than the 12 previous months, you can be denied coverage for a preexisting condition for up to 12 months, but credit must be given for the number of months that you did have coverage. Ideally, you should know about waiting periods and preexisting conditions *before* you enroll in the plan. Whenever possible, choose the plan with the least restrictive criteria, even if that means paying a little more for your coverage. Add your plan's waiting periods and preexisting condition restrictions to your list.

• **Identify your health plan's claim denial appeals process.** All health plans have some process for appealing a denied claim. A description of this process should appear in the contract. (If it does not, call the insurance company and ask about it.) Although you do not want to start out assuming that you will have to use your health plan's appeals process, it is a good idea to know what it requires. Most health plans conduct appeals in writing—you send a letter, along with copies of any medical records you feel support your position, and the company responds with a written decision. Even if you have made it all the way through your health insurance contract and you are overjoyed that it covers the infertility services you are considering, document everything. Ask your physician for full descriptions of everything he or she is proposing, and take notes. Document who says what in telephone calls. Keep a paper trail, just in case. (More on actually filing an appeal later in this chapter.)

## Confirm Your Benefits Before You Seek Infertility Diagnosis or Treatment

Once you have identified your health plan's benefits, limitations and restrictions (including waiting periods and preexisting conditions), and exclusions, compare your list with the services your physician recommended. Summarize your list in a letter to your health plan, asking for confirmation that your interpretations are correct. This is called a letter of "predetermination" of benefits. Address your letter to a person, by name, at the health plan (your benefits coordinator or the insurance company should be able to direct you to the appropriate individual). If you do not receive a response within 2 weeks, telephone the person. Politely ask when you might expect a return letter—and make it clear that you want a response in writing, even if the person gives you an answer over the phone. When you receive your letter, make photocopies for your physician's office to keep on file (never give anyone else your original letter).

### *Drafting a Letter of Predetermination of Benefits*

Be sure to include these elements in a letter of predetermination of benefits, addressed directly to a contact person you have identified in your insurance company, if possible:

- Patient identifiers: name, name of insured group and group number, patient identification number.
- The procedure you are considering; for example: IVF, GIFT, intrauterine insemination (IUI) with ovulation medication.

- The reasons the procedures are necessary, for example, blocked fallopian tubes, male factor infertility, unexplained infertility.
- The fee schedule from your physician, if available.

Questions you should ask in the letter include:

- Are the procedures covered under my policy?
- Are there limits to coverage (dollar amounts or number of attempts)?
- If there are limits, are any portions of the procedures covered (for example, monitoring with ultrasound and blood analysis for medicated cycles, prescriptions, laboratory work)?
- If a procedure is not covered, please provide the section of the contract that specifically excludes coverage, or I will assume that it is covered.

Request a reply as soon as possible or within a reasonable amount of time.

## Keep a Paper Trail

Continue your paper trail after you begin infertility treatment, too. Write down who you talk to, when you talked, whether by phone or in person, and what was said. This is particularly important when your health plan pays for some services but not others or imposes limitations.

### Voices

*As a diethylstilbestrol (DES) daughter, Evi moved from a state that mandated health insurance coverage for infertility to one that did not. After two unsuccessful IVFs, the third time was the proverbial charm. Once Evi became pregnant, her health plan started paying for her obstetrical care. However, what should have been smooth sailing soon turned into stormy seas.*

*"My doctor wants weekly ultrasounds to monitor for incompetent cervix, but my insurance company is balking at paying for them because it doesn't want to classify me as high risk," says Evi. "It doesn't consider you high risk with an incompetent cervix unless you've lost three pregnancies! I've already lost one, and my mother lost six for the same reason. I can't afford to lose another, either in terms of money or time."*

*With each ultrasound, Evi's insurance company asks her physician to document the medical reasons. Just over 6 months into her pregnancy, Evi wonders what else the insurance company will question. Ironically, the same health plan unhesitatingly paid for two surgeries for her husband's problems, a varicocele repair and a subsequent exploratory surgery.*

*"I never thought I'd be going through stuff like this," Evi says. "I now know a lot of people continue going to their regular OB-Gyn to avoid alerting their insurance companies to the true nature of their problems. I consider myself very fortunate that I've gotten this far."*

## Coordination of Benefits (COB)

Some couples address the insurance situation by each enrolling in a different type of plan. Each receives care under his or her own plan. Couples also can choose to enroll as dependents on each other's plans, if they meet the eligibility requirements (usually marriage, sometimes domestic partners). In such situations, the two health plans then engage in a practice called coordination of benefits—known in the industry as COB. When a claim's payment is coordinated, the subscriber's plan pays its benefit first. This is the primary coverage. Then the plan on which the person is the dependent pays its benefit. This is the secondary coverage. Generally the most the secondary plan will pay is the balance of costs; you do not get money back.

### Voices

*Teresa and Dwight chose to have separate plans without enrolling as dependents on each other's plan. "That way there are no coordination of benefits issues," explains Teresa. "He goes under his plan for what relates to him, and I go under my plan for what relates to me."*

*Teresa was fortunate that she had once worked in a physician's office and knew how health insurance worked from the "inside." She was able to use her knowledge to help her and her husband make insurance decisions that best met their needs. COB, she knew, was for the benefit of insurance companies, not patients. It was a process that involved time and paperwork, and often physicians' offices would try to collect payment from the patient while the insurance companies haggled over which would pay how much.*

*"Most of the time, people don't know how the system works," Teresa says. "You have to call the insurance companies to find out what they'll pay for and what they won't, and who will pay."*

If you are the only person on your health plan, you do not need to worry about COB. Your plan will pay for all covered services. Some couples intentionally choose plans with different benefits, using one as a fallback for the other.

This works if you carefully analyze your benefits compared with your anticipated needs. It is easy to get caught in the middle, however. Not all insurance companies follow the same procedures. It is best to get a letter of coverage, in writing and in advance, before entering into potentially expensive testing or treatment.

## State Mandates

Many individuals and couples believe laws should compel insurance companies to cover infertility treatment. Finally, state governments seem to be taking heed. There are two kinds of laws that address infertility services:

- **Mandate to cover**—laws requiring insurance companies *to cover* infertility treatment in every health plan. Premiums include the added cost of this coverage.
- **Mandate to offer**—laws requiring insurance companies *to offer*, for additional purchase, coverage for infertility treatment. Employers are not required, however, to purchase this additional coverage.

The following states have passed *mandates to cover* infertility benefits as of the publication of this book. Benefits included in required coverage vary significantly from state to state. Contact your state's insurance commissioner's office for a copy of the law that mandates coverage and any regulations passed to implement it:

*Arkansas*
*Hawaii*
*Illinois*
*Maryland*
*Massachusetts*
*Montana*
*New York*
*Ohio*
*Rhode Island*
*West Virginia*

These states have passed *mandates to offer* infertility benefits:

*California*
*Connecticut*
*Texas*

In 2000, ten states had mandates to cover infertility treatments, and three had mandates to offer such coverage. Because this list can change as quickly as states can pass laws, check to be sure whether your state's position has changed (your state insurance commissioner can tell you—see the Resource Section for contact information for the National Association of Insurance Commissioners). Also check whether your health plan is self-insured, sometimes referred to as an ERISA plan. Short for Employees' Retirement Income Security Act, ERISA is the federal law that governs self-insured health plans. ERISA plans are not subject to state laws. Even if you live in a state that mandates infertility coverage, if your employer self-insures your health plan, your health plan does not have to include coverage for infertility services.

Insurance companies have numerous explanations for why they do not routinely cover infertility. Outcomes are neither guaranteed nor predictable. Technology is continually changing, often blurring the line between cutting edge and experimental. Sometimes moral views enter into the debate, much the same as they do for reproductive services aimed at preventing or ending pregnancy, causing insurance companies to include potentially controversial benefits only when required to do so. Costs are high, and health insurance was never intended to cover *everything*.

Many of these reasons are fragile at best. Outcomes are not guaranteed for any medical treatment, and predictability is little more than an exercise in statistics whether you are considering heart surgery or IVF. Predictability also takes time—it took more than a decade for heart transplants to become covered procedures, for example (in part, charge critics, because the lack of coverage curtailed the number of transplantations surgeons could perform). Evolving technology reshapes the practice of medicine faster than books can be written about it in all areas, not just reproductive health. Why should one moral view prevent those with opposing views from receiving desired services? When health insurance first came into existence, it did cover just about everything that was possible at the time. True, those early health insurance plans were called "catastrophic major medical." But nearly any medical problem had great potential to be catastrophic in a time when antibiotics and vaccines were not widely available. As times have changed, though, so has knowledge. Far more treatment is commonplace today than anyone ever imagined 50 years ago. And yes, infertility services can be expensive. Coronary artery bypass surgery is far more expensive, yet it has become the most commonly performed surgery in the United States.

### Voices

*Most certainly, infertility issues are deeply personal. But they are also widespread. "People should confront these issues and press for changes in laws. Infertility was a horrible thing for me at first," Julia says. "I was from a small town in the Midwest, and it was kind of a shameful thing. But people need to talk about infertility. We need legislation to deal with it. Lack of insurance coverage makes people take unrealistic chances."*

# FINANCIAL PLANNING

Your available resources shape the direction of your efforts to resolve your infertility. But many people do not shop around to compare options and costs. This can turn out to be expensive, both in terms of time and money. Treatment costs can range from several hundred dollars (hormonal imbalance that responds to simple drug therapy) to thousands of dollars (IVF averages $10,000 an attempt). It is easy to get involved in infertility testing and treatment without realizing how much you are spending until you have depleted your resources. A little planning can help you avoid that experience.

## Make Decisions Based on Knowledge, Not Emotion

Many people do not discover they have infertility problems until they decide, after building careers or finding their partners, that they are now ready to start a family. Time becomes an instant enemy. Make the most of your time by making informed decisions. Know what approaches are possible for your condition or situation. Then find out about your physician's experience in using them.

### Voices

*"I didn't know being a DES daughter would cause infertility problems until I attempted to conceive," says Lavonne, who was 40 years old when she married and decided to have a family. "I wasted time, mostly because I didn't know what I wanted except to get pregnant. I didn't know what questions to ask, or what to expect. We tried IVF once with my eggs, then twice with eggs donated by my sister, without success. Then I had to wait until we had the money to try donor egg again. I feel I would've had a biological child 3 or 4 years ago had I known more about my options."*

## Know What You Are Getting

It is tempting to make dollar-based decisions, especially if your budget is already strained. It is more important to look at what you get when you write that check, however. The least expensive alternatives may turn out to be the least effective. If they work for you, that is great. But if they do not, the costs can quickly add up to equal or exceed what you would have paid for more expensive, although more effective, treatment. It is a lesson many people learn the hard way.

---

### Voices

*"We've spent close to $10,000 over the past 18 months just to get to where we are, yet the procedures we've gone through so far have been minimal and had a low probability of success," says Danielle. "What I wish I would've done is educate myself better on the broad spectrum of fertility problems, and try to find other people who had similar problems so I could talk with them about what worked for them and what didn't. I would've talked more with the first doctor about his success rate and about different procedures, rather than just jumping in. Because I didn't, now we're pretty much starting over again."*

---

## Know When It Is Time to See Someone Else or Try Something Else

It is easy to "go with the flow" when it comes to your insurance. Many people see physicians and seek treatments that their health plans cover, without really thinking about whether those are the most appropriate choices for their particular situations.

---

### Voices

*"We selected the first specialist because he was the only one covered under the PPO," recalls Teresa. The health plan's willingness to pay in part for treatment was encouraging—for a while. Teresa began to wonder how long that willingness would last. She and Dwight began to have doubts about the course of their treatment. "If we had continued, would they have continued to pay? We found the insurance company would do that with a lot of things, go along for a while and then put their finger on it and say, that's all!"*

*Finally Teresa and Dwight decided enough is enough. Teresa credits her experience working in a physician's office with helping her to realize she and Dwight needed to get a second opinion. They did, from an infertility specialist who uses state-of-the-art methods. "The second doctor spent a lot of time talking with us," says Teresa.*

---

*"He asked about our problems and what we'd tried so far. Then he talked about what he knew to be the best options for our situation. Now we're talking about elective infertility treatments, and insurance covers none of it," she says. "The general price tag is $12,000, so now we do have to wait until we have enough money. We both work full-time, and even though we pay dearly for our insurance, it doesn't help us in this area."*

Recognize, however, that more is not always better. Just because something is expensive does not mean it is the right answer for you. It is important to make decisions based on all the factors. Help yourself establish boundaries by discussing both treatment options and finances with your physician before you begin treatment. This gives you a framework for making objective decisions, especially if things do not go the way you hope they will. When emotions are intense, such decisions are all the more difficult to make.

### Identify Possible Expenses

Before you can do any effective planning, you need to know what you are facing. It often helps to set guidelines and boundaries early in your treatment about the options you want to consider and how far you want to go with them.

- Which tests are necessary, and which simply add more information? Which tests must be repeated, and how often? What do you learn from the results? Eliminating unnecessary procedures reduces your costs.
- Enlist your physician's assistance to help you get the most from your insurance benefits, particularly if you have limited or no coverage for infertility. Whether or not your insurance company pays for procedures often depends on how accurately the physician's office codes them.

## Have a Plan for How Far You Will Go, Both in Treatment and Expenses

Whether you are willing to mortgage the house and sell the furniture or whether you refuse to make any lifestyle changes at all, the "how far" and "how much" decisions are easier to make *before* you start infertility treatments. Your checkbook will frame many decisions, of course. Even so, there are numerous factors to consider. Are you willing to give up vacations, forego a new or second car, rent a small apartment instead of buying a house, take out a second mortgage on a house you already own? Will you work a second job, or try to borrow money from family or friends? Whatever your available options and choices, looking at infertility services through your wallet can strain any relationship.

### Voices

*"I've been very lucky that my husband gets an annual bonus," says Evi, who estimates her current pregnancy has cost more than $60,000 so far. "We don't have much furniture in our house, and we don't take vacations. But it's been very trying, very difficult. Now that I'm pregnant, we have no problems in our relationship. Before, we fought all the time about the infertility, mostly about the money."*

*Teresa and Dwight figure it will be 3 years or more before they can afford to try again to conceive. They live frugally, keeping their entertainment expenses to a minimum and buying only items that they absolutely need. They have considered withdrawing money from their retirement funds, but the financial penalties for doing so mean they would lose nearly half of what they could draw out.*

*"Unfortunately, we don't have parents or other relatives who can loan us this kind of money," Teresa says. "The doctor's office has a medical loan package, but we don't qualify because we did recently buy a house. Even if we did qualify, we wouldn't be able to make the payments after I had a baby, because I would take at least 3 months off from work."*

Some people can turn to family and friends for financial assistance. Others take out loans or extend their credit card limits. Although these options are tempting, they come with consequences that could be trouble down the road. When borrowing from family or friends, be sure to clearly establish the terms of the loan—then live up to them. Little comes between loved ones faster than money. Write and sign a simple contract, and keep it in a safe place. If a relative or close friend gives you money as a gift, ask for a short note that says this is the person's intent. Getting everything in writing prevents future misunderstandings. If you go the more formal route of taking a loan or extending your credit, read the fine print before you sign on the dotted line. Be sure you understand what interest rate you will be paying and how long it will take you to pay off the amount if you only make the minimum payments. Consider how your financial situation might change over that time—job, relationship, housing. If you conceive or adopt, will you continue working? Will your partner be able to contribute financially? Will you need to move to a bigger apartment or house? It may seem cold and even harsh to scrutinize your financial situation in such detail. But you cannot avoid it. The more complete your plans are, the less likely it is that you will find yourself confronting unpleasant surprises.

# LEGAL MATTERS

Sometimes it becomes necessary to deal with legal aspects of insurance coverage and even financial matters.

## Disputing an Insurance Claim Denial

Insurance companies are required to have procedures in place for people to dispute denied claims. This information probably appears in condensed form in your benefits booklet or brochure, and should appear in full detail in your health plan contract. If it does not, contact your state's insurance commissioner for guidance.

Generally, you must appeal a denied claim in writing. You might just need to send a letter, or your insurance company may have forms that you need to complete. In either case, keep copies of everything you send to your insurance company, and consider sending documents certified mail, return receipt requested. That way, you will have proof of the company's dated receipt of your appeal, and you will know what you sent if someone from your health plan calls you. You also have a paper trail, in case your insurance company misplaces your request for reconsideration.

Do not be too discouraged with an initial denial for services you thought (or hoped) your health plan would cover. Most health plans have a fairly automated process for reviewing and paying claims. Many automatically reject claims that do not fit the criteria. A few conduct a cursory investigation before taking any action.

• **Verify that your physician's office submitted the claim correctly.** All medical procedures are assigned code numbers that identify them to your insurance company's computer systems. Your physician's office translates the services you received into these codes, which then move on to your insurance company as your claim. Usually, although not always, your health plan sends a rejection to your physician's office as well. Let your physician's office know that you have received a rejection, and ask them to double-check the codes.

• **Verify that the service should be covered.** Check the description of services against your list of covered benefits and exclusions. Do you have a response from your insurance company to your predetermination letter, stating what is covered and what is not? If so, and the rejected claim appears to fall in the "covered" category, send copies of the claim and the letter to your insurance company.

• **Ask your insurance company for a written, detailed explanation of the**

**denial.** Sometimes the reason your health plan has denied payment is not clear, or you are not certain whether the service should be covered. Most denials include a brief reason that does not really explain why the claim is not covered.

• **Initiate a formal appeal through your insurance company's procedures.** If your health plan reviews your claim and denies it a second time, you can ask for a formal review. Sometimes the insurance company may ask your physician for copies of your medical records.

## Doing Battle with Your Insurance Company

If you are not getting anywhere with your insurance company and you believe you have a valid grievance, you can move your dispute to the next level by contacting your state's insurance commissioner. Each state has an insurance commissioner, who oversees the activities of insurance companies and health plans in your state. Most states require health plans to submit their contracts and rates for approval and have strict guidelines for how insurance companies can change benefits. Before you contact your insurance commissioner, however, read your contract carefully! Let knowledge, not emotion, guide your efforts. Remember, challenging your health plan through the insurance commissioner is a legal process. You may believe it is unfair that your health plan does not cover ART, but if the contract and its administration are within the bounds of the law, about all the insurance commissioner can offer is sympathy.

If the insurance commissioner agrees that your claim should be paid but your insurance company still refuses, consider contacting your employer for additional support. If you are not comfortable doing this, or your employer refuses, you will need to talk with an attorney about pursuing the matter through the courts. Court battles are often long, costly, and unsuccessful, however.

## Doing Battle with Your Employer

For the most part, employers comply with what they understand the laws and regulations about insurance to be. Insurance is a complex and ever-changing beast, however, and their knowledge is not always complete or even accurate. If you feel your employer is violating either a state or ERISA mandate regarding health plan coverage for infertility services, present your concerns (in writing) to your benefits administrator. Ask for a written response within a reasonable amount of time (10 working days is usually sufficient to research your concerns and write a response). If you are right, your employer should tell you what the company plans to do to correct the problem. If your employer agrees with you but offers no remedy, ask for one specifically. Most companies, when they realize they are in error, will move quickly to make things right. It just takes a phone call to have the health plan draft an amendment to the company's policy. Be aware, however, that if adding coverage for infertility services raises the premiums (which is nearly always the case), your employer will likely pass that increase on to you and everyone else who has healthcare insurance. In states where infertility coverage is mandatory, this increase in premiums often has proved to be nominal.

If your employer disagrees with you, or refuses to take corrective action, you will probably need to seek advice from an attorney as to whether you have a strong enough case to push further.

### Voices

*Cheri is undergoing intrauterine insemination (IUI) with medication to stimulate her ovaries. "Instead of writing to a congressman," Cheri asserts, "I think a more effective approach to changing insurance policies is to talk to employers. As an employee, if I write to my CEO, they owe me an explanation. My insurance pays 50 percent of infertility treatments, but totally excludes IVF, GIFT, and ZIFT. I was fortunate because my problems didn't involve that treatment, but others do need it. It does mean going 'public' with the boss about your infertility struggle—but nothing will change until employers are more aware that there's a real need."*

## Filing a Discrimination Claim

Depending on your situation, you could press an employer who is reluctant to offer a health plan that covers infertility services with a discrimination claim. Some court decisions in the 1990s supported discrimination claims on the basis of the Americans with Disabilities Act (ADA) and the Pregnancy Discrimination Act (PDA). These federal laws prohibit employers from discriminating against individuals with disabilities (ADA) or because of pregnancy-related conditions (PDA). Some courts have held infertility to be a disability. However, neither the ADA nor the PDA requires employers to offer health insurance that covers infertility. Whether you have grounds to file a discrimination claim depends on your specific circumstances, and only an attorney can advise you. If you choose to consult an attorney, select one with experience in these kinds of cases. Your local RESOLVE chapter may be able to provide you with additional resources.

## POSITIVE STEPS YOU CAN TAKE FROM CHAPTER 14

**Get the big picture of your financial resources to pursue family building.** Advance planning can help you stay in control and improve your decision making.

**Set the groundwork for using all your available health insurance coverage.** Read your insurance contract closely; protect yourself with a predetermination of benefits letter before you begin treatment; and research the company's appeal process before you may need it.

**Recognize that dealing with insurance and financial decisions in the midst of the infertility crisis can be very distressing.** Many people feel like they have assumed a second job. It is normal to feel stressed by this process. See chapters 11 and 12, "Staying Centered" and "Staying Healthy," for help with managing stress.

# 15 Exploring Other Family-Building Options:
## Adoption, Donors and Surrogacy, Living Childfree, and Resolving as a Stepfamily

In the early stages of the infertility experience, most decisions center around diagnostic testing. As the various tests and procedures narrow the potential causes, the emphasis shifts to treatment. Many couples wind their way through several protocols, often starting with medications and progressing to more sophisticated and expensive procedures such as intrauterine insemination (IUI), in vitro fertilization (IVF), and gamete intrafallopian transfer (GIFT).

Some people enter into infertility treatment with a clear idea of how far they will go and what paths they are willing to follow. If this proves a difficult juncture for you, a careful evaluation of what continued treatment can offer is imperative. Consider enlisting the help of your physician and perhaps an infertility therapist to provide some objective review.

### Voices

*"From the start, we decided we'd do three cycles of IVF and that would be it," says Kirsten. "By the time the third one failed, it no longer fazed me. In fact, it was kind of a relief." Other people are less certain about how far to go with treatment. "I don't know when I'll stop," says Debbie. "I thought I'd do everything until I knew it was too much. Each one of us knows when that is."*

## DECISIONS, DECISIONS: WHEN IS ENOUGH, ENOUGH?

When the dream of having children begins to evolve, and the prospect of conceiving and carrying a biological child of both partners seems unlikely, couples may evaluate whether they want to end treatment entirely or consider options such as donor gamete (sperm, egg, or embryo) or surrogacy. For those who decide clearly to move away from the treatment roller coaster, adoption and resolving without children become important avenues for research. Each option offers risks and benefits, pros and cons. Which path is right for you, and when, depends on your circumstances—your treatment analysis, finances, beliefs, emotions, and your needs.

No matter how rational you are, decisions involving infertility are emotional. Although certainly you would not want to make such significant choices without emotion, you also do not want to make them solely on the basis of emotion. People who are nearing the end of treatment typically are dealing with two separate, yet interwoven, issues—letting go and moving on. It can be terrifying: You may know you are nearing the end of your emotional, and maybe financial, reserves, yet you are afraid to take the next step to investigate a new path.

It is important to recognize that this is a normal feeling. First, you must make the decision to stop treatment toward your goal of having a pregnancy and a child of shared biology (or accept the fact that you must), then you must say good-bye to a dream you have cherished, perhaps most of your life.

For couples, it is especially important to enter the decision-making process as a team. Set aside whatever decisions you have made before, and focus on getting to know as much about each of the options as you can. Many fertility specialists recommend seeing an infertility counselor before making a final decision, to be sure you have considered all aspects and understand all ramifications of the choices you are making.

This chapter offers only a brief overview of family-building alternatives. "Next step" resolutions vary depending on infertility diagnosis and individual choice, of course, and they are not presented in a particular order. The decision tree at the end of this chapter offers a sample road map a couple might follow as they make their way through their options. In general, both you and your partner might want to take the following steps:

- Write a list of what appeals to you and what does not appeal to you for each option.
- Note any options that are completely unacceptable, and write a brief explanation of why.
- Prioritize your options in order of acceptance.
- Itemize what you would have to do, and by when, to make your top choice

become a reality. Then do the same for the remaining options, even if they do not appeal to you at the moment.

- Create a plan of action to make your choice become reality.

You and your partner can go through this exercise independently and then compare responses, or work your way through the process together. If you have widely differing priorities, consider consulting an infertility therapist, particularly if you have become "stuck" in your positions. Most important, though, work as a team in search of your common goal. The challenge is not to make the "right" decision, but to make a reasoned decision for which you can both eventually claim ownership.

# ADOPTION

Adoption is a joyful resolution for many people who cannot conceive, and for some who choose not to try to conceive, a biological child. With adoption, prospective parents can often choose whether to welcome an infant, toddler, or older child to their families, and sometimes whether the child will be a boy or a girl. With adoption, of course, there is no genetic link to the child. Many worries people have when considering adoption turn out to be myths and stereotypes:

- Is it too expensive for us?
- Can we really love a child who is not biologically connected to us?
- What if the child has, or develops, medical or emotional problems?
- Are the birth parents likely to interfere later?

There are ways to make adoption more affordable, and the vast majority of adoptions are enormously satisfying experiences for both parents and children. The best way to ensure a legally safe adoption is to work with a reputable agency and/or through an attorney who specializes in adoptions. Adoption "disruptions" through birth family intervention, for example, are rare, and most occur early, often before the prospective parents have met the child.

### Voices

*"Adoption," Erica asserts, "is not a cure for infertility; it's a cure for parenting. Some couples decide to adopt a child, while continuing with infertility treatments. We decided to get out of the ovarian Olympics. Parenting is what's most important to us."*

The following section is meant to serve only as an overview of adoption. Some of the best ways to explore adoption further are through the literature and through networking with adoptive or pre-adoptive parents in a RESOLVE chapter support group or another provided in your community (see the Resources at the back of this book for a number of adoption support organizations).

## Questions to Answer Before Proceeding

**Should you go through an agency or adopt privately through an attorney?** Many people believe an agency adoption is "safer" and less expensive than an adoption arranged privately through an attorney. This is not always the case. A reputable attorney who specializes in adoptions and family law might be able to arrange the adoption you desire at a price you can afford, with few risks of trouble in the future. An agency might accomplish the same mission. Again, the best choice is the one that meets your needs. Whichever route you select, however, check references. Both agencies and attorneys should be willing to provide you with the names of other clients who would talk with you about their experiences.

This would be a good time to attend an adoption conference or join an adoption support and networking group to begin to understand your options. For example, states' laws vary widely on the availability of, and legal requirements for, privately arranged adoption.

**Do you want an open or closed adoption?** Despite its history of secrecy, adoption is becoming a more open process. The birth mother sometimes wants to know the family that will love and raise the child she brought into the world. Families sometimes want to know their child's full background, beyond the adoption profile. When both parties agree, an open adoption can be successful for all involved. Other families and birth mothers prefer not to know about each other.

**How can you know whether the child has problems?** Prenatal care can be a concern to pre-adoptive parents. In adoptions handled through reputable agencies and experienced attorneys, however, there is generally some information about the birth mother and the pregnancy. If you are adopting an older child, find out as much as you can about the child's early years to prepare for any learning disabilities, health risks, and other challenges. Of course, challenges and risks accompany childrearing regardless of how families are built, but the more you know, the better your decisions and preparations will be.

**What kind of adoption best meets your needs and interests?** There are many factors to consider when thinking about whether to welcome an infant or an older child, or whether you could parent a child with special needs. Some older couples decide to adopt older children, looking ahead to the child's future needs and their ability to meet them. Waiting times for infants can be long.

## Choosing an Adoption Resource

Once again, reputation and experience are key when you are selecting an agency or attorney to handle your adoption. (If you use both, be sure the attorney reviewing documentation is not the same one handling the agency's legal work). Some general factors to consider with agency adoption include:

- What kinds of adoption does the agency offer? What services does the agency provide to prospective adoptive parents, and are all services included in the quoted fees?
- Is the agency registered with the state department or division responsible for overseeing adoption in your state (usually the department of social services)? Are there any complaints about the agency on record?
- What are the agency's fees and when are they payable? (Be cautious about paying a lump sum before services are rendered.) What amounts are refundable should something go wrong? Does the agency provide itemized statements?
- How long has the agency been in business? How many children does the agency place each year? Has the agency had disrupted adoptions?
- What restrictions and requirements does the agency have for prospective adoptive parents? How long does the adoption process typically take?
- What are the responsibilities and roles of the agency's attorney? What is the attorney's experience with adoptions?

Many of the above questions may also apply to attorney-facilitated adoption, depending on whether the attorney handles the entire adoption process or just reviews the documentation and legal papers.

### Voices

*Martha is a DES-daughter; her uterus is small and her cervix is compromised. Martha has tried three cycles of IVF; all have failed. Martha says, "I don't know what my plan is now. I'm pretty much making it up as I go along. Though I know because of the person I am, I'll do everything I'm supposed to do and fool myself into thinking I'm debating it. I may look into adoption sooner than later. My husband isn't sold on adoption, but I think he'd do it for me. He just feels like we wouldn't know what we're getting. I can understand and I agree with him. If I were to adopt, I'd do foreign. I may look into foreign adoption sooner than later."*

## International Adoption

If you are considering this option, assemble a list of agencies that specialize and inquire about the countries from which they make placements. Attend agency seminars to learn of the adoption laws and procedures that prevail in those countries, and consider these factors:

- Will you have to travel to the country of origin to pick up the child and complete the adoption process, or does the agency with which you are working provide an escort service to bring the child to the United States?
- What are your total costs, and when does your financial responsibility begin? Are there likely to be additional expenses, such as transportation and accommodations?
- If the adoption takes place in the child's country of origin, how long does the process take? For what steps must you be present?
- Are there language barriers and cultural differences that may make if difficult to obtain accurate health information about a child? (Children in other countries may have health problems that are rare in America, such as scurvy—caused by vitamin C deficiency.) Does the agency offer assistance with these issues, such as an escort with medical training?
- Do you have the name of a pediatrician who is knowledgeable about international health issues, should you need that expertise?

If you will be traveling to the child's country, familiarize yourself with local customs. Travel to some countries may require a valid visa, which can take a month or longer to obtain. If you do not know the language, make sure there will be someone available to translate for you.

## Independent Adoption

Some people opt for independent adoption, also called parent-initiated adoption. One advantage to this approach is that it is direct. You (or an intermediary working on your behalf, such as a physician, social worker, or clergy) locate an available child, nearly always an unborn child for whom the birth mother has made an adoption plan. Independent adoptions are not legal in every state, and carry a somewhat greater risk of falling through. By following the same precautions you would use in adopting through an agency, however, independent adoption can be successful, as well as fast and affordable. Be certain you fully understand the adoption laws in your state, and you should work with an experienced attorney who specializes in adoptions.

## Legal Considerations

Adoption issues have become quite complex: adoption laws and procedures vary considerably among states, and adoption law has become a specialty within the bar. Couples considering adoption sometimes worry that a birth parent will resurface some years down the road and attempt to regain custody. This is rare, but it occasionally happens. Most such situations involve questionable circumstances under which the child was separated from the birth mother. The courts are unlikely to negate an adoption that was legal and aboveboard at the time it took place. Thus the skill and knowledge of your legal team is of critical importance.

# DONOR INSEMINATION (DI)

Donor insemination (DI) involves the continuation of treatment, but using sperm from a donor. It is a common way to address male factor infertility; more than a million American children have been conceived this way. DI has a fairly high success rate, with the procedure resulting in pregnancy about 75 percent of the time. This is an overall average; the likelihood of conception is highest among women younger than 35 years of age who have no fertility problems themselves. However, regardless of medical circumstances, it may take several cycles of insemination to produce pregnancy (three to four cycles is not uncommon if you are a woman under 35 years). DI is less expensive than other options such as adoption or ART with ICSI. Although DI has the perception of being modern technology, it has actually been practiced for decades.

Many people do not give genetics a second thought until considering a family-building option that involves going outside their own gene pools to create a child. This can be an extremely emotional issue for couples. Accepting DI means half your baby's genetic material comes from the "outside." Grieving the loss of the male partner's contribution is important. It forces you both to think about traits he will not be able to pass on to your child. This can be a painful exercise, but it is necessary before embracing the new option. Talk through your feelings and concerns with each other, perhaps also with your physician or a counselor.

> ### *Voices*
>
> *One of the reasons Peggy and Darin chose DI over adoption was Peggy's desire to be pregnant and give birth. In the end, this took precedence over the loss of Darin's genetic contribution. "It was so important to me to feel those connections as a mother. I realize that not everyone needs the pregnancy and birth to feel connected, but when I look at my child and remember that I gave her life, that I nurtured her for 9 months, that I felt her first movements. . . . It is an incredible feeling. It's a combination of awe, joy, and actually, a feeling of power—that my body did that.*
>
> *"On another level, it was important to Darin and me that the child fulfill our obligation to the Jewish religion to bring more Jewish people into the world. Actually, though raised Jewish, I was the ultimate agnostic! But the whole infertility journey to having our child made me feel more comfortable with the idea of God, that there is a higher power involved. Darin and I are closer for the experience."*

Sometimes men feel left out of a pregnancy, no matter how diligent the woman is about including her husband or partner. After all, only one of you actually experiences being pregnant! It is important to do as much as you can to share the pregnancy. Do as much together as possible, from going to physician's visits to making the important decisions described below.

## Questions to Answer Before Proceeding

**Can both partners accept a child produced through DI as their own?** It can be difficult for some couples to accept a child as "theirs" when they know half of its genetic material is not theirs. Men often struggle more with this aspect of DI than do women, although the issue can trouble women as well. A related issue is the secrecy that shrouds male infertility. Many couples find it difficult to talk with family members and friends about their fertility problems. It is especially hard for some men to acknowledge the "fault" lies with them, as if doing so exposes a weakness. (A good infertility therapist can help you disentangle the separate issues of fertility and masculinity.) Having the husband or partner present during insemination is often an important psychological factor. This emphasizes the joint participation of the couple in both the decision and the process.

When most couples think of starting a family, they think of bringing new lives into the world that represent pieces of each of them. It is not easy to give up the idea of offspring in this genetic-sharing manner. It is normal to feel anger, sadness, and grief when it becomes clear having a genetically shared child is not likely. And it is important to let yourself feel these emotions, to talk about your feelings with your partner, and to accept your sense of loss. This is a normal part of "moving on" when resolving a life crisis.

Genetic composition does influence many characteristics—hair and eye color, height and body type, the shapes of fingers and toes. Environment, however, also greatly shapes and influences who an individual becomes. Many childcare experts strongly believe that how a child is raised is far more important than genetic makeup. For DI to be a successful family-building option for you, however, you must believe so as well.

**What is your potential for multiple gestation pregnancy?** If you have been taking drugs to stimulate ovulation, and particularly the injectable medications, there is a possibility of multiple eggs being released. This increases the chance of a multiple gestation pregnancy with DI. It is a good idea to discuss the possibility that this could happen to you, and make decisions in advance about how you would handle such a situation (see Chapter 16, "Surviving Infertility and Moving Forward").

**Should you tell your child he or she is a child of DI?** There is no clear answer to this question. It may seem premature to decide what you will tell your child at this early stage. As is the case with many moral and ethical dilemmas, what is "right" may differ among families. Again, a counselor can help you see your situation objectively and work through your options. If you think you may choose not to tell your child of his or her genetic origins, then do not tell anyone else, even now as you are considering your options. If there are others who know, the odds are great that your child will eventually find out. Some people advocate for honesty and openness, supporting a child's right to know his or her genetic heritage. Others point out that contemporary society is still not entirely comfortable with procedures such as DI, and support the need to protect the child. Couples who decide to be open with their children explain conception as a biological function, and stress how much they wanted a child. Some couples walk the middle of the road, deciding they will tell their children at some point but not while they are very young. Talk with others who have chosen DI to get a variety of views and experiences. (RESOLVE offers connection to members willing to speak with others on these issues.) Whatever you choose to do, you should both support the decision.

### Voices

*Becoming pregnant through donor egg raises the same questions about what to tell your child as choosing DI to become pregnant. Chi-Lin says, "Hisa and I decided to keep this not quite a secret but very private. Even my best friend doesn't know we did this through donor egg. Somewhere along the way we decided it was really the child's story. Why have that be a part of her life at a young age, where people would go around calling her the 'miracle baby.' She shouldn't have to hear that. We feel we owe our child some privacy."*

## Choosing a Donor

Start your quest to build a family with DI by choosing an infertility specialist who offers this option. If you live in a rural area, you may find you have fewer choices than if you live in or near a city, and you may have to travel for treatment. Most specialists work regularly with certain sperm banks, and can usually recommend at least two reputable banks for you to consider. Even if you select a sperm bank that is geographically distant, proper handling and storage makes it possible to transport specimens over great distances.

Sperm banks and infertility centers should have established standardized procedures for specimen collection, testing, storage, and transportation. Donors should be carefully screened for diseases and high-risk lifestyles. The American Society for Reproductive Medicine (ASRM) recommends, for protection against the spread of the human immunodeficiency virus (HIV), that:

- The donor test negative for HIV before the sample is procured;
- The sample be frozen for 6 months;
- The donor retest negative for HIV before the sample is released.

Although some donor profiles contain just basic physical descriptions such as height, weight, and hair and eye color, most feature more extensive information such as donor age, occupation, education, and family background to help you choose a good match.

Your physician or RESOLVE can give you a comprehensive checklist of questions to ask sperm banks about DI. Some general factors to consider when choosing a sperm bank include the following:

- What are the maximum and minimum ages of donors?
- How does the sperm bank screen donors and verify donor information? What information does the sperm bank make available to prospective recipients?
- For what diseases does the sperm bank test donors or specimens, and when? Does the sperm bank conduct any genetic screening or testing on donors? Any psychological testing?

- Does the sperm bank follow the ASRM recommendations for collecting, testing, handling, and storing specimens?
- Can you reserve or prepurchase sperm from the same donor to use if you want a second child? What are the costs and procedures for storing these specimens, and for how long will the sperm bank keep them?
- How long does the sperm bank keep donor medical records? Can adult children conceived through DI access donor medical records, if necessary? Are there donors who are willing to be identified to adult children?
- What are the sperm bank's procedures when the specimen has inadequate quality after thawing (such as low sperm count or low motility)?
- What legal documentation does the sperm bank have the donor complete and sign? Are documents notarized? For how long, and where, are they kept on file?

The vast majority of donors are anonymous. You select a donor profile that most closely matches your background and your preferences. Some general factors you may also want to consider when selecting a donor include the following:

- What are the donor's age, ethnic and cultural background, and physical characteristics?
- What is the donor's educational background, his religious background, and his career or profession?
- How frequently are the donor's specimens used, and does the bank track how often they produce pregnancies? (There may be a rare case of half siblings being born in the same area.)

Occasionally a couple may request a known donor for genetic or personal reasons. If you choose to use a donor you know, consult with your physician about procedures and testing. Also, you may want to consult with an infertility counselor who can assist you with some of the potential emotional/psychological issues that can arise with a known donor. It is especially important to have a clear understanding of the donor's role after a child is born, and to establish this in writing. You might want to consult with an attorney who specializes in adoption and other family-building agreements and cases before proceeding.

### The DI Procedure

DI may be done through cervical insemination or IUI. (For more about IUI, see chapter 7, "The Female: Structural Problems, Age-Related Factors, and Treatment.") Both insemination procedures are timed to coincide with your ovulation and are usually painless, although IUI can sometimes cause discomfort if you have a very narrow cervical opening.

With cervical insemination, the physician inserts a soft catheter through a speculum to rest near your cervix, and then allows the sperm to flow through the catheter. The woman usually stays lying on her back for 20 minutes or so to let the sperm begin their journey through the cervix and into the uterus.

In the IUI procedure, the physician passes a thin, flexible catheter through your cervix into your uterus, then injects the sperm directly into your uterus. Before IUI, the specimen is processed to remove the seminal fluid from around the sperm. This significantly reduces the chance of any cramping or allergic response. (With cervical insemination, your natural body fluids neutralize the semen as it flows into your uterus so this separation process is not necessary.)

If you do not become pregnant after several cycles of insemination, your physician will continue your infertility work-up. Your physician may prescribe medication, such as clomiphene citrate, to be used with IUI to help stimulate release of an egg(s) with ovulation (see chapter 6, "The Female: Hormonal Disorders and Treatment," for more information about fertility drugs). DI may also be combined with IVF using your eggs or donor eggs (see chapter 9, "Assisted Reproductive Technology [ART]").

## Legal Considerations

Legal matters involving anonymous sperm donors are fairly clear-cut. Often both the sperm bank and the infertility specialist will have forms for you to sign, legal documents that specify the roles and responsibilities of all parties and the limitations of the procedure. In most cases, the anonymous donor never knows who gets his sperm, and you never learn his identity. Any child that results from your DI treatment is legally yours. An anonymous donor has no parental rights or obligations, and signs a contract with the sperm bank to this effect, which you should verify before accepting the specimen.

Although DI is a straightforward process, you may want to talk with an attorney about the forms before you sign them, especially if you have questions or concerns. It can bring you great peace of mind, even when you do not antici-pate any problems. There are two circumstances in which you definitely should consult with an attorney before proceeding with DI: when the donor is some-one you know and in same-sex partnerships.

When you use a known donor, especially if you expect the donor will con-tinue to have contact with your family after your child's birth, it is prudent to consult with an attorney to clarify everyone's roles and responsibilities. Although this may seem unnecessary now, it can save much heartache and expense down the road should circumstances change.

---

### Voices

*Some lesbian couples use a combination of DI, donor egg, and IVF. One partner donates the eggs, which are fertilized in vitro using donor sperm. The embryo(s) are then transferred to the other partner's uterus. "The non–birth parent becomes the adoptive parent, and the birth parent retains her parental rights," explains Clarisse, who is pregnant as the result of such a procedure. "Diane is the biological mother, and I am the birth mother. Working with our attorney, we will do what needs to be done to clearly establish both of our parental rights."*

---

## DONOR EGG (DE)

When egg production or quality is the problem, egg donation (also called ovum donation) can be the solution for some couples. Donor egg (DE) pregnancy is often a successful option for women whose ovaries do not function properly—they may have premature ovarian failure (POF) or premature menopause, have had their ovaries surgically removed, or have other problems that keep them from releasing healthy eggs at ovulation. The process is more complex for both donors and recipients than is DI, and perhaps because it is a newer technology and a more expensive one, it is less common. Most donors remain anonymous, although some couples select known donors or will choose to meet the donor if given a choice.

DE involves retrieving eggs from a donor, fertilizing the eggs through IVF using either your partner's or donor sperm, and transferring embryos into the birthing parent's uterus. Donor eggs are not frozen, although the embryos that result from their fertilization may be frozen and stored for future use. About 39 percent of DE attempts reported (fresh embryo transfers for 1996 cycles) to the U.S. Centers for Disease Control and Prevention (CDC) through the Society for Assisted Reproductive Technology culminate in the birth of a child, although success rates vary widely among fertility clinics that perform the procedure. The donor faces the same risks as any woman undergoing ovulatory stimulation and egg retrieval for IVF. A younger donor has a higher likelihood of hyperstimulation of the ovaries from medication, and close monitoring is essential. The recipient faces no greater health risks than those for pregnant women in her age category.

As with DI, couples often face significant emotional issues when they choose to try DE. It is a choice they typically reach when other options prove unsuccessful. And because they may have been on a roller coaster of emotion for quite some time, it is often hard to enjoy a pregnancy for fear it will abruptly end and dash their hopes once again.

### Voices

*"Even now, I look for blood every time I go to the bathroom," says Claudia, who is 7 months into her DE pregnancy after four failed IVFs using her own eggs. "I won't be sure of a happy ending until I hold a breathing, moving baby in my arms."*

## Questions to Answer Before Proceeding

**Can you both accept a child produced through egg donation as your own?** As is the case with DI, it can be difficult for some women and couples to envision a child as "theirs" when they know half of its genetic material is not. For many other women, having the joy of experiencing pregnancy and childbirth when they had lost that hope makes acceptance relatively easy.

### Voices

*"I really wanted adoption so we could be on equal footing with this child," admits Michele, who finally opted for egg donation after other infertility treatments failed to result in the pregnancy she and her husband wanted. Although counseling is helping her to put her fears and feelings in perspective, she still harbors a sense of frustration about her situation. "Now I question, will I feel the same connection to this child as my husband? I'm in counseling right now for that."*

**How would you handle a multiple gestation pregnancy?** Because DE often involves transferring more than one embryo, multiple gestation pregnancy is a clear risk. It is important to understand this potential, and to have a plan for managing it. Address the issue of multiple gestation pregnancy with your physician before considering or undergoing DE. ASRM recommends that clinics transfer only the number of embryos appropriate to the *donor's* age, not to the age of the recipient. In most cases, this would not exceed three, and with the advent of blastocyst transfer technology, it would be safer and perhaps just as effective to transfer fewer.

### Voices

*"We never wanted five children; that was a shock," says Hugh, whose wife Moira conceived, and at 20 weeks lost, quintuplets. "We were given the opportunity to reduce but*

*we decided against it. Not that we're opposed to that for others, but it wasn't right for us. When we lost the quints, we didn't think about who was to blame, not ourselves or the physicians. We just thought that was how it was supposed to be. For men, this is difficult because you do your part early in the process, with the sperm, and after that all you can do is give your support."*

## Choosing a Donor

Most donor eggs are available through DE programs. Many are affiliated with infertility clinics; some are businesses that provide egg donor matches. Unlike sperm donors, who can donate frequently for decades, egg donors are limited in the frequency they can donate. Most DE programs seek women in their mid-20s who are in excellent physical and mental health. Procedures vary among programs. Some ART clinics use only anonymous donors, whereas others allow couples to choose a known donor if they prefer. When using DE, the success of the ART cycle is linked to the age of the donor, the woman who supplies the egg.

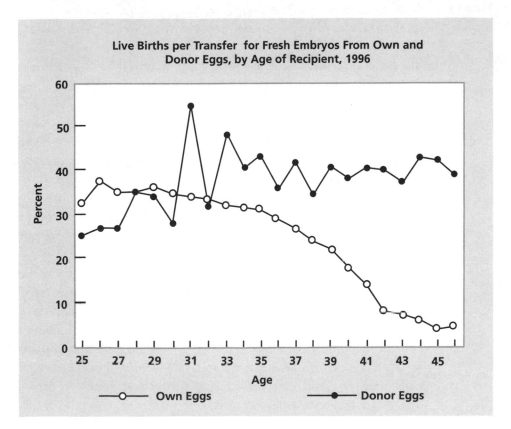

Live Births per Transfer for Fresh Embryos From Own and Donor Eggs, by Age of Recipient, 1996

The process of donating eggs is physically and emotionally more challenging than is the process of donating sperm. Most DE programs require counseling for donors before egg retrieval. Most egg donors come through the process just fine, many ready to do it again. They find it strongly satisfying to give such a gift to others.

Most couples choose a donor who has physical characteristics similar to the woman's, such as race and ethnic background, hair and eye color, and height and weight. Many also like to know more about the donor's religious and educational background, career or profession, and personality traits.

### Voices

*"When we picked the donor, we decided we wanted her to look like my husband," says Holly. "Every other recipient had wanted the donor to look like the wife, so the clinic really gave me a hard time. I was past the point of caring about my own genetics. We wanted a donor who was married and had children already, and somebody who had already donated and had donor egg children so that even if the laws changed to allow it, she probably wouldn't ever come looking for ours. Morally, ethically, because infertility had been a big part of our lives, we wanted someone who'd already had children."*

Some general factors to consider when choosing a DE program include the following:

- How does the DE program select its donors? What screening procedures does the program follow, and how consistently does it follow them? How much does the program know about a donor, and what information will the program share with you?
- What medical tests does the program conduct on the donor? How long does the program keep the donor's medical records? Will the program allow an adult child conceived through DE to access the donor's medical records if necessary?
- How old is the donor of the eggs you will receive, and how many times has she donated? If she has donated before, how many pregnancies have resulted? (Not all programs will reveal this information. Because of the relative scarcity of egg donors, however, there may be cases of half siblings being born in the same geographic area. This is also a consideration in practices in which eggs from one donor are split between two recipient couples.)
- Does one recipient receive all the eggs from one donor, or are the eggs divided among recipients?

- Does the program freeze embryos? If so, who retains the rights to their use, and what happens if you choose not to use any more of yours?
- Does your contract guarantee the number of eggs you will receive, and what happens if the retrieval produces fewer eggs than that amount?
- Could you use the same donor again if you wanted to have another child? Does the program stay in touch with its donors?
- Does the program adequately advise donors of all risks, including that of hyperstimulation of the ovaries?
- For which expenses are you responsible, and when do you pay them? What happens if the donor eggs fail to fertilize? Who pays for any unexpected donor medical expenses?

Because your intent is to become pregnant, it is important to evaluate your health and any potential problems that could occur during pregnancy. Older women (those older than 40) are more prone to certain pregnancy complications such as gestational diabetes and high blood pressure.

- Get a pre-pregnancy physical examination, including complete blood count, Rh factor, and screening tests for HIV, hepatitis, rubella, toxoplasmosis, and cytomegalovirus (CMV).
- Determine how many embryos will be transferred, and what you will do if multiple gestation pregnancy occurs.
- Talk with your obstetrician about the general risks of pregnancy and any that are particularly relevant for you.
- Begin taking prenatal vitamins, even if you feel you eat a balanced diet. There is strong evidence that the folic acid and B vitamins in standard prenatal vitamin preparations reduce your risk for certain kinds of birth defects.
- Decide, with your physician and your partner, whether you will have an amniocentesis and what you will do if the results show serious birth defects. Discuss with your partner what you will do if your child is born with birth defects not detected before birth.
- Ask to see samples of the informed consent and release forms donors typically sign and what steps the program takes to assure the donor fully understands what she is doing, such as predonation counseling.

**Choosing an anonymous donor.** About 80 percent of couples use anonymous donors. Selection of a donor is based on the characteristics and information in the donor profile. Some couples feel anonymous donation minimizes the likelihood of any potential legal issues down the road. It also helps keep the procedure totally confidential, if that is what you want to do.

### Voices

*"We were very careful to choose a donor who had other donor egg children and children of her own for two reasons: greater success and less vested rights issues," says Nadia. "We feel that the laws pertaining to donors may change in the next 10 years, and we wanted our donor to have as few ties to our child emotionally as she could possibly have. By choosing the donor we did, it would be clear to any court that she was informed about the procedure, knew the value of motherhood, and accepted that she had no more rights to our son than to her other donor egg children."*

**Choosing a known donor.** Some couples prefer a donor that they know, some use a relative, either for genetic reasons or because they feel they want to know the woman who is making such a significant contribution to their lives. If you choose to use a known donor, be sure you all agree on what role the donor will have in your child's life and what your child will be told about her. It is helpful to include these kinds of details in a written document, not so much for any sort of legal protection but to maintain a written record of the agreements among you. Consult an infertility therapist to help you consider other possible issues. (For example, what if the donor later develops infertility and is unable to have a biological child herself?)

### The DE Procedure

Most DE programs follow the same general protocols. After a donor completes all the screenings and health tests, her profile goes into the program's data bank. Prospective recipients review donor profiles. Once a recipient makes a choice, the program contacts the donor to be sure she is still available. If so, the program provides the donor with the drugs she will take to stimulate egg production, just as if she were undergoing IVF, and monitors her cycle. (For more information about IVF and other ART procedures, see chapter 9, "Assisted Reproductive Technology [ART].") When the time is right, the eggs are harvested by transvaginal ultrasound retrieval. This procedure uses ultrasound to locate the eggs, then to guide the physician in inserting a needle from inside the vagina into the ovarian follicles to retrieve them (the procedure is performed in a sterile environment with intravenous [IV] sedation to keep the donor comfortable).

Once the physician retrieves the eggs, they are fertilized with husband, partner, or donor sperm. After growing for 3 to 5 days in the laboratory, the embryos are ready for transfer. Before transfer, the recipient might take estrogen and progesterone to help prime the endometrium (the lining of the uterus) for receiving the embryos. Physicians typically transfer several embryos, but usually not more than three, to improve the odds that at least one will implant. (The age of the *donor* normally determines the quality of the embryos and influences the decision on the number of embryos to transfer; younger donors' embryos are more likely to survive and implant.) If you have decided to transfer more than one embryo, it is very important to discuss with your partner and your physician what you will do if multiple gestation pregnancy occurs.

It generally takes a week or so to determine whether the recipient has become pregnant. If so, donor egg pregnancy follows the usual course of pregnancy unless the recipient has specific circumstances that identify her as high risk, such as age (older than 40) or certain medical conditions, or if there is a multiple gestation pregnancy.

## Legal Considerations

DE, particularly with an anonymous donor, can be as straightforward from a legal perspective as DI. Most programs have an interest in safeguarding themselves against potential problems and liabilities, and have stringent standards and guidelines in place. There should be a signed contract between the program and the donor. Ask to see a blank sample contract, or a photocopy of the actual donor contract with the identifying information masked off. Because the egg donor faces some medical risks, the contract should identify who has responsibility for any adverse medical situations that develop as a direct or an indirect result of the egg donation process. There should also be a signed contract between the couple and the DE program. The contract should clearly specify the roles and responsibilities of all parties, including the program. If your IVF clinic also freezes and stores embryos, be sure your contract stipulates ownership of the embryos and what will happen to them if you choose not to use them.

It is a good idea to have an independent attorney look over both your contract and the contract the program has with the donor (even just your blank sample copy). If you use a known donor, it is essential that you each consult with an attorney (use different attorneys) to be sure you adequately protect your rights and establish your responsibilities. Look at this not as courting future trouble but as laying the groundwork for preventing it. Use an attorney who has experience with family-building issues and with drafting related agreements, for example in adoption and surrogacy matters.

## DONOR EMBRYO

Another family-building option that is emerging for couples who have both male and female factor infertility problems, or failed IVF attempts with their own gametes, for example, is embryo donation. There are thousands of frozen embryos that have been created through ART and that may be released by couples who have completed their families and have chosen to donate their embryos to others wishing for families. Many of the same issues regarding donor sperm and donor egg are relevant for the option of donor embryo pregnancy. Legal issues must be carefully considered, as well as the possibility of present or eventual contact with donors. Some ART clinics are beginning to offer donor embryo programs under carefully considered guidelines and consent procedures. The practice is relatively new, and success rates and financial arrangements should be reviewed with the clinic; consider addressing legal concerns with a qualified attorney and emotional issues with an infertility therapist or counselor.

## SURROGACY

Sometimes a woman cannot carry a pregnancy. She might have an abnormal uterus, or may have had a hysterectomy. In such situations, a surrogate—a woman who agrees to carry a pregnancy for another couple—may be a solution. Traditional surrogacy involves insemination using the couple's sperm and the surrogate's egg. Another type of surrogacy, called gestational surrogacy or gestational carrier, occurs when the couple, the "intended parents," creates an embryo(s) through IVF, and the embryo(s) is transferred to another woman's (the surrogate's) uterus for gestation.

Most surrogates are women who have children of their own. Often, the surrogate and the couple meet, although a few surrogate pregnancies take place with the surrogate remaining anonymous. Some attorneys who specialize in adoptions also handle surrogacy arrangements. There are also independent agencies that facilitate such arrangements.

Of all the infertility treatment options available, surrogacy is perhaps the one most shrouded in misunderstanding. It is often difficult for those not dealing with infertility issues to comprehend why a woman would put herself through a pregnancy to help an infertile couple achieve their dream of a child. Sometimes even those for whom surrogacy is an ideal option find it hard to understand a surrogate's motives. The surrogate's primary motivation is usually simple and straightforward. She has previously experienced, and enjoyed, pregnancy, already has at least one child, understands the joy of parenthood, and feels this is a way she can give someone else that joy. Although surrogates do get paid for their services, the amount they receive—typically between $12,500 and $18,500—is not really sufficient as the sole motivating factor.

Some general factors to consider when choosing a surrogacy program include the following:

- How long has the agency or program been in business? What is its success rate?
- How does the agency or program select surrogates? Does it use psychological screenings such as the MMPI (Minnesota Multiphasic Personality Inventory) to help determine a potential surrogate's motivation and emotional stability? Does the agency or program also conduct a psychological interview with the potential surrogate's husband or partner? (Some programs require the surrogate's family, including children who are old enough to understand pregnancy, to be involved in psychological screening.)
- What medical testing does the agency or program conduct to determine the surrogate's physical health?
- What legal documentation does the agency or program require between itself and the surrogate? Between itself and you?
- Does the agency or program encourage open relationships between couples and surrogates? Does it support closed relationships if that is what either side wants?
- What are the total fees, and what does your payment cover? Are services priced as a package, or will you have a continuous stream of expenses?
- What happens if the child has a serious birth defect? Who decides how to handle multiple gestation pregnancy? Who makes any other medical decisions that arise during pregnancy and delivery?
- How are parental rights finalized?

## Questions to Answer Before Proceeding

Many of the issues that surface with DI and DE are relevant with surrogacy as well. For example, how would you and your surrogate handle multiple gestation pregnancy? In addition, you will face questions specific to surrogacy.

**Do you and your partner fully agree on the decision to use a surrogate?** It can be both financially and emotionally draining to go through a surrogate pregnancy. Seeing another woman carrying your child can cause a flood of feelings you did not know you had or thought you had resolved. If you have an open relationship with your surrogate, you will both give support to and receive support from her. You may feel as though you have added a third person to your marriage or partnership. And if you have decided to have an anonymous or very limited relationship with your surrogate, you may feel frustrated by not knowing what is going on with her health and the baby's.

**If you have decided to keep private your decision to use a surrogate, how will you introduce your new baby to family and friends?** If you choose surrogacy, this may seem like an issue that is far away, but it will be in front of you before you know it. Are you planning to take maternity and paternity leave from work? You will need to file paperwork and provide evidence of your baby's birth to do so in most companies.

## Legal Considerations

Most surrogate pregnancies, when entered into with caution and appropriate legal protections, are positive experiences for both the surrogate and the new parents. The cases that do not work out get national media attention, are very high profile, and strike fear into the hearts of couples considering surrogacy. The risk for problems with surrogacy is greater than with DI or DE because the surrogate carries and delivers the child, which creates the potential for an emotional attachment that typically does not become a factor with sperm or egg donation. This makes it all the more important to select your surrogate carefully and to establish a strong contract that clearly states everyone's roles and responsibilities.

It would be unwise to enter into a surrogacy arrangement without the guidance of an independent attorney (one not affiliated with the agency that handles the surrogacy) to adequately protect the legal rights of all parties. Seek advice from an attorney who specializes in such matters. This is an increasingly complicated area of law, and the legal system has not quite caught up with technology. Although surrogacy contracts are not valid in some states, the practice may be either highly regulated or not regulated at all in others.

### Voices

*"We had an attorney draw up the contract," says Maryalice. "Our attorney was very thorough and addressed issues you wouldn't even think of, like expenses for time off work and travel for going to the physician."*

At the very least, your contract with a surrogate should specify the following information:

- How much money you pay the surrogate, when you make payments, and specifically what costs you are expected to cover.
- Whether you have any financial responsibility for other expenses, such as time off work or job loss, transportation for healthcare services, and child care for other children the surrogate may have.
- How you will handle unanticipated expenses.
- What responsibilities, obligations, and rights the surrogate has, and when her role ends.
- What responsibilities, obligations, and rights you have.
- The process you will enter into to resolve any legal problems that arise.
- What arrangements would be outlined in the legal contract about custody of the baby in the event of divorce or separation of the intended parents while the surrogate is pregnant.

## Considering Costs

A typical surrogacy arrangement costs around $50,000 for the whole package—from the fee to the surrogate to agency/legal fees, medical costs, and other costs, although it can range from as low as $30,000 to as high as $80,000 or more. What you pay depends on the role the agency or program plays, and whether you are seeking a conventional or gestational surrogacy. At the high end of the scale, you should expect the agency or program to handle just about everything. At the low end, you should expect to take care of many matters yourself. (Remember, though, good legal advice is key, and this should not be an area for economizing.) As well, there can be additional unexpected costs for complications during pregnancy or delivery, although such problems are fortunately not common. Be sure to review contractual expenses for medical procedures. Gestational surrogacy must be performed at an ART clinic or facility. Are all associated costs for ovulatory medication and monitoring, egg retrieval, sperm preparation, IVF, and embryo transfer included?

Using a surrogate who is someone you know and who does not expect payment may also entail expenses. Although your surrogate may have health insurance that will pay for the pregnancy and delivery, there are likely to be uncovered expenses that would be your responsibility to pick up. These could range from several hundred dollars in co-payments and deductibles to thousands of dollars for tests and procedures you want the surrogate to have to assure the baby's health, which the insurance company determines are not medically necessary (and therefore not covered). And if your surrogate is paying her own health insurance premiums, it may be appropriate for you to cover those payments for at least the duration of the pregnancy and its aftercare.

The legal concerns in a surrogate relationship are paramount. You should consult with an attorney to draw up a contract that is acceptable to you, your surrogate and her partner/husband, and her attorney. Although someone who has volunteered to be your surrogate might initially take offense at this recommendation, it really is the only way to protect you both.

## Choosing a Surrogate

Agencies who handle surrogacy typically have profiles on record for the women actively in their systems. For a traditional surrogacy (in which the male partner will provide the sperm and the surrogate will provide the egg), couples may try to match the surrogate's characteristics with the woman's to produce a child who appears physically to be a blend of the couple. For a gestational surrogacy, these factors are not an issue because the child will not have the surrogate's genetic material.

Some general factors to consider when choosing a surrogate include the following:

- Review the complete medical and psychological profiles of the surrogates you are considering, rather than just summaries. The agency or program should provide these for you, with identifying information masked.
- Has the agency or program ever had a couple change their minds after entering into a surrogate pregnancy? A surrogate change her mind? If so, how did the agency resolve the situation?
- Review the contract the agency signs with the surrogate, and any contract that would be signed between you and the agency. Is there also a contract directly between you and the surrogate? Have an independent attorney review all documents before you sign them.
- How old is the surrogate, and has she participated in a surrogate pregnancy before? How many times has she been pregnant, and how many children resulted from those pregnancies?
- Do you have the option of meeting the surrogate, and becoming involved with the pregnancy and delivery?

## Anonymous or Known Surrogate

Using a known surrogate fosters a stronger sense of relationship among all of you, allows you to be involved in the prenatal visits, and establishes a bond with your unborn child as much as this is possible. For many couples and surrogates, this becomes a relationship that extends far beyond the pregnancy as they find themselves inextricably linked by this event that has drawn them together. Some couples prefer to know as little as possible about the surrogate, but this is by far the exception and not the rule.

Whether and what you plan to tell your child about his or her origins may influence your choice about using a known or anonymous surrogate, too. If you do not want your child to know he or she came into this world with the help of a surrogate (or at least want to delay your child's knowledge of this), you will have to decide with your surrogate how best to handle the situation. Whether and what you tell is not nearly as important as all of you agreeing on how to proceed. Be clear on what you and your partner want. If you want to get to know the surrogate and keep her in your child's life but do not want to tell your child of her role until your child is older, agree to present her as a special friend. If you want to remain distanced from the surrogate and have no contact after your child's birth, then agree to this at the very beginning.

## Pregnancy and Delivery

The surrogate should receive regular prenatal care. Because surrogates enter into surrogacy arrangements voluntarily, they are typically highly motivated to eat properly and nutritiously, exercise regularly, and in general take good care of themselves and the pregnancy. If you have entered into an open relationship with your surrogate and are actively involved with the pregnancy, you can monitor how she cares for herself. If you are going to do anonymous surrogacy, you will have to rely on the agency to monitor the surrogate's and the baby's health and well-being. The physician and agency should make arrangements with the hospital, which should know the delivering woman is a surrogate and you are the baby's intended parents.

The issues of legal parenthood, names on birth certificate, and possible need for adoption proceedings after the birth of a baby from a surrogacy arrangement are matters of state law, if they have been addressed at all through case law or legislation in the state. Be sure you cover these issues with your attorney and the agency well in advance of the birth.

Because surrogacy is a relatively novel path to family building, networking with others who have chosen it can be an important way to evaluate its appeal for you. See the Resources appendix for referral to the Organization of Parents Through Surrogacy (OPTS).

## LIVING CHILDFREE: RESOLVING WITHOUT PARENTING

At first, living childfree appears to be the decision of default—the path taken when all other options fail—to most couples considering it as an option. They often view themselves as "childless," implying that they are lacking in some way, rather than "childfree," which connotes a chosen alternative. To consider this decision as "resolving without parenting" is perhaps more accurate, since it acknowledges that you will continue somehow to have children in your life. If you make a successful, well-reasoned transition to a life in which you are not raising children, it will feel very different from feeling childless during the infertility crisis. One of the nicest surprises will be the enjoyment of children again. You may also reconnect with friends whose children are older and whose lives are less child-centered.

### Voices

*For some couples, the transition from one perspective to the other is both dramatic and satisfying. "I would see some couples that didn't have children and seemed happy," says Prue. "Over time, Jerry and I decided to think more about the good life we did have. We could work on our careers, we could go on vacations, we have free time, and we really have fun together. We have friends who rush around trying to work and have a family, who can't go out over the weekend because they feel bad leaving their kids all week. It's not that I didn't want that life, but I was beginning to see that there was a trade-off. It was a very slow transition over a year and a half or so. But being able to realize we really did enjoy being able to travel and having our own lives, and that we wouldn't be giving that up—that felt pretty good."*

Unlike the fulfilled decision to have or adopt a child, the decision to resolve without parenting is not irreversible. As older parenthood has become more accepted and avenues to achieve it have widened, reaching closure on the parenting role in life has become elusive. (Even menopause no longer signals that day.) Some emerging from the infertility crisis may decide to "try on" childfree living for a period of time, like the fictional couple in the decision tree at the end of this chapter. This is *not* to suggest that a childfree decision should serve as an interim one on the way to your *real* goal—only that these decisions are complex and not always reached quickly. To be at peace with your resolution, you and your partner must embrace it fully. If you have an infertility counselor, keep in touch, as there may be times when you need to revisit your choice and the decision tree that led you there.

## Managing Emotionally Difficult Situations

Even when you think you have made the adjustment to living childfree, holidays can be especially challenging. Many couples who choose not to parent make plans for "adult" activities during particularly stressful holidays such as Christmas or Hanukkah. You might plan a cruise, or a vacation to someplace it would be difficult to travel with children.

Maintain a support network to pull you through any tough times. If you found your local RESOLVE childfree group helpful, continue going to meetings. Consider starting your own support circle with others who have made the same choices you have, either in person or through periodic telephone or e-mail contact. Ask relatives not to bemoan your decision, especially in your presence. Sometimes reminding others, nondefensively, of your path to this decision and all that fills your life helps you to affirm your choice, too. Although it is hard to believe when your decision is still fresh, the hurt you feel when you view couples with children gradually will heal. You may remember the sharp pain you felt in such situations, but the memory will dull with time. If this seems impossible to you right now, you might consider counseling to help you understand and process your grief so you can move on.

## Finding Happiness as a Family of Two

It does seem that the world assumes happiness and fulfillment come when a marital union produces children. Even adults are encouraged to "get in touch with the child within" to keep fun and joy in their lives. So how can you find happiness as a family of two? Start by rediscovering each other. If you have spent years trying to become a family of three (or more), the transition back to focusing on just you two will take time and may even feel awkward for a while. Think of ways to have fun with each other again, perhaps returning to activities you loved before infertility treatment or support groups became your lives! Change the way you think of yourselves from "couple" to "family." Making such a conscious shift can alter your perception more than you thought possible. And remember that choosing to resolve without parenting does not mean excluding children from your life. There are many ways to become involved with children aside from raising them that can be very satisfying.

# RESOLVING AS A STEPFAMILY

A complicated challenge for a couple to face is infertility within a marriage in which a stepfamily has formed. A partner who has had children from a previous marriage or relationship may not share the driving motivation to conceive or adopt experienced by the partner without children. Conversely, the partner who has parented may feel a special urgency to share the experience of parenting with a partner who has not had children. Sometimes both partners have children from previous marriages, and the drive is to create a new "family" within the union. A couple may want to explore the resolution of infertility within a stepfamily marriage through a variety of paths, including treatment, adoption, donor pregnancy or surrogacy, and resolving without parenting *more* children.

Resolving without parenting in a stepfamily marriage seems impossible, because children, whether they are step or biological, are often such a central part of the union. But if one partner has not conceived or adopted, this resolution may feel like a childfree one to him or her. Grieving the child the new partners would have produced will be an essential part of moving to resolution. Approaching resolution as a couple is important under any circumstances, but it is particularly critical in a stepfamily union, especially if there is an imbalance in parenting experience. The value of good infertility counseling cannot be overstated when these decisions are being made.

All families evolve with time; your relationship with your own parents now that you are an adult is probably very different from the one you had with them when you were a child. So, too, do stepfamilies evolve. Successful stepfamilies often create their own traditions and family language over time. Resolving as a stepfamily may take plenty of time and the help of good and frequent counseling. If you choose this path, you may find that many of the rewards of family life, such as nurturing children and potential grandparenting, are available to the stepparent as well.

Pressures within stepfamilies can be enormous without the added dimension of infertility, and the full dynamics of stepfamily living are well beyond the scope of this book. If you face these challenges, see the Resources appendix at the back of this book for stepfamily reference.

## WHEN IS ENOUGH, ENOUGH?

We have created the following decision tree, using the fictional couple Anik and Jake, to help you explore other family-building options, and to decide "when is enough, *enough?*"

Anik is 41 and her husband, Jake, is 39. Their careers are thriving, and both travel extensively for their work. They began trying to conceive 3 years ago.

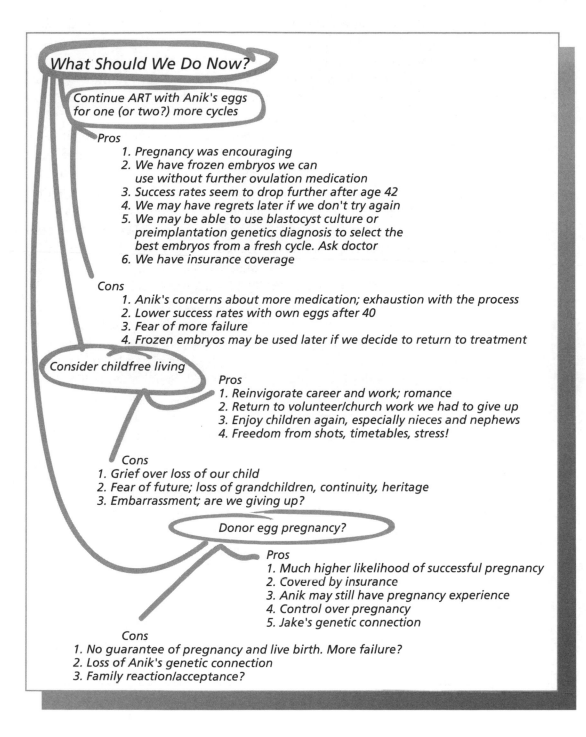

**What Should We Do Now?**

**Continue ART with Anik's eggs for one (or two?) more cycles**

*Pros*
1. Pregnancy was encouraging
2. We have frozen embryos we can use without further ovulation medication
3. Success rates seem to drop further after age 42
4. We may have regrets later if we don't try again
5. We may be able to use blastocyst culture or preimplantation genetics diagnosis to select the best embryos from a fresh cycle. Ask doctor
6. We have insurance coverage

*Cons*
1. Anik's concerns about more medication; exhaustion with the process
2. Lower success rates with own eggs after 40
3. Fear of more failure
4. Frozen embryos may be used later if we decide to return to treatment

**Consider childfree living**

*Pros*
1. Reinvigorate career and work; romance
2. Return to volunteer/church work we had to give up
3. Enjoy children again, especially nieces and nephews
4. Freedom from shots, timetables, stress!

*Cons*
1. Grief over loss of our child
2. Fear of future; loss of grandchildren, continuity, heritage
3. Embarrassment; are we giving up?

**Donor egg pregnancy?**

*Pros*
1. Much higher likelihood of successful pregnancy
2. Covered by insurance
3. Anik may still have pregnancy experience
4. Control over pregnancy
5. Jake's genetic connection

*Cons*
1. No guarantee of pregnancy and live birth. More failure?
2. Loss of Anik's genetic connection
3. Family reaction/acceptance?

When pregnancy did not occur in 6 months, the couple consulted an infertility specialist. They are fortunate to live in a state that mandates comprehensive insurance coverage for infertility treatment, and they have undergone two IVF cycles, with two fresh embryo transfers and one thawed embryo transfer. They had one biochemical pregnancy, after the thaw cycle, but Anik miscarried. They have three frozen embryos stored at the clinic.

Anik and Jake were both shocked at how treatment consumed their lives. The stress of travel, work, and treatment has been enormous, and their RESOLVE support group meetings became their "lifeline." Anik wants to consider stopping treatment; Jake is encouraged by the pregnancy and feels they should keep trying. Take a look at the options the couple has outlined and the decision they have made as a result (see chapter 7, "The Female: Structural Problems, Age-Related Factors, and Treatment," for a decision tree involving surrogacy and chapters 8 and 9, "The Male: Diagnosis and Treatment" and "Assisted Reproductive Technology [ART]," for adoption decisions).

**Decision:** Just looking at the tree calmed Jake's anxiety. He is willing to talk with the couple's infertility therapist about at least taking a break and attending the RESOLVE chapter's childfree group—"trying on" the option—because he knows he and Anik have further treatment options. Anik feels great relief at not having to darken the door of the clinic again, at least for a while. They both realize they may be giving up their dream of a biological child and will need to begin to grieve that loss. They are considering using contraception to make sure they are off the roller coaster of hope and despair while they explore this territory.

## Accepting Your Decision

It is natural to wonder, at times, whether the decision you have made is indeed the right one. Eventually, you will realize you have accepted that it is. Sometimes others will question you as well. Such questioning can be disconcerting. It can cause you to question yourself, even after you thought you were comfortable with your decision. Being prepared for this is the best way to deal with it. As you go through your decision-making process, create your own decision tree and write down your thoughts and reasons for the choices you make in your infertility journal. Then, when you find yourself questioning whether you have made the right decisions, you have an objective record of why you made them. Odds are, if you have given the process the appropriate level of attention and careful thought, your writings will affirm your decision.

## POSITIVE STEPS YOU CAN TAKE FROM CHAPTER 15

**Take the time you need to reach your decision.** The decision to stop infertility treatment to reach your original dream may be a difficult and painful one, and may involve a grieving process. The resolution of infertility, however, offers many wonderful paths in addition to traditional biological parenting. As you consider which path to choose, read about, talk about, and explore it as thoroughly as possible to improve the quality of your decisions.

**Nurture your support network.** Maintain connection and support as you make alternative decisions, and maybe for years after they are made, to help you and perhaps your children find community.

**Welcome resolution.** Infertility is a life crisis through which you will pass. You may hear faint echoes of the experience later in time, but the intense feelings and sorrow will fade after you have resolved the crisis. Find strength in believing that you will emerge from it, perhaps with a different understanding of family and maybe stronger than when you began.

# 16 Surviving Infertility and Moving Forward

There is life after infertility. It may not be the life you imagined you would have—infertility changes you, regardless of the outcome. You know, first-hand, the frailty of dreams, the randomness of success, and the legacy of loss. You have had to readjust your view of what it means to be and have a family. And you know life goes on. Your mission is to make that life as fulfilling as possible.

## REACHING FOR RESOLUTION: MAKING YOUR DECISION

Resolving infertility is a process. You may have tried years of treatment or decided to move right to options such as adoption or living childfree. Many people feel enormous relief when they have made a decision and can now move forward.

For some, of course, events determine decisions. This is most definitely the case when a successful pregnancy occurs.

## PREGNANCY AFTER INFERTILITY

After years of struggling with infertility, being pregnant may feel joyful, sad, and frightening. Along with the profound relief at finally achieving pregnancy comes the anxiety: Will the pregnancy go well? Will the delivery be medically uneventful? Will the baby be healthy? Many questions swirl through the minds of parents-to-be, who had nearly given up the dream of a biological child. Many emotions surface—feelings of celebration and happiness alternate with fears and worries. This is a time of great transition.

For those who have miscarried in the past, perhaps multiple times, being pregnant may be very stressful. Each day focuses on searching for signs that this pregnancy, too, may fail. Every twinge, every ache, every cramp becomes a sign of potential trouble.

---

### Voices

*Claire, a 37-year-old woman who is pregnant after a long struggle with infertility, says, "Now that I am pregnant, infertility is still having an effect on me. It is hard to trust what is so clearly there. I have pregnancy symptoms. I have a picture of the embryo. I have blood work that says that everything is normal. And yet, I still can't trust it. And I am not alone. My good friend who also dealt with years of infertility is pregnant (what a gift!) and she feels the same way. So instead of thinking of names and planning the nursery, I wait for some magical number of weeks to go by so I feel safe. I thought that was 8 weeks (I am there) but now I think it's 12 or 14 weeks. I don't think that'll do it either. Infertility has changed me."*

---

Some who have found support and empathy in a group or with others experiencing infertility may suddenly feel cast out and abandoned, as if they had crossed over to the fertile world. Many couples who are newly pregnant feel that they have received a temporary visa, at best, and reports of women experiencing disbelief right up to delivery are not uncommon. This is a time when connection with those who are pregnant after infertility can be comforting. Check with your local RESOLVE chapter for referral to a support group or to receive a member contact.

## Prenatal Tests

The most pressing need during pregnancy is to maintain the health and well-being of both the growing fetus and the mother. Fortunately, the vast majority of pregnancies produce normal, healthy babies. There are a number of prenatal tests used, however, to detect potential structural and chromosomal abnormalities. In some cases, deciding whether to have these tests means also deciding what you will do if the results indicate a problem, especially as test results are not always conclusive.

It is nearly an unbearable thought for many couples to consider that the child they have desired for so long may have a birth defect that could threaten its ability to survive or quality of life after birth. This is a particularly stressful time for the older woman. Older mothers are statistically at greater risk for a number of birth defects in their children, including Down syndrome. The older the genetic mother, the more likely it is the obstetrician will order prenatal tests. (These concerns may not apply to an older woman pregnant through *donor* egg or embryo, as it is the age of the donor that influences the quality of the egg.)

Blood tests can provide information about the mother's health, and the baby's health to some extent. Routine blood testing can determine the presence of conditions such as anemia (insufficient iron in the blood) or toxoplasmosis (a parasitic infection that, if untreated, can cause blindness or brain damage to the baby). A blood test called MSAFP (maternal serum alpha-fetoprotein) performed between 16 and 18 weeks from the last menstrual period can indicate possible neural tube defects and other abnormalities. Although high or low AFP levels can be present in a normal pregnancy, they warrant further investigation through additional tests.

Ultrasound provides a noninvasive way to "see" inside the uterus using high-frequency sound waves to create visual images. Ultrasound can often detect major problems such as spina bifida (an opening in the spinal column) and anencephaly (inadequately small or absent brain), and it provides a way to measure the size and position of the fetus.

Amniocentesis and chorionic villi sampling (CVS) are other commonly used prenatal tests. Because they are invasive procedures, they carry a slight risk of complications. Of course, detection of life-threatening or major problems may mean an agonizing decision about pregnancy termination.

Amniocentesis is usually performed between 15 and 17 weeks of pregnancy. The physician uses ultrasound to locate the position of the fetus and placenta, inserts a thin, hollow needle through the woman's abdomen into her uterus, well away from the fetus, and withdraws about a tablespoon of amniotic fluid for analysis. Amniocentesis detects a wide range of chromosomal disorders including Down syndrome, Tay-Sachs disease, sickle cell anemia, hemophilia, and muscular dystrophy. It can also provide information about the baby's sex, which can be an important factor if either partner is a carrier for a sex-linked disorder.

During CVS, usually done during week 10 of pregnancy, the physician inserts a thin needle through the cervix into the uterus. Instead of sampling amniotic fluid, a few of the tiny hairlike projections, or villi, that are part of the developing placenta are withdrawn. These villi contain fetal cells that can be analyzed for the presence of many genetic abnormalities, and some chromosomal disorders. Rarely, amniocentesis may be required later to verify the results of CVS testing. CVS will not provide results for some conditions, such as neural tube defects.

## The Risks of Multiple Gestation Pregnancy and the Difficult Choices to Make

At this point in your journey—after trying so long and so hard to have a baby—it may seem incredible to have to consider what will happen if you get pregnant with multiple fetuses. You may even consider multiples a "bonus." But the fact is that assisted reproductive technology (ART) procedures have resulted in multiple gestation pregnancy (42.9 percent of ART pregnancies achieved in women younger than 35 years were reported as multiple gestation pregnancy in the *1996 ART Success Rates Report*, see "Resources"), posing high risks to mothers and infants. Multiple gestation pregnancy also may occur in non-ART cycles in which the woman takes ovulatory medication and conceives either through sexual intercourse or with intrauterine insemination (IUI) (see chapter 6, "The Female: Hormonal Disorders and Treatment," for information on the monitoring of these cycles).

The risks to a woman carrying multiple fetuses (even twins) include high blood pressure, gestational diabetes, increased risk of bleeding, premature labor, and cesarean section birth. Risks to the infants include prematurity, low birth weight, and respiratory and eye complications. Premature infants are at higher risk for congenital abnormalities and learning disabilities.

Unfortunately, the risks for maternal and fetal complications increase dramatically with the number of fetuses carried. For this reason, couples with a multiple gestation pregnancy of three or more fetuses may consider a procedure called multiple gestation reduction (MGR), which involves reducing the number of fetal sacs to improve the chance of having a healthy pregnancy—and a healthy baby. Approximately 2,000 of these procedures have been performed in the United States since the early 1980s.

The decision of whether or not to undergo a reduction procedure is an individual one, based on ethical, moral, and personal beliefs as well as medical facts. After gathering all available information, it is up to you and your partner to do what is best for you. You may find it helpful to seek support and advice from outside your family and your medical team. Ask your physician for the names of other patients who have experienced MGR and would be willing to talk with you. Ask them about their physical as well as emotional experience. Talk with a mental health professional who will help you analyze some of the emotional issues that arise with a multiple gestation pregnancy and the decision of whether to reduce. You may wish to seek counsel from your clergy or rabbi to help you arrive at the decision that is right for you.

## The Reduction Procedure

If you and your partner decide to do MGR, first find an experienced physician to do the procedure. It is important to discuss the associated miscarriage and complication rates. If you live in a rural area or far from a major medical center, you may have to travel to a large hospital for the procedure.

There are two techniques used in MGR: transvaginal or transabdominal. Both procedures are performed on an outpatient basis. Transvaginal reductions are done at 8 to 10 weeks after your last period. They involve using ultrasound to guide the insertion of a needle through the vagina to the sac. Transabdominal reduction is done at 10 to 12 weeks after your last period and involves using ultrasound to guide the needle through the abdomen into the sac. In both procedures, potassium chloride is injected. The reduced sac will become smaller and disappear.

The main risk of reduction is the loss of the entire pregnancy. This risk can vary from 2 to 15 percent depending on the number of fetal sacs, their locations, and the experience of the center doing the procedure. There is also a slight risk for intrauterine infection; some doctors prescribe antibiotics for several days after the procedure. After a reduction, your obstetrician will follow the pregnancy as with any single or twin pregnancy. A pregnancy reduced to twin gestation may still deliver early, but likely with the babies' weights higher than if it had not been reduced.

You may feel encouraged by two studies that showed most women who underwent MGR said that they never regretted their decision, even though they felt depressed and sad after the procedure. Furthermore, they reported that they sometimes thought about their loss, but that having healthy babies made their medical decision right for them.

## Dealing with Friends from the Infertility Journey

If you are now pregnant or parenting, it may be hard to know how to share your joy with those who are still struggling. Psychologists sometimes refer to such feelings as survivor's guilt. Because there often is no real explanation for why one person is successful and someone else is not, the ones who are successful may feel guilty for their good luck. Such feelings are normal, particularly if your struggle seems less difficult or traumatic than someone else's experience. It is important to acknowledge your feelings, both of joy and of guilt. Your "good luck" in conceiving, adopting, or otherwise building your family has nothing to do with the continued infertility of others, and there is nothing you can do to change circumstances for others. To deprive yourselves of enjoying your child because others may resent that it is you and not they who have become parents is not fair to you or your child. Yes, your infertility experiences have changed you. And just as your circle of friends shifted when you began your struggle to overcome your infertility, again you will find the focus of your life changing. This does not mean you have to give up the friendships you formed when infertility drew you together. It just means that you may have to dig deeper to find common bonds.

### Voices

*"Now that I am a mom, I feel really sad about the distance between me and the friends in RESOLVE I left behind," says Shirley. "I never know what to say or how to make it okay with them. I know they realize how much I deserve and enjoy my new son, but if I celebrate too much with them, I know it is hurtful. If I downplay my joy, it seems ungrateful. I suffer from lots of guilt in having serendipity, in having good luck.*

*"I have become more careful about what I say in public," Shirley continues. "It's amazing how invisible infertility is. I always want to explain my situation, the infertility, so I don't appear to be gloating in front of an unidentified infertile person. Having been there, I know how hard and important it is to do the right thing, to act the right way."*

## PARENTING AFTER INFERTILITY

For those who thought they would never experience parenting, a child's presence in the family is absolutely wondrous. Often years of hopes, prayers, treatments, and waiting precede the birth or adoption. This child, whose existence was desired for so long, is finally here. After the excitement settles into a daily routine, expectation runs head-on into reality. New anxiety may enter your life. Parenting is difficult; it is perfectly normal to feel overwhelmed sometimes. Most new parents feel some uncertainty about their parenting skills. Overprotection of this miracle baby is a common fear of parents emerging from the experience of infertility. Parenting classes and post-adoption parent groups can help you establish healthy parenting practices.

### Voices

*Parenting after infertility raises some unique issues for single women. "I think my biggest fear is my child being angry about not having a father," says Linda, who con-*

*ceived a child through donor insemination (DI) after several years of infertility treatment. "I really thought about my decision before moving forward, and I know my family will help with this. Still, I think it could get really hard during the teenage years. My deepest hope is that my child will be happy to be here."*

If your child was conceived through ART procedures, surrogacy, or donor gamete(s), you will need to decide what, how much, and when to tell your child. It helps to have a general plan in mind so you are prepared when the time comes to address any questions. Some people decide to be open with their children from the start, emphasizing how much they desired and love them. Others decide to "play it by ear" or wait until the child seems ready. Again, professional counseling and networking with other parents who have blazed the trail can help you make your decisions.

Decisions about disclosure of infertility resolution are deeply personal. Some child development specialists advocate for openness, believing it is important to share even difficult information with children and that children have a deep capacity to understand complex information. Others believe it is important for the child to feel "the same" as his or her peers and perhaps siblings, and that giving a child too much information too early creates confusion and uncertainty for the child. However, a child who has a genetic background different from yours (as a result of donor insemination, egg, or embryo) may at some point have a need (and some would argue a right) to know this fact for medical purposes.

The issue of disclosure is much more settled, of course, in the world of adoption. There are many resources within the adoption community for speaking with young children about the adoption journey to family. Many parents introduce the concept of adoption to their children as soon as language permits.

### Voices

*"I'll never forget the day Jason and I began to tell our 3-year-old son of his adoption story," says Susan. "He took off running excitedly around the house squealing 'I'm a doctor, I'm a doctor!' "*

## Special Challenges of Secondary Infertility

Secondary infertility is defined as having difficulty conceiving or carrying a pregnancy to term after already having had at least one successful pregnancy and delivery. For some, secondary infertility is a complete shock, as pregnancy may have come easily before. For others, it represents a trip back into the painful land of infertility in which they have already traveled. Because most infertility support services are geared toward couples who have no children, those dealing with secondary infertility may feel isolated and lacking the support they need.

Although secondary infertility is more common than primary infertility, more people decide not to enter into medical treatment. *We succeeded so easily the first time*, couples may reason, *so if we just keep trying, we can do it again.* It is hard to believe, but there may be little connection between having conceived in the past and being able to conceive now. Age and subsequent medical problems can take their toll on fertility for both men and women, and it is important for those experiencing secondary infertility to undergo thorough medical evaluation in order to make good decisions about treatment or alternatives.

### Voices

*Stacey and Ross are experiencing secondary infertility. This time, as with their first child, the couple will be using sperm from an anonymous donor, because of Ross's male factor infertility problems. Stacey remembers, "During the course of treatment with my second child, I was taking a longer time to get pregnant than the first time, and I was getting very concerned that something was wrong. I called my doctor when one particular cycle did not work and complained that I was having 'bad luck.' The doctor said to me, 'No Stacey. The first time you got pregnant right away with the donor was good luck. Now you're just having "regular luck." ' That kept it in perspective for me."*

Secondary infertility can affect family dynamics. Sometimes, one partner becomes consumed by the issues of secondary infertility, while the other remains ambivalent or even nonsupportive. And although primary infertility typically involves just the individual or couple, secondary infertility can affect the child (or children) already in the family. The child may want a sibling, or may wonder why its parents want another child so much. Play groups in which other mothers are experiencing their second and third pregnancies may become painful events, and parents may feel guilty not being able to provide their child a sibling when all the other kids have one or two.

In addition, parents struggling with secondary infertility often feel isolated and find less support among family and friends, and even healthcare providers. But having one child may not diminish the sense of loss people experience in not being able to have another. For some, secondary infertility can be just as emotionally traumatic as primary infertility.

It is important for couples to approach secondary infertility and its resolution as a partnership. RESOLVE chapters often provide secondary infertility support groups, and there are therapists who specialize in this area of infertility counseling. This is also a time when some couples weigh the treatment and adoption options carefully, and some proceed to create "blended families" with children welcomed both by birth and adoption.

### Parenting in a One-Child Family

After resolving infertility through successful treatment or adoption, some individuals and couples are content with a one-child family. Many decide to stop treatment or not to pursue adoption for a second child, to live as a family of three, and to welcome another pregnancy only if it is spontaneous. Some couples even eliminate the possibility of pregnancy by using birth control. This may not be an easy choice for some, as family members and friends may hint, or openly suggest, that a sibling for your child would be so wonderful, or that you are somehow selfish for not pursuing another pregnancy. These hurtful comments may make you question your resolution; again, the guidance of an infertility therapist could be useful at these times.

## LONG-TERM EFFECTS OF THE EXPERIENCE OF INFERTILITY

Regardless of outcome, the infertility experience may continue to affect your life. You may wonder what would have happened had you chosen another alternative. You may think about what the child you did not have or adopt would have been like. Anniversaries such as the loss of a pregnancy may be painful. Family and friends may not understand.

Infertility may feel like a loss of innocence. You may no longer assume that life is easy or fair. It may take some time to recover your self-esteem or to feel good about your body again. Infertility is a life crisis; it usually takes time to heal from this experience.

Infertility may change your relationships, too. Those who share as much of the experience of infertility as possible seem to draw strength from their sharing, regardless of the outcome. Many couples find that their relationship strengthens and their commitment to each other deepens, with a new understanding. The infertility experience may be destructive of a relationship, as well. The toll it takes on intimacy is often heavy, but restoring bonds is usually possible with time and professional guidance.

## Menopause and Beyond

Menopause traditionally marks the conclusion of a woman's childbearing ability. It can be a particularly difficult milestone for women who had infertility treatment without success. A woman's menopause normally occurs somewhere between her early 40s and mid-50s and represents a critical life passage for many women. If menopause occurs prematurely, as it does in a small percentage of women, this early and unexpected conclusion of the body's reproductive function is a traumatic shock. At a time when friends and siblings are pregnant and having children, the woman with premature menopause may be experiencing hot flashes and other menopausal symptoms. Although adoption and donor egg pregnancy are wonderful potential paths to parenthood, grief for this loss can be profound.

It is important to recognize the significance of this life passage whenever it occurs, and to grieve the losses it represents. It is also important to realize that menopause is only the end of reproductivity, not the end of life. New research and literature on the menopause years and beyond, in fact, are exploding some of the old myths. Many women are finding new vigor at this time of life and looking forward to new adventures, new nurturing or volunteer opportunities, and perhaps new careers thanks to a longer life expectancy than past generations enjoyed.

# MOVING FORWARD

For most people, it is a relief to be moving beyond infertility. You will start to feel more in control of your life. There can be a process of reconnecting with yourself and with your partner, no matter how you choose to resolve your infertility, and a sense of satisfaction that comes with it. Yet there is often also a sense of sadness and of loss, because to move forward you must leave something behind. Infertility consumes your life like few other experiences. The decision to put infertility behind you represents a major life change.

Many people develop a close bond to the friends they have made through participation in infertility support groups and RESOLVE chapters. Moving forward can mean leaving these friendships behind. This can be difficult and painful, because you have shared your most intimate dreams and frustrations with each other, perhaps for years.

### Voices

*"I wish more than anything we could stay friends and stay connected," says Judith of the friends she has made through RESOLVE. Despite her determination to remain connected to those who have shared so much of her anguish and her hopes through the years, Judith now finds the birth of her son is reweaving the fabric of her life in ways she did not expect. "I am so quickly becoming encultured into parenthood, and it's becoming harder and harder to understand and know how to behave with my RESOLVE friends who are not pregnant or parenting."*

Friendships formed around infertility, however, often do survive beyond resolution. Finding and nurturing a common bond, whether it be parenting or shared hobbies and activities, can sustain the friendship even when resolution takes different paths. Reports of former support group members' tenth, even twentieth annual reunions are not uncommon.

One surprising consequence of moving forward may be the rekindling of friendships you had before infertility took center stage in your life. Many of the friends who drifted away as they had babies and started families may no longer be so consumed by the demands of parenting. Their children are older now, with lives of their own that often do not include their parents. If you have resolved without parenting, the path of friendship may circle back to reconnect you with these friends and the interests you once shared.

## POSTCARDS

No matter which path you take, the infertility experience may echo down the years for you, and you may occasionally receive an old "postcard" from the journey. The old, too-familiar reminder of infertility may occur when you reflect on the years lost to you, and perhaps to your aging parents, in enjoying your young family. Or it may arrive when your friends begin to welcome grandchildren into their families, or you realize you may not see your own grandchildren because of late parenting. Parents happily raising children adopted or conceived through donor gametes may receive a message or two, as their children begin to explore identity or reach milestones such as puberty or giving birth themselves.

Resolving infertility is a lifelong process. Careful mapping of the journey, using the tools in this book and others you discovered along the way, will mean that the postcards you receive from the past, while poignant, will be faded.

# Glossary

**Abortion** Premature termination of a pregnancy.

**Abortion, spontaneous (miscarriage)** The unintended ending of a pregnancy before the first 20 to 24 weeks of gestation.

**Abortion, complete** A miscarriage in which the embryo or fetus and all tissues produced as a result of pregnancy are expelled from the uterus.

**Abortion, incomplete** A miscarriage in which the contents of the uterus are not completely expelled, and some tissue is left behind.

**Abortion, missed** A miscarriage in which the fetus dies in the uterus, but is not expelled.

**Acrosome** A membrane covering the head of a sperm cell that when activated enables the sperm to penetrate the egg, leading to fertilization.

**Acrosome reaction** The activation of the acrosome, which allows the sperm cell to penetrate the egg for fertilization.

**Adenomyosis** The abnormal growth of tissue from the uterine lining (endometrium) into the muscle of the uterine wall (myometrium). This is different from endometriosis, in which tissue from the endometrium grows outside of the uterus.

**Adenosis** Abnormal growth of glandular tissue, which can occur on the outside of the cervix in diethylstilbestrol-exposed (DES-exposed) women.

**Adhesions** Rubbery bands of fibrous scar tissue that form on, in, or around reproductive organs and can bind the surface of one organ to another.

**Adrenocorticotropic hormone (ACTH)** Pituitary hormone that, when secreted, triggers the release of other hormones by the adrenal cortex. Also called *adrenocorticotropin.*

**Agglutination** The clumping together of cells; can inhibit sperm motility (ability of sperm to swim) and interfere with fertilization.

**Agonist** A drug that has the same properties and produces the same results as a natural chemical found in the body.

**Antagonist** A drug that counteracts the action of a natural chemical found in the body.

**Allopathic disorder** A condition in which

immune system cells attack newly formed cells in the body; when embryonic or placental cells are attacked, a miscarriage results.

**Amenorrhea** A condition in which menstruation does not occur. A woman who has never menstruated has *primary amenorrhea,* which is very rare. A woman who menstruated at one time but has stopped for at least four consecutive months has *secondary amenorrhea.*

**Amniocentesis** A test performed between 15 and 17 weeks of pregnancy to detect chromosomal disorders in the developing fetus. See CHORIONIC VILLI SAMPLING.

**Ampulla** The widest portion of the fallopian tube in a woman or the widest section of the vas deferens in a man.

**Anabolic steroids** Group of drugs that produce effects similar to those of the male sex hormone testosterone; it may lower sperm count.

**Androgens** Male sex hormones necessary for the development of male secondary sex characteristics, such as a deep voice and facial hair. They are chiefly produced in the testes and in small amounts in the ovaries and adrenal glands of women. The primary androgen is testosterone.

**Andrologist** An M.D. or Ph.D. who specializes in the study of male reproduction and fertility.

**Anovulation** The absence of ovulation. A woman may still menstruate, even if ovulation does not occur.

**Antinuclear antibody (ANA)** Protein substance made by the immune system that attacks the nucleus, or center, of cells; when cells involved in reproduction are attacked, miscarriage ensues.

**Antiphospholipid antibody (APA)** Substance produced by the immune system that destroys cells necessary for the growth and development of the placenta;

may cause a blood clotting problem at the site of placental attachment.

**Antiprostaglandin medication** Drugs that relieve cramping and muscle spasms in the reproductive organs that can occur as a result of endometriosis.

**Antisperm antibodies** Antibodies produced by the immune system of a man or woman that attack sperm, causing them to clump (agglutinate).

**Antithyroid antibodies** See THYROID PEROXIDASE ANTIBODIES.

**Arterial embolization** A procedure performed by a radiologist to block the blood flow to vessels that feed tumors, such as uterine fibroids.

**Artifical insemination (AI)** Procedure in which healthy sperm are deposited directly into the woman's vagina, cervix, uterus (intrauterine insemination), or fallopian tubes via a catheter or syringe instead of by sexual intercourse.

**Artificial insemination, donor (DI)** Insemination with the sperm of a donor, either known or anonymous.

**Artificial insemination, husband (AIH)** Insemination with husband or partner sperm.

**Asherman syndrome** Condition that is characterized by scar tissue within the uterine cavity, typically as a result of an infection, or after an abortion or overscraping of the uterine lining during a dilation and curettage (D&C).

**Aspermia** Condition in which a man does not ejaculate semen. It is usually the result of a problem with the prostate gland and the seminal vesicles, which produce most of the components of semen.

**Assisted hatching** An ART micromanipulation technique in which a tiny opening is made in the embryo's zona pellucida (outer layer) to facilitate implantation in the uterine lining (endometrium).

**Assisted reproductive technology (ART)** A group of procedures in which fertilization of a woman's egg by a man's sperm occurs without sexual intercourse. These procedures include in vitro fertilization (IVF), gamete intrafallopian transfer (GIFT), and zygote intrafallopian transfer (ZIFT).

**Asthenospermia** A condition in which the sperm demonstrate low motility and/or poor velocity (forward progression).

**Atresia** An ongoing process in which ovarian follicles and the eggs they contain begin to develop but do not mature; they are then absorbed back into the ovary.

**Autoimmune disorder** Condition in which the body's immune system malfunctions and produces antibodies that destroy the body's own tissues and cells.

**Azoospermia** Absence of sperm in semen caused by a malfunction of the testes or a blockage that prevents the sperm from traveling out of the testes.

**Balanced translocation** A process in which genetic material from two chromosomes is transposed, or switched. Individuals with this condition are physically normal, but there is a high probability that they will pass a defective chromosome on to their offspring, which may result in miscarriage in affected pregnancies.

**Basal body temperature (BBT)** The body's temperature when the individual is at rest, measured typically in the morning upon waking. *Monophasic basal body temperature* refers to a consistent reading of temperature throughout the menstrual cycle, indicating an absence of ovulation. *Biphasic body temperature* refers to a slight rise in body temperature in the last half of the menstrual cycle, which indicates that a woman is ovulating.

**β-human chorionic gonadotropin (β-hCG) test** A blood test that measures precisely the level of placental hormone, or *human chorionic gonadotropin;* may be measured 10 to12 days after embryo implantation to detect pregnancy.

**Bicornate uterus** A congenital defect that results in a muscular wall that divides the uterus into two separate cavities. Often, one uterine cavity is larger than the other.

**Blastocyst** Occurring near the 5th day after fertilization, the embryonic stage during which the embryo implants in the uterine lining (endometrium).

**Blighted ovum** A fertilized egg (embryo) that does not divide or develop owing to an abnormality in the sperm, egg, or embryo.

**Bromocriptine mesylate (Parlodel)** Drug used to regulate the production of prolactin by the pituitary gland. Prolactin is normally released to stimulate lactation in women who are breastfeeding and occasionally rises in women trying to conceive. Abnormal levels can affect ovulation and/or the luteal phase of the cycle.

**Cabergoline (Dostinex)** Drug used to regulate the production of prolactin by the pituitary gland.

**Capacitation** Transformation of the sperm cell that facilitates its ability to penetrate and fertilize the egg.

**Catheter** A thin, flexible tube used to add or remove liquid from the body.

**Cerclage** Surgical procedure that involves placing a stitch in the cervix to keep it closed during pregnancy.

**Cervical hypoplasia** A result of diethylstilbestrol (DES) exposure, this condition is characterized by weak muscle tone that prevents the cervix from staying closed during pregnancy.

**Cervical mucus** Secreted by the cervix, this normally thick fluid changes composition a few days before ovulation owing to elevated estrogen levels, enabling sperm cells to penetrate the cervical canal and move toward the uterus.

**Cervical stenosis** A blockage or narrowing of the cervical canal that can be congenital or the result of surgery.

**Cervix** Located at the entrance to the uterus, this fibrous ring of tissue provides a passageway between the vaginal canal and the uterus. The cervix remains closed during pregnancy to protect the developing fetus and opens, or dilates, during labor.

*Chlamydia trachomatis* A bacterium, which is sexually transmitted, that can lead to infection and is frequently the cause of pelvic inflammatory disease (PID).

**Chocolate cysts** Ovarian cysts, containing old blood, that develop when endometriosis spreads to the ovaries; the tissue bleeds, creating pockets of blood that are not absorbed by the body.

**Chorionic villi sampling (CVS)** Test performed about week 10 of pregnancy to examine the villi, tiny hairlike projections of the developing placenta, to reveal genetic abnormalities or chromosomal disorders in the developing fetus.

**Chromosomes** Tiny structures in the nucleus of each cell that carry all the individual's genetic information. In humans, the egg and the sperm each contributes 23 chromosomes to the embryo, to make a total of 46.

**Cilia** Small, hairlike structures that line the fallopian tubes and, with a sweeping motion, help move the egg through the tube toward the uterus.

**Clomiphene citrate (Clomid, Serophene)** Synthetic oral fertility drug that stimulates the release of follicle-stimulating hormone (FSH) and luteinizing hormone (LH) from the pituitary gland, which in turn stimulate ovarian function in women and the production of sperm in men.

**Computer-assisted semen analysis (CASA)** A test that evaluates the number, motility (ability to swim), velocity (speed), and morphology (size and shape) of sperm cells via a computer-programmed instrument.

**Computerized axial tomography (CAT) scan** Diagnostic test used to obtain images of the inside of the body to help identify structural abnormalities, especially tumors. See MAGNETIC RESONANCE IMAGING.

**Conception** Process by which an egg is fertilized by a sperm cell and an embryo is formed.

**Cone biopsy** A cone-shaped portion of tissue is surgically removed for examination under a microscope; used to obtain cervical cells when Pap smear results are abnormal.

**Congenital** Term used to describe a condition present at birth.

**Congenital absence of the vas deferens (CAVD)** A rare condition that prevents sperm from leaving the body because of the absence of the vasa deferentia, the tubes that carry the sperm from the epididymis (where the sperm are stored before ejaculation) to the ejaculatory duct in the prostate gland.

**Controlled ovarian hyperstimulation (COH)** Stimulation of the ovaries using fertility drugs such as follicle-stimulating hormone (FSH) and human menopausal gonadotropin (hMG) to produce multiple follicles and eggs and to stimulate ovulation. Also called *superovulation*.

**Corpora cavernosa** Two rod-shaped bundles of muscle on either side of the penis that relax and fill with blood upon sexual stimulation, causing erection and allowing the penis to penetrate the vagina during sexual intercourse.

**Corpus albicans** Scar tissue on the surface of an ovary that occurs when an immature follicle is reabsorbed by the ovary.

**Corpus luteum** A small cyst that forms in the empty ovarian follicle after an egg is released during ovulation. It produces progesterone, which is critical to the development of the endometrium and will help support a pregnancy for 8 to 10 weeks; then progesterone comes primarily from the placenta.

**Cowper's glands** Two very small glands in the urethra that produce lubricant to nourish and support sperm cells and help them exit the body during ejaculation.

**Cryocautery** A surgical technique that destroys tissues by freezing them by application of a substance such as solid carbon dioxide.

**Cryomyolysis** A technique used to destroy, for example, fibroid tumors by freezing them.

**Cryopreservation** The process of freezing cells, such as embryos or sperm, for future use.

**Cryptorchidism** See UNDESCENDED TESTICLES.

**Cumulus mass** Protective layer of cells around the ovum that the sperm must penetrate for fertilization to take place.

**Cytokines** A group of proteins produced by cells that can either activate or suppress the growth of new cells, including embryos.

**Cytomegalovirus** A virus that may cause miscarriage.

**Cytoplasm** The thick liquid material within a cell that plays a key role in determining how that cell functions.

**Danazol (Danocrine)** A synthetic male hormone used to treat endometriosis by inhibiting the production of the pituitary hormones follicle-stimulating hormone (FSH) and luteinizing hormone (LH), thereby inhibiting estrogen production in the ovaries.

**Dehydroepiandrosterone sulfate (DHEAS)** Adrenal gland hormone that produces the same effects as male hormones (androgens); when produced at high levels may cause fertility problems in both men and women. Also called *adrenal androgens*.

**Deoxyribonucleic acid (DNA)** Located in the nucleus of a cell, this substance carries the specific genetic information for each person.

**Dexamethasone** Type of oral steroid used to treat polycystic ovarian syndrome (PCOS) by decreasing testosterone levels, which may be high in some women who have this condition.

**Diethylstilbestrol (DES)** Synthetic estrogen prescribed for pregnant women in the 1950s and 1960s to prevent miscarriage. DES exposure in utero caused numerous abnormalities in the reproductive organs of both males and females that affect fertility.

**Dilation and curettage (D&C)** Surgical procedure in which the cervix is dilated and the lining of the uterus is scraped or suctioned to remove tissue remaining after an incomplete or missed abortion.

**Distal tubal blockage** Blockage of fallopian tubes that involves the fimbriated end, the end of the tubes closest to the ovaries.

**Dominant follicle** The follicle that will produce the egg upon ovulation, and will produce progesterone (as the corpus luteum) for the remainder of the cycle and through the first trimester, if pregnancy occurs.

**Donor sperm** Sperm produced by someone other than the husband or male partner.

**Down regulation** Gonadotropin-releasing hormone (GnRH) agonists are given in the cycle before controlled ovarian hyperstimulation (COH) begins to cause the ovaries to cease follicular development.

**Dysgenesis** Abnormal formation of organs and/or cells, especially during embryonic development.

**Dysplasia** Abnormalities in tissues; dysplasia of the cervix can usually be detected by a Pap smear.

**Ectopic pregnancy** Pregnancy in which the implantation of an egg takes place outside of the uterus, usually in the fallopian tubes; it may also (rarely) occur in the cervix, ovary, or abdominal cavity.

**Egg aspiration** Process by which eggs are removed from mature follicles during in vitro fertilization (IVF).

**Ejaculatory ducts** See VAS DEFERENS.

**Embryo** Term used to describe a fertilized egg from fertilization until the 8th week of pregnancy, after which it is referred to as a fetus.

**Embryologist** An M.D. or Ph.D. who specializes in laboratory work with egg, sperm and embryos.

**Embryo toxicity assay (ETA)** Diagnostic test used to identify protein cells that may be toxic to embryos (cytokines).

**Endometrial biopsy** Diagnostic procedure done after day 21 in the cycle that involves taking a sample of tissue from the endometrium for close analysis to see if the effects of natural ovulation and estrogen and progesterone stimulation are working to prepare the uterus for the implantation of an egg.

**Endometrioma** Uterine tissues growing on the ovary, caused by endometriosis; see CHOCOLATE CYSTS.

**Endometriosis** Condition in which cells that normally line the uterine cavity (endometrium) grow outside of the uterus, usually on reproductive organs, causing adhesions, irritation, and inflammation and often leading to painful menstruation and infertility. Although it usually affects organs in the pelvic cavity, in rare cases, it can be found in the abdominal wall, the lungs, and the brain.

**Endometritis** Inflammation of the endometrium (uterine lining) caused by a bacterial infection that interferes with the normal implantation of a fertilized egg.

**Endometrium** The inner lining of the uterus where embryos implant and are nourished during pregnancy. The endometrium is shed from the body during menstruation when implantation does not occur.

**Enzyme-linked immunosorbent assays (ELISAs)** Laboratory tests used to reveal the presence of antithyroid antibodies, substances produced by the immune system that interfere with the proper functioning of the thyroid gland in women. Also called *gel agglutination tests.*

**Epididymis** Elongated, tubular organ that is attached to the testes and stores sperm while they mature and develop before they travel to the ejaculatory ducts of the prostate gland.

**Erectile dysfunction** Impotence or the inability to achieve or maintain an erection during sexual intercourse.

**Estradiol ($E_2$)** A type of estrogen produced by the ovaries that stimulates follicle growth and ovulation and, along with progesterone, helps prepare the uterine lining for the implantation of a fertilized egg. It is also the form of estrogen that is responsible for the development of secondary female sex characteristics.

**Estrogen** The most important female sex hormone, chiefly produced by the ovaries from the time of puberty until menopause. It is responsible for female secondary sex characteristics.

**Estrogen replacement therapy (ERT)** Prescribed to menopausal women to replace the estrogen their ovaries no longer produce. ERT, or hormone replacement therapy (HRT), often involves a combination of estrogen and progesterone.

**Fallopian tubes** Two hollow, muscular tubes that transport the ovum (egg) from the ovaries to the uterus. The egg normally meets the sperm in one of the fallopian tubes (called the ampulla), where fertilization usually takes place.

**Falloposcopy** A procedure that allows visual examination of the inside of the fallopian tubes and the uterus without the use of x-rays.

**Fertilization** The penetration of a sperm into the egg (ovum), usually in the fallopian tube, that results in an embryo.

**Fetus** Term used to describe the developing baby in utero from the 9th week of pregnancy until birth.

**Fibriolysis** Surgical removal of scar tissue.

**Fibroid** Noncancerous growth, or tumor, made of fibrous and muscular tissue that usually develops in or on the uterine wall. A fibroid may cause no symptoms or problems with conception, or it may disrupt egg fertilization or embryo implantation.

**Fimbria** Long, thin projections at the entrance to the fallopian tubes that catch the egg as it is released from the ovary during ovulation and move it into the fallopian tube.

**Fimbrioplasty** Surgical procedure that corrects abnormalities in the fimbria, located at the end of the fallopian tubes.

**Follicles** Small fluid-filled sacs in the ovary that contain maturing eggs that are released during ovulation.

**Follicle-stimulating hormone (FSH)** Hormone produced by the pituitary gland that stimulates the growth of ovarian follicles in women and sperm production in men. FSH is also a component of some of ovulatory-stimulating drugs, including Follistim, Gonal F, Fertinex, and Metrodin.

**Follicular phase** Precedes ovulation and is characterized by the development of follicles and the thickening of the lining of the uterus, both stimulated by high levels of estrogen.

**Follitropin (Gonal F, Follistim)** Synthetic drug that contains pure follicle-stimulating hormone (FSH) and is used to stimulate the ovaries. Urofollitropins (Fertinex, Metrodin), also FSH, are extracted from human urine.

**Gametes** Reproductive cells produced by both males (sperm) and females (eggs).

**Gamete intrafallopian transfer (GIFT)** A procedure in which egg and sperm are placed into the fallopian tubes for fertilization. A laparoscopy is necessary to do GIFT.

**GAST test** A test to evaluate ovarian response after giving a woman gonadotropin-releasing hormone (GnRH) agonists, such as Lupron and Synarel.

**Geneticist** A physician or Ph.D. who studies the expression and transmission of genetic material. Also used to refer to a genetic counselor.

**Germ cell** The first stage of a cell's development when it is at its most immature state.

**Gestation** Period of time in which the embryo and fetus develop, from the moment of conception until birth.

**Gestational surrogacy** Placing an embryo into the uterus of a genetically unrelated woman, who will carry the pregnancy to term for an infertile couple.

**Gonadotropins** Hormones (follicle-stimulating hormone [FSH], human menopausal gonadotropin [hMG], and luteinizing hormone [LH]) produced by the pituitary gland that stimulate either the ovaries to produce eggs or the testes to produce sperm.

**Gonadotropin-releasing hormone (GnRH)** Released by the hypothalamus in both men and women, it stimulates the pituitary gland to produce follicle-stimulating hormone (FSH) and luteinizing hormone (LH), which in turn stimulate ovulation in women and the production of sperm in men.

**Gonadotropin-releasing hormone (GnRH) agonists (Lupron, Synarel)** Class of drugs used to treat endometriosis and small uterine fibroids and to prepare women for ovulatory-stimulating drugs in an assisted reproductive technology (ART) cycle.

**Gonadotropin-releasing hormone (GnRH) antagonist (Antagon)** This class of drug recently has been introduced to inhibit premature surge of luteinizing hormone (LH).

**Gonads** Term used to describe the sex glands: the testicles in men, which produce sperm and testosterone, and the ovaries in women, which produce eggs and estrogen.

**Gonorrhea** A sexually transmitted disease (STD) that may cause infertility in both men and women.

**Granulosa cells** Ovarian cells that produce the hormones estrogen and progesterone.

**Hamster egg test** See SPERM PENETRATION ASSAY (SPA).

**Hatching** Process by which the protective outer layer of the egg (zona pellucida) breaks open, allowing the embryo to implant in the uterus.

**Hemizona assay test** Laboratory test used to measure the ability of sperm to penetrate the outer membrane of an egg.

**Heparin** Medication taken by subcutaneous injection to thin the blood; it is used to treat recurrent miscarriages caused by antibodies that attack cells in the uterus and placenta that are needed for implantation of the fertilized egg and nurturing of the fetus.

**Herpes simplex** A viral infection that may cause problems in the newborn if vaginal herpes is acute during labor.

**Hormones** Chemicals secreted by endocrine glands that travel through the bloodstream to control all of the body's functions.

**Human chorionic gonadotropin (hCG) (Novarel, Pregnyl, Profasi)** Produced by the placenta, this hormone helps support the corpus luteum, which produces estrogen and progesterone needed to sustain a pregnancy. To determine if a woman is pregnant, the level of this hormone is measured. Also called the *pregnancy hormone*.

**Human menopausal gonadotropin (hMG) (Humegon, Pergonal, Repronex)** A natural substance that contains follicle-stimulating hormone (FSH) and luteinizing hormone (LH) taken from the urine of postmenopausal women and used to stimulate ovulation.

**Hydatidiform mole** See MOLAR PREGNANCY.

**Hydrocele** A fluid-filled swelling around the testes that is a rare complication of surgery for varicose veins in the testes (varicocele); it occurs when one of the lymph ducts located very close to the veins is closed off.

**Hydrosalpinx** A fluid-filled bulge in the fallopian tubes that is caused by blockage at the end of the fallopian tube.

**Hyperprolactinemia** Condition characterized by excessive production of the pituitary hormone prolactin, which can interfere with normal ovulation in women and may reduce testosterone levels and sperm count in men.

**Hyperthyroidism** Condition caused by an overproduction of thyroxine, a hormone produced by the thyroid gland that affects fertility by interfering with normal ovulation.

**Hypoplastic uterus** A uterine abnormality in which the muscle tissue of the uterus is weak, which inhibits proper functioning.

**Hypospadias** A structural abnormality of the penis in which the urethral opening is not at the end of the penis but, most commonly, on the underside or (rarely) as far away as the scrotum.

**Hypothalamic amenorrhea** Cessation of menstruation owing to a decrease in the production of gonadotropin-releasing hormone (GnRH) from the hypothalamus gland.

**Hypothalamic anovulation** Cessation of ovulation owing to reduced production of gonadotropin-releasing hormone (GnRH) from the hypothalamus gland.

**Hypothalamus** Endocrine gland located in the brain that secretes gonadotropin-releasing hormone (GnRH), which regulates the production of the pituitary hormones luteinizing hormone (LH) and follicle-stimulating hormone (FSH).

**Hypothyroidism** Underproduction of the thyroid hormone thyroxine, which can interfere with normal ovulation.

**Hysterectomy** Surgical procedure in which the uterus is removed owing to a structural or functional abnormality that may adversely affect a woman's health. Total hysterectomy includes removal of the ovaries (oophorectomy) as well.

**Hysterosalpingogram (HSG)** A diagnostic procedure used to examine the uterus and fallopian tubes for abnormalities that may affect fertility. A special dye is injected into the uterine cavity and fallopian tubes, which are then examined via x-ray images to make sure the uterus is properly shaped and there are no obstructions in the tubes.

**Hysteroscopy** A test used to examine the inside of the uterus for abnormalities or growths, such as polyps or fibroids. A very small telescope with a light attached to it, called a hysteroscope, is inserted into the cervix and moved through to the uterus to get a clear picture of the uterine cavity.

**Immunobead binding assay (IBD)** A comprehensive test that identifies the presence of antisperm antibodies attached to sperm cells.

**Implantation** Process by which an embryo attaches itself to the lining of the uterus (endometrium).

**Impotence** See ERECTILE DYSFUNCTION.

**Incompetent cervix** A cervix with a structural abnormality that interferes with a woman's ability to carry a pregnancy.

**Intracytoplasmic sperm injection (ICSI)** A microsurgical technique done during in vitro fertilization (IVF) in which a single sperm cell is injected into the egg to enhance fertilization. Also called *intracytoplasmic sperm insemination.*

**Intramuscular injections** Shots that are administered by inserting the needle into a muscle.

**Intrauterine device (IUD)** Method of contraception using a plastic or copper device in the uterus to prevent implantation of a fertilized egg.

**Intrauterine insemination (IUI)** Procedure in which specially prepared sperm are deposited directly into the uterus at the time of ovulation.

**In vitro fertilization (IVF)** Procedure in which an egg is fertilized in a laboratory dish, rather than inside of a woman's body (called in vivo fertilization). The newly formed embryo is then placed in the woman's uterus. Also called *test tube baby procedure.*

**Isthmus** The thin section of the fallopian tube that connects to the uterus; the proximal end.

**Kallmann's syndrome** A congenital disorder of the hypothalamus in men in which gonadotropin-releasing hormone (GnRH), needed for the manufacturing of sperm and secondary sex characteristics, is not being produced.

**Karyotyping** Evaluation and analysis of the chromosomes to determine if any abnormalities are present.

**Klinefelter's syndrome** A congenital chromosomal abnormality in men that results in permanent infertility.

**Laparoscopy** Surgical procedure in which a small telescope is inserted through a tiny incision made in the abdominal wall just below the navel to examine the pelvic organs, such as the ovaries, uterus, and fallopian tubes. If endometriosis, adhesions, or polycystic ovaries are found, they can be treated using laser surgery and other surgical tools during a laparoscopic examination. This procedure is done in a day surgery unit.

**Laparotomy** Surgical procedure in which a

large horizontal incision is made in the abdomen to allow visualization and access to the pelvic organs. This procedure requires hospitalization.

**Leydig cells** Located in the testicles, these cells produce the male hormone testosterone when stimulated by luteinizing hormone (LH), which is released by the pituitary gland.

**Liquefaction** The process by which liquid semen, upon ejaculation, coagulates into a gel-like substance. This coagulation is caused by proteins produced by the seminal vesicles.

**Luteal phase** Occurs after ovulation and lasts until menstruation begins. In this phase of the woman's cycle, the corpus luteum in the ovaries produces progesterone to prepare the uterine lining for implantation of the embryo. When the uterine lining is shed at the start of menstruation, the luteal phase is over.

**Luteal phase defect (LPD)** Dysfunction in the corpus luteum that inhibits the production of progesterone, which affects the uterine lining and may prevent implantation.

**Luteinized unruptured follicle (LUF) syndrome** Condition in which the egg is not released from the follicle but all other indications of ovulation are present, such as the surge of luteinizing hormone (LH) and a rise in basal body temperature (BBT).

**Luteinizing hormone (LH)** Manufactured and released by the pituitary gland in both men and women, this hormone stimulates the ovaries to produce estrogen and to release mature eggs from ovarian follicles during ovulation and stimulates the testes to produce sperm.

**Luteinizing hormone (LH) surge** A sharp increase in women in the production of luteinizing hormone (LH) by the pituitary gland, normally resulting in ovulation.

**Macrophages** White blood cells that produce an autoimmune response. Women with endometriosis may have higher than normal levels of macrophages in their pelvic fluid.

**Magnetic resonance imaging (MRI)** Imaging technique that uses sound waves and magnetic fields to obtain a picture of internal organs and structures.

**Maternal serum alpha-fetoprotein (MSAFP)** A blood test performed between 16 and 18 weeks from the last menstrual period that can indicate possible neural tube defects and other abnormalities.

**Meiosis** Process by which the reproductive cells, ova (eggs) and spermatids (immature sperm cells), divide so that each one has 23 chromosomes. When the sperm and egg join during fertilization, under normal circumstances they will produce an embryo that has 46 chromosomes.

**Menarche** Time at which a young woman begins to menstruate.

**Menses** The monthly shedding of the uterine lining by bleeding that occurs when there is no pregnancy. Also called *menstruation*.

**Micromanipulation** A technique that uses magnification and tiny instruments to enhance fertilization or implantation. See INTRACYTOPLASMIC SPERM INJECTION (ICSI) and ASSISTED HATCHING.

**Microsurgery** Delicate surgical procedure that uses very small instruments and magnification.

**Microsurgical epididymal sperm aspiration (MESA)** The removal of sperm from the epididymis to be used for intracytoplasmic sperm injection (ICSI).

**Miscarriage, clinical** Premature ending of a pregnancy after the gestational sac has been identified and a fetal heartbeat has been heard.

**Miscarriage, inevitable** Premature ending of a pregnancy signaled by increased bleeding, cramping, and an open cervix.

**Miscarriage, multiple** Occurrence of three or more miscarriages in a row. Also called *recurrent miscarriage.*

**Miscarriage, subclinical** A very early pregnancy loss that occurs after a small gestational sac has been found on ultrasound; may result in a heavy and long menstrual bleed.

**Miscarriage, threatened** A pregnancy that is in danger, indicated by spotting or very light bleeding and sometimes low back pain, even though the cervix is still closed.

**Mitochondria** Pockets of stored energy within cells; in sperm cells, they control motility, enabling they to swim quickly and in the right direction.

**Mittelschmerz** Discomfort associated with ovulation that occurs on one side of the lower abdomen and includes cramping, painful twinges, and low back pain.

**Molar pregnancy** Rare condition in which fetal tissue is not seen on ultrasound examination, but placental tissue continues to grow in an abnormal way. After a dilation and curettage (D&C), careful monitoring of β-human chorionic gonadotropin (β-hCG) levels is done for 6 weeks to 6 months until levels are back to normal. Also called *trophoblastic disease* and *hydatidiform mole.*

**Müllerian ducts** Tubular structures that join together in the developing fetus to form the uterus. If they do not develop normally and attach properly, the reproductive organs may be malformed.

**Multiple gestation pregnancy** More than one fetus are implanted and growing in the uterus.

**Multiple gestation reduction (MGR)** Procedure to reduce the number of fetal sacs in multiple gestation pregnancy. Also called *multiple-fetal pregnancy reduction.*

**Myolysis** Laparoscopic technique used to destroy fibroid tumors by heating or freezing them.

**Myomectomy** The surgical removal of uterine fibroids usually through laparotomy.

**Myometrium** The muscular wall of the uterus.

**Nucleus** The center and most important part of a cell; the part of the cell that is responsible for replication and cellular development.

**Oligomenorrhea** A condition characterized by irregular menstrual cycles.

**Oligospermia** A condition characterized by poor sperm quality and low sperm count.

**Oocyte** Egg, or ovum.

**Oogenesis** The formation of eggs in the ovaries of female fetuses, which occurs at about 14 to 16 weeks' gestation.

**Ovarian drilling** A surgical procedure in which a laparoscope is used to puncture the outer membrane of ovarian cysts.

**Ovarian dysgenesis** Congenital chromosomal defect in females in which one of the X chromosomes is abnormal, resulting in ovaries that do not contain eggs or follicles. Women with this condition do, however, have a uterus.

**Ovarian hyperstimulation syndrome (OHSS)** Overstimulation of the ovaries caused by fertility drugs.

**Ovarian reserve** The ability of the ovaries to produce good-quality eggs and good-quality embryos that will implant well.

**Ovaries** The two small circular female sex glands that produce mature eggs (ova) and secrete the female hormones estrogen and progesterone.

**Ovulation** The process by which a mature egg is released from an ovary once every month or so, approximately 14 days after the start of menstruation.

**Ovulation induction** The use of fertility drugs to stimulate the woman's ovaries to release a ripened egg for fertilization.

**Ovum** Ripened egg produced by the ovaries.

**Pap smear** Test that involves scraping a small piece of tissue from the surface of the cervix to screen for cancer.

**Pelvic inflammatory disease (PID)** An infection of the female pelvic organs that can cause blockages in the fallopian tubes and scarring in the pelvic cavity.

**Perimenopause** Changes prior to the onset of menopause, including any or all of the following: rising cycle day 3 follicle-stimulating hormone (FSH) and estradiol levels, irregular periods, decreased ovulation, and more estrogen in relation to progesterone than at an earlier age.

**Pituitary gland** Small round endocrine gland located at the base of the brain that controls and regulates all hormonal functions, including those related to fertility and reproduction. Among the hormones produced by the pituitary gland are luteinizing hormone (LH), follicle-stimulating hormone (FSH), thyroid-stimulating hormone (TSH), and prolactin.

**Placenta** Vascular, membranous organ that develops in the uterus during pregnancy and envelops the fetus; it connects with the fetus through the umbilical cord, which carries nourishment and oxygen from the woman to the fetus, promoting normal growth and development.

**Plasma progesterone level** The amount of progesterone in the blood.

**Polycystic ovarian syndrome (PCOS)** Common condition of the ovaries characterized by the development of a large number of ovarian cysts, or follicles, caused by a hormonal imbalance that affects ovarian function and fertility. PCOS is also characterized by overproduction of androgens (male sex hormones). Also called *hyperandrogenic chronic anovulation, polycystic ovarian disease (PCOD), and Stein-Leventhal syndrome.*

**Polyp** Small growth of tissue that is almost always noncancerous. It is commonly found on the internal surface of the uterus or cervix.

**Polyploidy** Abnormality in the amount of chromosome present in an embryo.

**Postcoital test (PCT)** Analysis of cervical mucus performed a few hours after sexual intercourse and as close to ovulation as possible. A sample of the mucus is examined to determine its ability to sustain live sperm and to evaluate sperm motility and sperm count. Also called the *Sims Huhner test.*

**Premature ovarian failure (POF)** Failure of the ovaries to produce follicles or eggs and the cessation of menstrual periods prior to the age of 40.

**Premenstrual syndrome (PMS)** Symptoms such as headaches, breast tenderness, irritability, and weight gain that may occur before the beginning of menstruation as a result of hormonal changes.

**Presacral neurectomy** Procedure used to alleviate chronic pelvic pain by cutting off the nerves that sensitize the area; often used for severe endometriosis.

**Primary ovarian failure** Congenital condition in which the ovaries do not function properly. Women who have primary ovarian failure have never ovulated and do not produce the hormones responsible for female secondary sex characteristics.

**Progesterone** Female hormone produced by the corpus luteum (in the ovaries) after ovulation has occurred; it stimulates changes in the endometrium (uterine lining) that will prepare it for the implantation of a fertilized egg. Progesterone also sustains the newly formed placenta, enabling the embryo to grow and develop during the early stages of pregnancy.

**Prolactin** Pituitary hormone that stimulates the breasts to produce milk for breastfeeding; it usually prevents pregnancy during this time by disrupting ovulation patterns.

**Prostaglandins** Chemical substances that function like hormones and are important for mediating many physiologic processes.

Those produced in the pelvic cavity can cause uterine cramping and muscle spasms.

**Prostate gland** Located at the base of the bladder and encircling the urethra in men, it produces an important component of seminal fluid that helps sustain the sperm. It also produces prostaglandins.

**Prostatitis** Inflammation of the prostate that is usually caused by an infection. Sperm motility and sperm count may decrease while the infection is active.

**Proximal tubal obstruction** A blockage of the fallopian tubes at the proximal end, or the end that connects to the uterus (uterotubal junction).

**Pseudomenopause** Condition induced by the gonadotropin-releasing hormone (GnRH) agonist drugs (Lupron, Synarel), which are used to treat endometriosis and to shrink fibroid tumors. These medications produce a menopause-like state by dramatically lowering estrogen levels. Hot flashes, vaginal dryness, and mood swings are common.

**Reproductive endocrinologist (RE), board certified** An obstetrician-gynecologist (OB-Gyn) who has taken a 2-year fellowship in reproductive medicine, and passed oral and written exams to become certified.

**Reproductive immunologist** An M.D. or scientist who specializes in diagnosing and treating problems of the immune system that affect reproduction.

**Resectoscope** Surgical instrument used to remove adhesions in the uterine cavity by applying electrical current directly to the scar tissue.

**Retrograde ejaculation** Condition in which semen does not leave the body through the penis during ejaculation, but flows backward into the bladder.

**Retrograde menstruation** Condition in which blood produced as a result of menstruation flows through the fallopian tubes back into the pelvic cavity, rather than leaving the body through the vagina.

**Retroverted uterus** Uterus that is tilted backwards.

**Salpingectomy** Surgical removal of one or both fallopian tubes.

**Salpingitis** Inflammation on the inside of one or both of the fallopian tubes, usually caused by a bacterial infection.

**Salpingitis isthmica nodosa (SIN)** Inflammation of the fallopian tubes that may prevent a fertilized egg from moving down into the uterus.

**Salpingography** Diagnostic test used to evaluate problems of the fallopian tubes. Thin, flexible catheters are inserted into the cervix and pushed through to the fallopian tubes; then dye is injected and x-ray images are taken to obtain clear pictures of possible abnormalities.

**Salpingolysis** The surgical removal of adhesions from one or both fallopian tubes.

**Salpingoscope** Small instrument used to magnify the ampullar portion (area closest to the ovaries) of the fallopian tubes during a diagnostic test, such as a salpingography, or during a surgical procedure, such as a laparoscopy.

**Salpingostomy** Surgical procedure that involves making a small cut into a fallopian tube to remove a blockage or to remove a tubal (ectopic) pregnancy.

**Salpingotomy** Incision of a fallopian tube.

**Scrotum** Sac of skin and muscle that contains the testes.

**Sedimentation rate** A blood test that indicates if the body has been fighting an infection.

**Semen analysis** Comprehensive diagnostic test that evaluates all functional and structural aspects of sperm cells. The test measures sperm count, ability of sperm to swim (motility), size and shape of sperm (morphology), total semen volume, and stickiness of seminal fluid (viscosity). Semen analysis also checks fructose levels and for the possible presence of infectious organisms or sperm antibodies. This analysis can be done using a microscope or a computer-assisted sperm analysis (CASA) machine.

**Seminal fructose** Sugar-like substance needed by sperm cells for nourishment and energy, produced by the seminal vesicles.

**Seminal vesicles** Two pouch-like glands located next to the prostate and connected to the vas deferens (ejaculatory duct) that produce most of the seminal fluid.

**Seminiferous tubules** Tiny testicular tubes in which sperm are produced and develop until they are ready to move to the epididymis to complete the maturation process.

**Septate uterus** A fibrous tissue wall that divides the uterine cavity. See UTERINE SEPTUM.

**Sertoli cell only syndrome** Congenital condition in which no sperm cells and only the Sertoli cells are present in the testicular biopsy.

**Sertoli cells** Cells produced in the testes that facilitate spermatogenesis and then nourish and support the developing sperm cells.

**Sexually transmitted diseases (STDs)** Diseases that are spread by sexual contact, usually an infection. The most common STDs are chlamydia and gonorrhea.

**Sonogram** See ULTRASOUND.

**Sonohysterography** Diagnostic ultrasound test using a saltwater (saline) solution to examine the uterus and fallopian tubes for structural abnormalities.

**Sperm morphology** The size and shape of sperm.

**Sperm motility** The ability of sperm to swim.

**Sperm penetration assay (SPA)** Sperm function test that determines the sperm's ability to penetrate the outer membrane of an egg for fertilization. Hamster eggs are used because, unlike the eggs of other animals, they can be penetrated by human sperm. Also called the *hamster egg test*.

**Sperm washing** Process by which healthy sperm are filtered out of the seminal fluid and concentrated together for use in in vitro fertilization (IVF) and intrauterine insemination (IUI). Sperm washing is necessary to remove substances from sperm that may cause severe uterine cramping.

**Spermatids** Immature sperm cells.

**Spermatocyte** Single sperm cell.

**Spermatogenesis** The production of sperm in the testes.

**Spinnbarkeit (SBK)** A type of cervical mucus that resembles stretchy egg white and should develop several days prior to ovulation.

**Stillbirth** Death of a fetus in utero after the 20th week of pregnancy.

**Subcutaneous injections** Injections in which the needle is inserted into the fatty layer directly below the skin that covers the front of the thighs or the underside of the upper arms. Examples of fertility drugs that are injected subcutaneously are Lupron, a gonadotropin-releasing hormone (GnRH) agonist used to treat endometriosis, and Follistim and Gonal F, urofollitropins used to stimulate ovulation and egg production.

**Superovulation** See CONTROLLED OVARIAN HYPERSTIMULATION (COH).

**Surrogacy** When a woman carries a fetus that does not have any of her genetic makeup.

**Testes** Male sex glands contained in the scrotum that produce the male hormone testosterone and sperm cells.

**Testicular failure, primary** Failure of normal testicular function due to abnormality in the testis itself.

**Testicular failure, secondary** Failure of normal testicular function, e.g., sperm production, due to abnormal hormone production from the pituitary gland and/or hypothalamus.

**Testicular sperm extraction (TESE)** Procedure used to obtain sperm from the testes or epididymis when there is no sperm in the ejaculate or when the sperm count is very low. Often used in conjunction with in vitro fertilization (IVF) and intracytoplasmic sperm injection (ICSI).

**Testosterone** Primary male sex hormone, produced by the testes, that is necessary for the production of sperm and responsible for male secondary sex characteristics. Also produced in small amounts by the female sex gland, the ovary.

**Thermogram** Instrument that helps locate varicoceles in the testicles by detecting areas of heat that often signal the presence of these testicular varicose veins.

**Thyroid gland** Butterfly-shaped endocrine gland in the lower part of the neck that produces thyroid hormones (including thyroxine) and regulates hormone use and balance in the body. Hyperthyroidism (an overactive thyroid) and hypothyroidism (an underactive thyroid) are thyroid disorders that can affect a woman's fertility.

**Thyroid peroxidase antibody (TPA)** Substance produced by the body's immune system that inhibits the proper functioning of the thyroid gland. Also called *antithyroid antibody.*

**Thyroid-stimulating hormone (TSH)** Pituitary hormone that stimulates the production of thyroxine in the thyroid gland.

**Thyroxine** Hormone secreted by the thyroid gland that is regulated by thyroid-stimulating hormone (TSH), which is produced by the pituitary gland.

**Toxoplasmosis** A bacterial infection that can cause miscarriage. The organism *Toxoplasma gondii* is often found in cat feces.

**Transvaginal ultrasound** See ULTRASOUND.

**Triploidy** Chromosomal abnormality in which an embryo receives an extra set of chromosomes, giving it a total of 69 instead of the usual 46.

**Trisomy** Genetic abnormality in which there is an extra copy of one of the chromosomes, often resulting in miscarriage of an affected pregnancy. Trisomy 21 (three copies of chromosome 21) results in Down syndrome.

**Trophoblastic disease** See MOLAR PREGNANCY.

**Tubal anastomosis** Surgical procedure that removes a blocked portion of the fallopian tube, leaving a clear passageway for eggs and sperm cells.

**Tubal cannulation** See TUBAL CATHETERIZATION.

**Tubal catheterization** Procedure that uses a catheter to remove a blockage at the proximal end of the fallopian tubes, closest to the uterus. Also called *tubal cannulation.*

**Tubal ligation** Surgical procedure that sterilizes a woman, and is used as a form of birth control, that involves taking out a portion of the fallopian tubes or burning the ends of the tubes. The ligation can sometimes be reversed with a procedure called *tubal reanastomosis.*

**Tubal pregnancy** See ECTOPIC PREGNANCY.

**Turner's syndrome** A congenital condition that occurs when a female has only one X chromosome instead of the normal two. Ovaries do not develop; therefore, ovulation does not occur and the female sex hormone estrogen is not produced.

**Ultrasound** Diagnostic test that uses high-frequency sound waves, rather than x-rays, to create pictures of internal organs and structures such as the ovaries, uterus, and fallopian tubes. Also called *sonogram.*

**Undescended testicle**s Anatomical abnormality, present at birth, in which one or both testes are missing or, as is usually the case, are present in the abdominal cavity. Also called *cryptorchidism.*

**Ureaplasma** Bacterium that may cause infection and early miscarriage.

**Urethra** In the male, the urethra is a thin tubular passageway in the penis that moves urine from the bladder to outside the body; it is also the conduit for semen, carrying it from the prostate and out through the penis. Infections in the urethra can be harmful to healthy sperm. In females, as in males, the urethra moves urine from the bladder to the outside.

**Urofollitropin (Fertinex, Metrodin)** A type of drug that contains pure follicle-stimulating hormone (FSH) made from the urine of postmenopausal women and used to stimulate the ovaries for normal ovulation and production of follicles and eggs.

**Urologist** An M.D. who diagnoses disorders of the male reproductive and urinary tracts.

**Uterine didelphys** A rare congenital abnormality of the uterus, in which a woman has two separate uteri. This occurs because the Müllerian wall that normally disintegrates to form one uterus, remains intact, forming two distinct uteri with a wall between them. With this condition, there are also two cervixes, and two vaginal canals.

**Uterine septum** Abnormal structure that partially or totally divides the uterine cavity. Circulation to a septum is poor; therefore, the chances of embryo implantation and successful pregnancy are low.

**Uterus** Hollow, pear-shaped, muscular female reproductive organ that holds and nurtures the developing embryo and fetus until birth.

**Vagina** Entrance to the vaginal canal.

**Vaginitis** Infections of the vagina, including yeast and bacterial infections, that can be harmful to sperm and interfere with their journey from the vaginal canal to the cervix.

**Varicoceles** Testicular abnormality in which there are dilated veins, or varicose veins, around the testes, usually on the left side, which raises the temperature of the testes and often causes infertility.

**Vas deferens** Two long, tubular ejaculatory ducts in the scrotum that move sperm from the epididymis in the testes to the ejaculatory ducts in the prostate gland, to the ejaculatory ducts in the penis.

**Vasectomy** Simple surgical procedure used as a male form of birth control. A portion of the vas deferens is removed; the ends are then closed, cutting off sperm supply from the testes and eliminating any sperm in the ejaculate.

**Vasogram** Diagnostic x-ray procedure that identifies blockages in the vas deferens that may be preventing the normal passage of sperm out of the testes.

**Vasovasostomy** Rejoining the surgically separated parts of the vas deferens to reverse a vasectomy.

**Venography** X-ray procedure used to evaluate venous blood flow, to identify a varicocele.

**Vitelline membrane** Located right under the protective outer layer of the egg (zona pellucida), this membrane surrounds and protects the egg and is the place where the sperm and the egg actually join together.

**X chromosome** The chromosome in sperm that carries the genetic code needed to create a female. All eggs carry one X chromosome, but only half of all sperm do. (The other half carry a Y chromosome.) When an egg and an X-chromosome sperm combine, a female is produced.

**Y chromosome** The chromosome in sperm that carries the genetic code needed to create a male. Eggs do not carry Y chromosomes, but half of all sperm do. When a Y-chromosome sperm joins with an egg (which carries an X chromosome), a male is produced.

**Zona pellucida** Tough, protective outer layer of the egg that must be penetrated by a sperm cell for fertilization to take place.

**Zygote** Term used to describe the fertilized egg in the earliest stages of development.

**Zygote intrafallopian transfer (ZIFT)**
Surgical procedure in which an egg is fertilized outside the woman's body in a laboratory dish; the next day, the zygote is deposited into a fallopian tube, from which it will move into the uterus.

## ACRONYMS AND ABBREVIATIONS

### Fertility Procedures

**AI** artificial insemination
**ART** assisted reproductive technologies
**COH** controlled ovarian hyperstimulation
**DI** donor insemination
**GIFT** gamete intrafallopian transfer
**ICSI** intracytoplasmic sperm injection (or insemination)
**IUI** intrauterine insemination
**IVF** in vitro fertilization
**IVIG** intravenous immunoglobulin therapy
**MESA** microsurgical epididymal sperm aspiration
**TESE** testicular sperm extraction
**ZIFT** zygote intrafallopian transfer

### Hormones

**DES** diethylstilbestrol
**DHEAS** dehydroepiandrosterone sulfate
**E₂** estradiol
**FSH** follicle-stimulating hormone
**GnRH** gonadotropin-releasing hormone
**hCG** human chorionic gonadotropin
**hMG** human menopausal gonadotropin
**LH** luteinizing hormone
**TSH** thyroid-stimulating hormone

### Diagnostic Tests

**CASA** computer-assisted semen analysis
**CAT** computerized axial tomography
**CVS** chorionic villi sampling
**ELISA** enzyme-linked immunosorbent assay
**ETA** embryo toxicity assay

**HSG** hysterosalpingogram
**IBD** immunobead binding assay
**MRI** magnetic resonance imaging
**MSAFP** maternal serum alpha-fetoprotein
**PCT** postcoital test
**SPA** sperm penetration assay (hamster egg test)

### Conditions

**CAVD** congenital absence of the vas deferens
**LPD** luteal phase defect
**LUF** luteinized unruptured follicle syndrome
**OHSS** ovarian hyperstimulation syndrome
**PCOS** polycystic ovarian syndrome (also called **PCOD**, polycystic ovarian disease)
**PID** pelvic inflammatory disease
**PMS** premenstrual syndrome
**POF** premature ovarian failure
**SIN** salpingitis isthmica nodosa
**STD** sexually transmitted disease

### Terms Related to Fertility and Reproduction

**AIH** artificial insemination husband
**ANA** antinuclear antibodies
**APA** antiphospholipid antibodies
**BBT** basal body temperature
**D&C** dilation and curettage
**DNA** deoxyribonucleic acid
**ERT** estrogen replacement therapy
**IUD** intrauterine device
**OC** oral contraceptive
**RE** reproductive endocrinologist
**TPA** thyroid peroxidase antibodies; antithyroid antibodies

## Insurance and Financial Planning

**ADA** Americans with Disabilities Act
**COB** coordination of benefits
**ERISA** Employee Retirement Income Security Act
**HIPAA** Health Insurance Portability and Accountability Act
**HMO** health maintenance organization
**PDA** Pregnancy Discrimination Act
**PPO** preferred (or participating) provider organization

## Organizations

**ASRM** American Society for Reproductive Medicine
**CDC** Centers for Disease Control and Prevention
**FDA** Food and Drug Administration
**SART** Society for Assisted Reproductive Technology

# RESOLVING Infertility Resource Guide

*The resources in this guide are unscreened by RESOLVE and offered for referral purposes only. Referrals should not be viewed as recommendations or endorsements, express or implied, by RESOLVE. The reader is advised to research the organization or service to make a determination of its personal usefulness.*

## Adoption

**American Academy of Adoption Attorneys**
PO Box 33053
Washington, DC 20033-0053
202-832-2222
**www.adoptionattorneys.org**
• National association of lawyers who specialize in adoption; directory available.

**Dave Thomas Foundation for Adoption**
PO Box 7164
Dublin, OH 43017
614-764-3009
• Public charity working to raise awareness about adoptable children. Offers *Beginners' Guide to Adoption* and *Employers' Guide to Adoption.*

**National Adoption Center/Faces of Adoption**
1500 Walnut Street, Suite 701

Philadelphia, PA 19102
800-862-3678; 215-735-9988
nac@adopt.org
www.adopt.org
• Referral for special needs children.

**National Adoption Information Clearinghouse**
330 C Street SW
Washington, DC 20447
888-251-0075; 703-352-3488
naic@calib.com
www.calib.com/naic
• NAIC is a service of the U.S. Department of Health and Human Services. Provides packet of information on adoption options, including infant, inter-country, and special needs; home study information; national adoption referrals; and comprehensive review of state laws on adoption.

**National Council for Adoption**
1930 17th Street, N.W.
Washington, DC  20009
202-328-1200
• Provides advocacy and information on adoption issues; offers monthly newsletter.

**North American Council on Adoptable Children (NACAC)**
970 Raymond Avenue, Suite 106
St. Paul, MN 55114
800-470-6665; 651-644-3036
nacac@aol.com
• Specializes in information and advocacy for placement of older and special needs children.

**U.S. State Department**
Bureau of Consular Affairs
Office of Children's Issues
International Adoption
202-736-7000
http://travel.state.gov/children's_ issues.html#adoption
• Offers wide range of information on international adoption, including safeguards for legal adoption, general, and country-specific information.

## Alternative Medicine

**American Association of Naturopathic Physicians**
601 Valley Street, Suite 105
Seattle, WA 98109
206-298-0126
• Provides referral to naturopathic doctors.

**National Certification Commission for Acupuncture and Oriental Medicine**
11 Canal Center Plaza, Suite 300
Alexandria, VA 22314
703-548-9004
**www.nccaom.org**
• Provides referrals; directory online.

**National Institutes of Health**
U.S. Department of Health and Human Services
Bethesda, MD 20892
**www.nih.gov**
• Provides extensive database for studies and articles on alternative medicine.

## Assisted Reproductive Technology (ART)

*Assisted Reproductive Technology Success Rates: National Summary and Fertility Clinic Reports*
U.S. Department of Health and Human Services
Centers for Disease Control and Prevention
For a free copy, call 770-488-5372
Available online at **www.cdc.gov/nccdphp/drh/art96/index.htm**
or through a link at **www.resolve.org**

## Condition/Disease-Related

**American Social Health Association**
P.O. Box 13827
Research Triangle Park, NC 27709-9940
919-361-8400
National STD Hotline: 800-227-8922
**www.ashastd.org**
• Offers advocacy, education and information on sexually transmitted diseases.

**D.E.S. Action**
1615 Broadway, Suite 510
Oakland, CA 94612
800-DES-9288
desact@well.com
www.desaction.org
• National, nonprofit consumer organization dedicated to informing about DES and helping DES-exposed individuals. Publishes the *DES Action Voice*; provides physician referral.

**Endometriosis Association**
8585 N. 76th Place
Milwaukee, WI 53223
800-992-3636; 414-355-2200
endo@endometriosisassn.org
www.endometriosisassn.org
• National, nonprofit, self-help organization dedicated to providing information and support to women and girls with endometriosis. Offers support groups and newsletters.

**The Gilda Radner Familial Ovarian Cancer Registry**
Roswell Park Cancer Institute
Elm and Carlton Streets
Buffalo, NY 14263
800-OVARIAN (800-682-7426)
• Provides packet of information on ovarian cancer warning signs, risk factors, and diagnostic testing.

**Polycystic Ovarian Syndrome Association**
PO Box 7007
Rosemont, IL 60018-7007
630-585-3690
info@pcosupport.org
www.pcosupport.org
• Seeks to promote awareness of PCOS and to serve as support and information system for women with PCOS.

## Lesbian Parenting

**National Center for Lesbian Rights**
870 Market Street, Suite 570

San Francisco, CA 94102
415-392-6257
info@nclrights.org
www.nclrights.org
• Feminist, multicultural legal center devoted to advancing rights and safety of lesbians and their families. Offers information regarding legal issues surrounding donor insemination.

## Miscarriage, Stillbirth, and Infant Loss

**Centering Corporation**
1531 N. Saddle Creek Road
Omaha, NE 68104
402-553-1200
• Offers written resources for coping with miscarriage and stillbirth.

**The Compassionate Friends, Inc.**
PO Box 3696
Oak Brook, IL 60522-3696
630-990-0010
tcf_national@prodigy.com
www.compassionatefriends.org
• National, nonprofit support organization for families grieving the death of a child of any age. Offers chapters across the United States; publishes a quarterly magazine.

**National Share Pregnancy and Infant Loss Support, Inc.**
300 First Capitol Drive
St. Charles, MO 63301-2893
800-821-6819; 636-947-6164
share@nationalshareoffice.com
www.nationalshareoffice.com
• International organization offers information and correspondence packets for parents bereaved through miscarriage, stillbirth, or newborn death. Over 130 chapters; publishes bimonthly newsletter.

**Pregnancy and Infant Loss Center**
1421 E. Wayzata Blvd., Suite 70
Wayzata, MN 55391
612-473-9372
• Publishes a newsletter.

## Multiple Gestation Pregnancy and Birth

### Mothers of Supertwins (MOST)
PO Box 951
Brentwood, NY 11717-0627
516-859-1110
maureen@mostonline.org
www.mostonline.org
• International nonprofit support network for families with or expecting triplets or more. Offers quarterly magazine and expectant parents' package.

### Sidelines National Support Network
PO Box 1808
Laguna Beach, CA 92652
949-497-2265
sidelines@sidelines.org
www.sidelines.org
• Network of support groups for women and families experiencing complicated pregnancies; publishes *Left Side Lines*, magazine for women with high-risk pregnancies, bed rest, etc.

### The Triplet Connection
PO Box 99571
Stockton, CA 95209
209-474-0885
tc@tripletconnection.org
www.tripletconnection.org
• Nonprofit organization for multiple birth families; provides information, encouragement, resources, quarterly newsletter.

## Pregnancy

### National Pregnancy/Environmental Hotline
800-322-5014 (in Massachusetts)
781-466-8474 (outside Massachusetts)
• Answers to questions about drugs and/or environmental exposure during pregnancy.

## Professional Organizations

### American Association of Tissue Banks
1350 Beverly Road, Suite 220 A

McLean, VA 22101
703-827-9582
**aatb@aatb.org**
**www.aatb.org**
• Scientific, nonprofit organization founded to facilitate provision of high-quality transplantable human tissue in quantities sufficient to meet national needs. Offers list of accredited sperm banks in the United States.

**The American College of Obstetricians and Gynecologists**
409 12th Street, S.W.
 P.O. Box 96920
Washington, DC 20090-6920
**www.acog.org**
• Provides a physician directory and multiple e-mail addresses for questions about a variety of women's health issues.

**American Society of Laser Medicine and Surgery**
2404 Stewart Square
Wausau, WI 54401
715-845-9283
**aslms@aslms.org**
**www.aslms.org**
• Dedicated to promoting research, education, and high standards of clinical care in medical-based laser applications. Will give consumers physician referral to local society members.

**American Society for Reproductive Medicine**
1209 Montgomery Highway
Birmingham, AL 35216-2809
205-978-5000
**asrm@asrm.org**
**www.asrm.org**
• Devoted to advancing knowledge and expertise in reproductive medicine and biology. Offers patient information booklets; office of government relations follows federal and state legislation and advocacy issues. Publishes *Fertility and Sterility* professional journal.

**National Association of Insurance Commissioners**
120 West Twelfth Street, Suite 1100
Kansas City, MO 64105-1925
816-842-3600

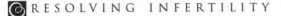

www.naic.org
• Organization of insurance regulators from the 50 states, the District of Columbia, and four U.S. territories (American Samoa, Guam, Puerto Rico, and the U.S. Virgin Islands). Offers contact information to insurance commissioners' offices at the Web site.

## Resolution Options/Support

**Childless by Choice**
PO Box 695
Leavenworth, WA 98826
509-763-2112
**76206.3216@compuserve.com**
**www.now2000.com/cbc**
• Information clearinghouse for those who have decided not to have children or are deciding whether to become parents.

**Donor Conceptions Support Group of Australia, Inc.**
PO Box 53
Georges Hall
New South Wales 2198
Australia
**warren@ozemail.com.au**
**www.ozemail.com.au/ ~ warrenh**
• Self-funded organization for people considering or using donor sperm, egg, or embryo; those who have children conceived with donor gametes; adult donors; and offspring. Offers bimonthly newsletter, telephone contacts, and consumer advocacy.

**Organization of Parents Through Surrogacy (OPTS)**
PO Box 611
Gurnee, IL 60031
847-782-0224
**director@opts.com**
**www.opts.com**
• Information, education, networking, support, and referral for those interested in surrogacy. Offers updated information on status of surrogacy laws by state.

**Stepfamily Association of America**
650 J Street, Suite 205
Lincoln, NE 68508
800-735-0329; 402-477-7837
**www.stepfam.org**

• Nonprofit organization providing information, education, and advocacy for stepfamilies and those who work with them. Offers quarterly publication, *Stepfamilies;* referrals to local professionals with training in working with stepfamily issues; local chapters for support.

## Single Women/Single Parenting

### Committee for Single Adoptive Parents
PO Box 15084
Chevy Chase, MD 20815
• Offers support and publications for those considering single parenthood through adoption.

### Single Mothers by Choice
PO Box 1642
Gracie Square Station
New York, NY 10028
212-988-0993
• Offers support and information for those who have chosen or are considering single motherhood.

## Therapist Referral/Counseling

### American Psychological Association
750 First Street, N.E.
Washington, DC 20002
202-336-5500
www.apa.org
• Scientific and professional organization representing psychology in the United States; offers a consumer help center and referral to qualified psychologists.

### American Society for Reproductive Medicine
Mental Health Professional Group
1209 Montgomery Highway
Birmingham, AL 35216-2809
205-978-5000
asrm@asrm.org
www.asrm.org
• Offers referral to qualified mental health professionals with experience and training in infertility issues.

**The National Association of Social Workers**
750 First Street NE, Suite 700
Washington, DC 20002-4241
202-408-8600; 800-227-3590 (to order Registry directory of social workers)
**info@naswdc.org**
**www.socialworkers.org**
• Provides online Register of Clinical Social Workers; may be searched by specialty, name, and location.

# Test Result Worksheets for Women and Men

The test result worksheets for women and men can help you keep track of the medical tests you undergo during infertility treatment and their results. We suggest you make photocopies of these worksheets, use a three-hole punch, and create a notebook that includes the worksheets and copies of confirming laboratory reports you receive from your physician.

The test result worksheets for women and men become an important complement to your journal and infertility decision tree worksheets, providing a record of what tests you have had should you change physicians. We have also included a page to record physician and clinic contact information and medication information; make as many copies for your notebook as you need.

As we discussed in chapter 4, "Choosing Your Medical Team," and chapter 5, "The Basic Infertility Work-up for Women and Men," your healthcare team includes two very important members: *you and your partner*. Take an active role in tracking your treatment progress by keeping your test result notebook current. Use the decision tree worksheets to help you work through the concerns, issues, and treatment options that arise as you move through the infertility resolution process.

Each test that appears on the test result worksheets for women and men is described in detail in the text of *Resolving Infertility*. You will find information that explains what the results mean and how they might affect various treatment options. Not every test is appropriate for every person, so do not worry if there are tests on the worksheets that your physician has not ordered for you or your partner. Here is how to use each column of the test result worksheets for women and men:

- In the **Date** column, write in the date you have the test performed. If you are doing a retest, write that in below the original test date or use a second copy of the worksheet to track retests.
- The **Test** column gives the medical name for the tests. As necessary, you will want to refer to the text discussion in *Resolving Infertility* for more information about each test and its range of results and treatment options.
- On the test result worksheet for women, the **Cycle Day** column identifies the point during your menstrual cycle when the test needs to be performed.
- The **Normal Range** column tells you the normal results for each test, when applicable.
- The **Results** column provides a place for you to write in the results of the tests your physician orders. Remember, not every test is appropriate for every individual, so there may be some empty spaces on your worksheet.
- The **Comments/Need to Retest** column provides a space for you to jot down any specific notes about what your physician tells you regarding your test results. On occasion, your physician may want you to repeat certain tests, often at specific intervals during your treatment or after specific procedures. Write down the date the test will be repeated and enter in the retest results when they are available. Photocopy additional worksheets for your notebook, if necessary, to add retest results.

Whenever you have tests and procedures done, ask your physician to provide you with copies of the full results. You can then log your results on your worksheet, and add photocopies of the test reports to your notebook for future reference.

# TEST RESULT WORKSHEET FOR WOMEN FOR _____

**Date** _____

| Test | Cycle Day | Normal Range | Results | Comments/Need to Retest |
|------|-----------|--------------|---------|-------------------------|
| Follicle-stimulating hormone (FSH) | 3 | < 10 mIU/mL * < 20 mIU/mL * *depending on laboratory | | |
| Estradiol | 3 | < 50 pg/mL | | |
| Progesterone | Midluteal: 7 days after luteinizing hormone (LH) surge | > 10 ng/mL | | |
| Prolactin | Any cycle day | < 25 ng/mL | | |
| Thyroid-stimulating hormone (TSH) | Any cycle day | 0.5–3.8 IU/mL | | |
| Total testosterone | Any cycle day | 6.0–8.6 ng/dL | | |
| Dehydroepiandros-terone sulfate (DHEAS) | Any cycle day | 35–350 mcg/dL | | |

mL, milliliters; mIU, milli-International Units; IU, international units; ng, nanograms;
dL, deciliters; pg, picograms; mcg, micrograms; > , more than; < , less than

# TEST RESULT WORKSHEET FOR WOMEN FOR _____

| Date | Test | Cycle Day | Normal Range | Results | Comments/Need to Retest |
|---|---|---|---|---|---|
| | Endometrial biopsy | After day 21 | Normal endometrium in phase with no lag | | |
| | Hysterosalpingogram* <br> *Antibiotic for several days after hysterosalpingogram | Before ovulation | Normal tubes and uterus | | |
| | Laparoscopy | Usually before ovulation | Normal pelvic organs, no adhesions or endometriosis | | |
| | Hysteroscopy | Usually before ovulation | Normal uterine cavity | | |
| | Postcoital | Close to ovulation time | 5–10 sperm per high-power field | | |
| | Ultrasound to check uterine lining | Just before injection of Human chorionic gonadotropin (hCG) | 8 mm or more | | |

mL, milliliters; mIU, milli-International Units; IU, international units; ng, nanograms; dL, deciliters; pg, picograms; mcg, micrograms; > , more than; < , less than

# TEST RESULT WORKSHEET FOR MEN FOR _____

| Date | Test | Normal Range | Results | Comments/Need to Retest |
|------|------|--------------|---------|-------------------------|
| | Semen analysis | 2–5 mL volume<br>Motility: >50%<br>Forward progression:<br>normal > 2.0<br>Sperm count:<br>>20 million/mL<br>White blood cells:<br>< 10 per high-<br>power field<br>Viscosity: normal<br>(totally fluid in consistency)<br>Clumping: none<br>Agglutination: none<br>Fructose: present<br>Pentrak score: > 30 mm | | |
| | Strict morphology:<br>Kruger test<br>World Health<br>Organization | > 4% normal forms<br>At least 30% normal forms | | |
| | Zona-free hamster<br>test | At least 15% of eggs penetrated<br>(original assay)<br>> 5 penetrations/egg (optimized<br>assay with egg yolk buffer) | | |

mL, milliliters; dL, deciliters; pg, picograms; mIU, milli-International Units; ng, nanograms; >, more than; <, less than.

# TEST RESULT WORKSHEET FOR MEN FOR _____

| Date | Test | Normal Range | Results | Comments/Need to Retest |
|------|------|--------------|---------|-------------------------|
| | Hypo-osmatic swelling test (sperm viability test) | 57.6 ± 7.9 | | |
| | Prolactin | < 20 ng/mL | | |
| | Testosterone | 300–1,111 ng/dL | Dependent on individual laboratory standards for normal range | |
| | Follicle-stimulating hormone (FSH) (FSH) | 4–10 mIU/mL 4–10 mIU/mL | | |
| | Luteinizing hormone (LH) | 6–19 mIU/mL | | |
| | Estradiol | < 60 pg/mL | | |
| | Vasography | Normal circulatory pattern documented | | |
| | Testicular biopsy | Normal sperm production documented | | |

mL, milliliters; dL, deciliters; pg, picograms; mIU, milli-International Units; ng, nanograms; >, more than; <, less than.

# PHYSICIAN AND CLINIC CONTACT SHEET
## FOR _____

*\*Make a photocopy of your insurance card and place it in your record-keeping notebook.*

## PRIMARY CARE PHYSICIAN

*Fill in your primary care physician contact information here.*

Physician name:

Address:


Telephone:

Fax:

E-mail:

## OB-GYN

*Fill in your ob-gyn contact information here.*

Physician name:

Address:


Telephone:

Fax:

E-mail:

## INFERTILITY CLINIC

*Fill in contact information here for your physician*

Physician Name:

Telephone (Direct line):

E-mail:


*Fill in clinic information here*

❖ Name of clinic:

   Address:


   Telephone:


❖ Insurance Coordinator:

   Telephone extension:

   E-mail:


❖ Nurse or physician assistant:

   Telephone extension:

   E-mail:

   Notes:

## INFERTILITY CLINIC

*Fill in contact information here for your physician*

Physician Name:

Telephone (Direct line):

E-mail:


*Fill in clinic information here*

❖ Name of clinic:

   Address:


   Telephone:


❖ Insurance Coordinator:

   Telephone extension:

   E-mail:


❖ Nurse or physician assistant:

   Telephone extension:

   E-mail:

   Notes:

# MEDICATION AND DOSAGE INFORMATION

*Use this space to record the names and dosages (amount of dose
and how often the dose is taken) of infertility medications prescribed
by your physician. Also record the date you started taking the medication
and the date you stopped.*

Medication name:

Dose:

How often taken:

Date started:

Date stopped:

Notes:


Medication name:

Dose:

How often taken:

Date started:

Date stopped:

Notes:


Medication name:

Dose:

How often taken:

Date started:

Date stopped:

Notes:


Medication name:

Dose:

How often taken:

Date started:

Date stopped:

Notes:


Medication name:

Dose:

How often taken:

Date started:

Date stopped:

Notes:


Medication name:

Dose:

How often taken:

Date started:

Date stopped:

Notes:

## About RESOLVE, the National Infertility Association

RESOLVE is a national nonprofit consumer organization serving the unique needs of individuals experiencing infertility and allied health professionals with support, education, and advocacy. Barbara Eck Menning founded RESOLVE in 1974.

## RESOLVE's Mission

The mission of RESOLVE is to provide timely, compassionate support and information to people who are experiencing infertility and to increase awareness of infertility issues through public education and advocacy.

## Members, Chapters, and Outreach

RESOLVE serves hundreds of thousands every year through the chapter network, national and chapter HelpLines, e-mail service, Web site, and national business office.

## Membership Services and Benefits

- RESOLVE National and Local Chapter Newsletters
- Telephone HelpLines
- Discounts on RESOLVE Publications
- Physician Referral Service
- Medical Call-In Hours
- Advocacy Alerts and Updates
- Member-to-Member Contact Systems
- Support Services Available Through Local Chapters

## Fact Sheets and Publications

Infertility, adoption, and resolving without parenting are among the topics covered in more than 50 Fact Sheets produced by the National RESOLVE office. RESOLVE publishes quarterly newsletters at the national level, and local chapter newsletters offering a variety of articles on medical updates, emotional issues, and more.

## Funding

Membership dues, publication sales, and tax-deductible contributions from concerned individuals, foundations, and corporations support RESOLVE.

## National Infertility Awareness Week (NIAW)

The goal of NIAW is to inform the general public about the medical and emotional issues faced by those experiencing infertility, as well as to highlight family-building options. It is recognized annually in the fall.

## Join RESOLVE today. . .

Start receiving National and Chapter newsletters, access to Medical Call-in HelpLine and Member-to-Member Contact Systems, and Advocacy for Legislative and Insurance Reform.

*In principle and practice, RESOLVE values and seeks a diverse membership. There shall be no barrier to full participation in this organization.*

See RESOLVE's Web site for a *complete list of publications*, full membership and benefits information, and sample newsletter articles: **www.resolve.org**

## Membership Form

Please send this form to:
RESOLVE, 1310 Broadway, Somerville MA  02144-1779,
or call the HelpLine: 617-623-0744
to join and order literature with VISA/MC.

## Membership—Annual Fee

❑ Basic $45                ❑ Supporting $75
❑ Contributing $65         ❑ Circle of Friends $100
❑ Professional $125        ❑ Limited Income $35

Membership is annual. Dues are shared equally between National RESOLVE and the local chapters. Services are the same in all categories.

Membership                       $_____
Tax-deductible contribution      $_____
Matching gift from my company    $_____

**TOTAL PAYMENT**                $_____

**FORM OF PAYMENT**
❑ Visa
❑ Mastercard
❑ Check (must be in U.S. dollars from a bank clearing funds through a U.S. bank)

Name_____    Credit Card #_____
Address_____    Expiration Date_____
_____    Phone(required for credit)_____
City, State, Zip                     Signature_____

# Index

Grateful acknowledgment is made to the following sources for permission to reproduce selected images in this book.

*Traditional pyramid model of aging* and *current pillar model of aging,* page 11. Reprinted with permission of Martha Farnsworth Riche, Ph.D., and the Communications Consortium Media Center.

*Ultrasound of an ovary under the influence of fertility medication,* page 73. Reprinted with permission of Reproductive Biology Associates.

*Hysterosalpingogram (HSG),* page 76. Reprinted with permission of Reproductive Biology Associates.

*Sonohysterography, normal and abnormal side view of uterus,* page 77. Reprinted with permission of Reproductive Biology Associates.

*Sperm in the counting chamber,* page 82. Reprinted by permission of Larry I. Lipshultz, MD, Baylor College of Medicine.

*Ultrasound of an ovary showing PCOS,* page 94. Reprinted with permission of Reproductive Biology Associates.

*Ultrasound images of normal and thin endometrial linings,* page 100. Reprinted with permission of Reproductive Biology Associates.

*Physician's ultrasound view of multiple follicles,* page 179. Reprinted with permission of Reproductive Biology Associates.

*Human embryo: blastocysts,* page 181. Reprinted with permission of Reproductive Biology Associates.

*Intracytoplasmic sperm injection (ICSI)* and *assisted hatching,* pages 186 and 187. Reprinted with permission of Reproductive Biology Associates.

*Pregnancy and live birth rates for fresh, nondonor ART cycles, by age of woman, 1996,* page 190. Reprinted from the *1996 Assisted Reproductive Technology Success Rates: National Summary and Fertility Clinic Reports,* U.S. Department of Health and Human Services, Centers for Disease Control and Prevention.

*Desired weights of women and men aged 25 and over,* page 235. Reprinted with permission of the Metropolitan Life Insurance Company, *Statistical Bulletin.*

*The food guide pyramid,* page 236. Reprinted courtesy of the USDA Center for Nutrition Policy and Promotion.

*Live births per transfer for fresh embryos from own and donor eggs, by age of recipient, 1996,* page 275. Reprinted from the *1996 Assisted Reproductive Technology Success Rates: National Summary and Fertility Clinic Reports,* U.S. Department of Health and Human Services, Centers for Disease Control and Prevention.